MEDICAL RADIOLOGY

Diagnostic Imaging and Radiation Oncology

Springer

Berlin
Heidelberg
New York
Barcelona
Budapest
Hong Kong
London
Milan
Paris
Santa Clara
Singapore
Tokyo

P. R. Algra · J. Valk · J. J. Heimans (Eds.)

Diagnosis and Therapy of Spinal Tumors

With Contributions by

P.R. Algra · J.L. Bloem · W. Boogerd · M.J. Donovan Post · C.F. Dowd · M.W. Fidler
K.W. Fraser · J.J. Heimans · J.W.H. Leer · P.M. Parizel · L.M.P. Ramos · J. Ratcliffe
C.A.F. Tulleken · J. Valk · M.A. Van Buchem · V.P.M. Van der Hulst · W.P. Vandertop
J. Weerts · J.T. Wilmink

Foreword by

A.L. Baert

With 141 Figures in 280 Separate Illustrations, Some in Color

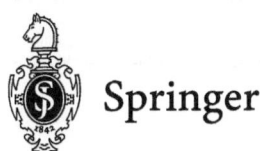 Springer

PAUL R. ALGRA, MD, PhD
Department of Radiology
Medical Center Alkmaar
Wilhelminalaan 12
P.O. Box 501
1800 Alkmaar
The Netherlands

JAAP VALK, MD,PhD
Department of Radiology
Free University Hospital
P.O. Box 7057
1007 MB Amsterdam
The Netherlands

JAN J. HEIMANS, MD, PhD
Department of Neurology
Free University Hospital
P.O. Box 7057
1007 MB Amsterdam
The Netherlands

MEDICAL RADIOLOGY · Diagnostic Imaging and Radiation Oncology

Continuation of
Handbuch der medizinischen Radiologie
Encyclopedia of Medical Radiology

ISSN 0942-5373
ISBN-13:978-3-642-64321-7   e-ISBN-13:978-3-642-60254-2
DOI: 10.1007/978-3-642-60254-2

Library of Congress Cataloging-in-Publication Data. Diagnosis and therapy of spinal tumors / P. R. Algra, J. Valk, J. J.
Heimans, (eds.) ; with contributions by P. R. Algra ... [et al.] ; foreword by A. L. Baert. p. cm. -- (Medical radiology)
Includes bibliographical references and index.
ISBN-13:978-3-642-64321-7 (alk. paper) 1. Spine--Tumors. I. Algra, P. R. II. Valk,
J. III. Heimans, Jan J. IV. Series [DNLM: 1. Spinal Neoplasms--diagnosis. 2. Spinal Neoplasms--therapy. 3. Diagnostic
Imaging. WE 725 D5359 1997] RC280.S72D53 1997 616.99'282--dc21 DNLM/DLC for Library of Congress 97-18905
CIP

© Springer-Verlag Berlin Heidelberg 1998
Softcover reprint of the hardcover 1st edition 1998

The use of general descriptive names, registered names, trademarks, etc. in this publication does not imply, even in the
absence of a specific statement, that such names are exempt from the relevant protective laws and regulations and
therefore free for general use.

Product liability: The publishers cannot guarantee the accuracy of any information about dosage and application contained in this book. In every individual case the user must check such information by consulting the relevant literature.

Cover design: de'blik, Berlin

Typesetting: Verlagsservice Teichmann, Mauer

SPIN: 10111594   21/3135 - 5 4 3 2 1 0 - Printed on acid-free paper

Foreword

Spinal Tumors are relatively rare conditions, but they present distinct and specific clinical and radiological features.

Modern radiological imaging techniques, especially the new cross-sectional methods such as CT and magnetic resonance imaging, allows us nowadays to depict the exact localization and extent of these lesions more clearly. Moreover, the specific findings of these different morphological diagnostic modalities yield deeper insight into the exact nature of these tumors and their differential diagnosis.

During the past few years, important progress in the therapy of spinal tumors has been achieved. Information about these new developments, however, is disseminated throughout the medical literature and scattered across the different medical disciplines. Furthermore, opinions regarding the best diagnostic approach and/or therapy are not always concordant.

The editors of this book should be congratulated to bringing together several international authorities with particular expertise in the diagnosis and the treatment of spinal tumors.

Together, these authors provide a complete overview of the currently prevailing diagnostic algorithms and therapeutic strategies for spinal tumors.

The book will therefore suit excellently the needs of all physicans involved in the management of patients which such tumors: neurologists, neurosurgeons, orthopedic surgeons and radiologists. It will be of particular interest to radiologists, who are nowadays responsible not only for the diagnosis of these tumors but also, in some cases, for their non-surgical treatment.

Leuven   ALBERT L. BAERT

Preface

Many different opinions exist on the diagnostic workup and, particularly, on the therapy of spinal tumors. For instance, there is no consensus on the optimal treatment of spinal compression caused by vertebral metastases.

With the advent of new imaging techniques (MRI) and therapeutic regimens, an up-to-date reference work is needed. This book is the first of its kind in that it offers an overview of the opinions of internationally renowned specialists. The editors hope this publication will help to establish rational imaging and therapy protocols for spinal tumors.

Alkmaar	PAUL R. ALGRA
Amsterdam	JAAP VALK
Amsterdam	JAN J. HEIMANS

Contents

1 Clinical Aspects of Spinal Tumors

J.J. HEIMANS

CONTENTS

1.1
Introduction

Spinal tumors can arise from each of the three compartments of the spine.

Tumors from the extradural space are mainly metastatic tumors, arising from the vertebrae. Benign and malignant primary bone tumors arising in the spine are relatively rare. These extradural tumors usually cause pain, but, in a later stage, may cause neurological symptoms due to compression of the spinal cord.

Tumors from the intradural extramedullary space are meningiomas, neurofibromas and leptomeningeal metastases. Intradural tumors lead eventually to

J.J. HEIMANS, MD, PhD, Department of Neurology, Free University Hospital, POB 7057, 1007 MB Amsterdam, The Netherlands

compression of the spinal cord within the vertebral canal. Especially when the tumor grows slowly, it may be a long time before neurological symptoms develop.

Tumors from the intramedullary space are almost always primary tumors of the spinal cord. There is a great variety of spinal cord tumors, most of them rare. Spinal cord metastases must also be considered very rare.

These three categories of spinal tumors have several clinical aspects in common, but there are also substantial differences. Therefore the three tumor locations will be discussed separately.

1.2
Tumors from the Extradural Space

1.2.1
Epidural Metastases

1.2.1.1
Epidemiological Aspects

Skeletal metastasis from primary tumors occurs most frequently in the vertebral column. The spine is involved in about 40% of patients who die of cancer (BYRNE and WAXMAN 1990). Epidural metastases involve the thoracic spinal column more frequently than the lumbar spinal column. This can be explained by the greater number of thoracic vertebrae: the thoracic and the lumbosacral vertebral levels are almost equally affected (BOOGERD and VAN DER SANDE 1993). Clinical signs of thoracic metastases may appear earlier than clinical signs of lumbar metastases, because the thoracic spinal canal is narrower. Lung cancer spreads more frequently to the thoracic levels, and prostate and colon cancer metastasize more often to the lumbar spine.

The most important clinical consequence of epidural metastasis is spinal cord compression or compression of the cauda equina. This condition should be recognized as soon as possible, because it eventually leads to paraplegia and sphincter dysfunction. Also in patients with metastasized cancer, spinal cord compression should be treated immediately.

In about 10% of patients epidural metastases are the first manifestation of malignant disease.

In approximately 85% of cases of spinal cord compression the compression results from metastases that are present in the vertebral column (BYRNE and WAXMAN; GILBERT et al. 1978). The vertebral body is the most frequent site of vertebral metastasis. In 10 %–15 %f cases compression is caused by metastases in the paravertebral space that extend into the epidural space through the intervertebral foramen. This is especially the case with lymphomas, metastases of renal cell carcinomas and Pancoast tumors. In only a small minority of patients are metastases located in the epidural space itself (ALGRA et al. 1992).

Primary tumors that lead most frequently to vertebral metastases are lung, breast and prostate cancer. But also other primary cancers, such as renal carcinoma, tumors of the gastro-intestinal tract, myeloma and lymphoma may give rise to epidural spinal cord compression. Especially in patients with breast and prostate cancer, metastases may develop in multiple vertebrae.

Vertebral metastases may grow into the spinal canal, thus leading to narrowing of the canal and eventually to cord compression. Compression of the spinal cord or the cauda equina may also result from a pathological fracture and subsequent collapse of a vertebra. In that case signs and symptoms may develop acutely.

1.2.1.2
Clinical Symptoms and Signs of Vertebral Metastases

Pain is almost always the first symptom of vertebral metastases, and in almost all cases pain precedes signs of spinal cord compression. Also when the patient presents with neurological dysfunction, retrospectively back pain will have been present for weeks in many cases. However, the diagnosis will often only be made when neurological signs are present. In rare cases spinal cord compression leads to gait ataxia without pain (HAINLINE et al. 1992).

In a very well documented series of 235 cases, 39 patients were paraplegic at the time of diagnosis (GILBERT et al. 1978). All these paraplegic patients had experienced pain prior to the onset of weakness. Paraparesis was present in 116 patients. Sensory loss was never a first symptom in this series of patients.

However, sensory abnormalities were present at neurological examination in 78% of patients. In the majority of these patients the upper limits of sensory deficit corresponded with the site of the lesion, and in only two patients was the sensory level far below the site of the lesion. The severity of the sensory loss usually corresponded well with the severity of motor dysfunction. Autonomic dysfunction was present in 57% of patients at the time they were first seen. The presence of urinary incontinence or retention was prognostically unfavorable with regard to motor function.

Back pain is often accompanied by radicular pain, especially when metastases are present in the lumbar spine. In a series of 153 patients with metastatic spinal cord compression, the median duration of symptoms before diagnosis was 40 days for radicular pain, 21 days for weakness of the legs, 14 days for sensory symptoms and 3 days for bladder disturbances (HELWEG-LARSEN and SØRENSEN 1994). These data indicate that neurological disturbances may develop gradually. On the other hand the neurological condition may worsen rapidly at any moment during the process, and because such a sudden deterioration cannot be predicted, therapy is usually indicated as soon as the diagnosis of epidural spinal cord compression has been established.

In most patients who are known to have a primary malignancy, treatment of epidural spinal cord compression will consist of radiotherapy in combination with corticosteroids. In a minority of patients who have a solitary vertebral metastasis and who are in a good clinical condition, surgical treatment is indicated (see Chap. 8).

Treatment has to be started as soon as possible, because patients who are still able to walk at the time of treatment will have a good chance of recovery, but patients who are paraplegic at the time of diagnosis will probably stay paraplegic. In patients who are not known to have a primary cancer, operation will be necessary in order to obtain a histological diagnosis.

1.2.2
Primary Vertebral Tumors.

Primary vertebral tumors can be subdivided into benign and malignant tumors.

1.2.2.1
Benign Tumors

The most important benign vertebral tumors are osteoid osteomas, osteoblastomas, aneurysmal bone cysts, hemangiomas and eosinophilic granulomas.

Osteoid osteomas of the spine occur mainly in children and young adults between 5 and 30 years of age (mean 14.5 years) (PETTINE and KLASSEN 1986). These small tumors occur in all parts of the spine and become manifest by pain in the back or the neck or painful scoliosis, in some cases in combination with radicular pain.

Osteoblastomas are larger in diameter than osteoid osteomas. The mean age of the patients is 23 years (PETTINE and KLASSEN 1986). Presenting symptoms do not differ from those in patients with osteoid osteomas. Both in patients with osteoid osteomas and in those with osteoblastomas neurological deficit may develop as a result of root compression. This will only be the case in a minority of patients.

Aneurysmal bone cysts are uncommon lesions which show a predilection for the lumbar spine, especially for the neural arch. The lesions can be confined to one vertebra but the majority of patients are affected at more than one level. The name is somewhat misleading because these lesions are neither aneurysms nor real cysts. Aneurysmal bone cysts occur mainly in the second decade. There is a slight predilection for females. Pain is one of the presenting symptoms but, in contrast to osteoid osteomas and osteoblastomas, these lesions may cause serious neurological deficit due to their aggressive behavior. These neurological signs vary from minor root symptoms to complete paraplegia (HAY et al. 1978).

Vertebral hemangioma is a common lesion with an estimated incidence of 10%–12% in the population (DAGI et al. 1990). These lesions can occur at all ages and are slightly more common in females than in males. In the vast majority of cases the lesions do not become manifest during life and are incidental findings. In a number of cases pain is the initial symptom, and in those cases development of neurologic deficit is an exception. Vertebral hemangioma as a cause of progressive spinal neurological deficit is rare. The cord may be compressed by epidural tissue as an extension from the vertebra, by expanded vascular bone, by epidural hematoma or by a fractured hemangiomatous vertebra (FOX and ONOFRIO 1993). In most cases of neurological deficit there is a gradual increase of symptoms, but the onset may also be acute.

Eosinophilic granuloma is a granulomatous, focal process of bone of unknown etiology. It is a rare condition with a strong childhood predominance, but occasionally also occurs in (young) adults. Pain is the usual presenting symptom, but neurological deficit may occasionally be found. Extracortical expansion of the tumor or collapse of the eroded vertebra is the cause of cord compression (GREEN et al. 1996)

Chondromas account for 2% of all spinal tumors. Pathologically these tumors may be classified also as osteochondromas, chondroblastomas and chondromyxoid fibromas. They may arise from the neural arch as well as from the vertebral body or the spinal process. Clinical presentation is usually with local swelling or local pain. Radicular pain is rare, and cord compression or cauda compression are also seldom observed (GAETANI et al. 1996).

1.2.2.2
Malignant Tumors

Malignant primary vertebral tumors are giant cell tumors, osteosarcomas, chondrosarcomas, chordomas, Ewing's sarcomas and angiosarcomas.

Giant cell tumors can occur in the cervical, the thoracic and the lumbar vertebrae. The tumors occur mainly in the second and third decade and are more common in females than in males (SANJAY et al. 1993). Back pain is the usual presenting symptom, but neurological deficit, due to either compression of nerve roots or compression of the spinal cord or cauda equina, occurs in a considerable proportion of cases.

Osteosarcoma of the spine is a rare condition. Only a small minority of all osteosarcomas originate in the vertebral column: 1122 patients with osteosarcoma were seen at the Mayo Clinic between 1909 and 1980, and in only 30 of them was the tumor located in the vertebrae (SHIVES et al. 1985). These 30 patients varied in age from 11 to 80 years; seven were older than 50 years. Pain is always the first symptom, but in the majority of patients neurological abnormalities can be demonstrated at presentation. The prognosis is poor despite surgery and radiotherapy.

Chondrosarcoma of the spine is about as rare as osteosarcoma of the spine. Patients are usually somewhat older than osteosarcoma patients: in a series reported by SHIVES et al. (1986), the mean age was 45 years with a range from 18 to 70. Presenting symptoms and signs are the same as in osteosarcoma: local pain is always present and may be accompanied by neurological deficit.

Chordomas of the spine occur more frequently than osteosarcomas and chondrosarcomas. Chordomas typically arise from the axial skeleton: about half of these tumors originate in the sacrum, 35% at the base of the skull and 15% in the vertebrae (SUNDARESAN 1986). This is a tumor that occurs mainly in the fifth, sixth and seventh decades, although isolated cases of childhood cases have been reported. The symptoms depend on the location of the tumor. In sacral tumors local nonspecific pain is the most frequent presenting symptom. Rectal dysfunction may also occur. A rectal examination in these patients a prevertebral mass can be palpated. Vertebral tumors may give rise to symptoms and signs of cord compression, which evolves subacutely. The prognosis is better than with osteosarcoma and chondosarcoma: median survival for all chordomas of the spine is about 5 years. Sacral tumors have a 10-year survival rate of 40%. (SUNDARESAN et al. 1979).

Ewing's sarcoma of the spine accounts for less than 10% of all primary Ewing's sarcomas. Spinal metastases of Ewing's sarcoma are much more common than primary tumors. In the literature there are mainly sporadic case reports, the largest series consisting of 22 patients (PILEPICH et al. 1981). Apart from local neck or back pain and neurological deficit, there may be a palpable mass at the level of the tumor. The results of chemotherapy or surgery followed by chemotherapy are better in the patients with a tumor in the cervical, thoracic or lumbar spine than in those with a tumor located in the sacrum (SHARAFUDDIN et al. 1992).

1.2.3
Other Spinal Abnormalities That Can Cause Compression of Spinal Cord or Cauda Equina

Protrusion of an intervertebral disk usually causes local back pain in combination with radicular pain or neurological deficit in the distribution area of the compressed nerve root. Obstruction of the spinal canal with subsequent compression of the spinal cord or the cauda equina can be considered an exception. Intervertebral disk disease of the low lumbar region is very common, intervertebral disk disease of the cervical spine less so. A herniated disk in the thoracic region, however, must be considered very rare.

Cervical myelopathy may be caused by spondylosis of the cervical spine. The condition is usually seen in elderly patients with a history of neck pain with or without brachialgia. Symptoms develop gradually and may consist of weakness of one or both legs and unsteadiness of gait. On examination

spasticity of the legs is usually prominent and plantar reflexes are extensor. Disturbed position sense is the most common sensory abnormality in this condition. Apart from spondylosis of the spine some other spinal abnormalities may cause myelopathy. Anomalies of the craniocervical junction, such as basilar invagination, platybasia and abnormalities of the odontoid process, are possible causes of cervical myelopathy, with spastic tetraparesis as the most prominent sign. Patients with rheumatoid disease may develop subluxation or dislocation of the upper cervical vertebrae with subsequent cervical myelopathy.

A cauda equina syndrome may be caused by *ankylosing spondylitis* of the lumbar spine.

Infective lesions of the spine, such as *extradural spinal abscess* or *vertebral osteomyelitis*, are uncommon conditions that require immediate surgical intervention. Extradural spinal abscesses occur mainly at the lumbar and thoracic levels and are in most cases located posterior to the spinal cord. They can give rise to myelopathic symptoms within a few days. Pyogenic vertebral osteomyelitis may be caused by staphylococci, streptococci and Escherichia coli. Both pyogenic and tuberculous osteomyelitis may lead to the formation of an extradural abscess. These abscesses are located anterior to the cord. The course in these patients will be less acute than in patients with primary extradural abscess.

Epidural spinal hematoma may be caused by trauma, but in a substantial proportion of cases no obvious trauma has taken place. Lumbar puncture may cause epidural spinal hematoma, especially in patients who use anticoagulant therapy. Usually pain and symptoms of myelopathy develop within 1–2 days.

1.3
Tumors from the Intradural Extramedullary Space

1.3.1
Neurofibromas

Neurofibromas represent about one fourth of spinal tumors. These benign tumors arise from the sheath of a spinal nerve root and therefore produce radicular pain as one of the first symptoms. However, also poorly localized pain may be present. A number of patients will complain of motor weakness or bladder dysfunction at first presentation. In a series of 66 cases (LEVY et al. 1986), only 10% of the patients had a completely normal neurological examination at the time of diagnosis. Motor dysfunction was present in 30% of the cases. The tumors may occur in any part of the spinal canal, with a certain predilection for the lumbar spine.

After surgical treatment, the majority of patients will have complaints such as local or irradiating pain, paraparesis, sensory deficit due to a spinal cord lesion or radicular deficit (SEPPALA et al. 1995).

Multiple tumors may be present, and this is often a sign of von Recklinghausen's disease. These neurofibromas may undergo malignant transformation in 20% of cases. The majority of neurofibromas are located intradurally, but in a number of cases, the tumors are located extradurally or extra- and intradurally (TÖNNIES et al. 1963). This latter category includes the so-called hourglass or dumbbell lesions: tumors that grow through the intervertebral foramen. The portion of the tumor located within the spinal canal is attached by a narrow sleeve of tissue via the foramen to the larger part outside the spinal canal.

1.3.2
Meningiomas

Meningiomas are somewhat less common than neurofibromas but represent the second most common intradural, extramedullary tumor. The ratio of intracranial to spinal meningiomas varies in the literature but is approximately 5:1 (SOUWEIDANE and BENJAMIN 1994). Spinal meningiomas occur much more frequently in women than in men: about 80% of the patients are women in their fourth or fifth decade. A review of six major series revealed that 80% of spinal meningiomas were located in the thoracic spine, 17% in the cervical region and only 3% at the lumbar level (SOUWEIDANE and BENJAMIN 1994). This predilection for the thoracic spine appeared only in female and not in male patients (LEVY et al. 1982).

The meningotheliomatous meningioma is the most common variety, followed by the transitional form (LEVY et al. 1982). Calcifications may be present, and in rare cases the tumor may become completely calcified (LUNARDI et al. 1992).

Spinal meningiomas arise most frequently in the approximation of the nerve roots, lateral to the spinal cord (SOLERO et al. 1989). The great majority are located completely intradural. However, extradural and intra-extradural locations may be found (SOLERO et al. 1989).

The tumors become manifest by symptoms and signs of a slowly progressive myelopathy. Back pain

and paresthesias in the legs are usually the first symptoms. The initial neurological examination may reveal motor weakness in a vast majority of patients (NAMER et al. 1987). A spastic paraparesis may be accompanied by sensory deficits in the lower extremities. Radicular symptoms and signs are not as common as in neurofibromas. A case has been reported in which paroxysmal sensorimotor attacks were the only manifestation of a thoracic spinal meningioma for several years (RUBINSTEIN and KURITZKY 1990).

The symptoms may be present for many months or even years before a diagnosis is made (LEVY et al. 1982). In this regard it is important to realize that the chances for complete restitution of neural function decrease with increasing duration of compression of the cord (CIAPETTA et al. 1988). Multiple spinal meningiomas have also been reported (KANDEL et al. 1989; PAGNI et al. 1990; WEIL et al. 1990; CHAPARRO et al. 1993). In rare instances spinal meningiomas may grow "en plaque", forming a diffuse collar-like mass around the spinal cord (STECHISON et al. 1987).

When spinal meningiomas are compared with spinal neurofibromas, there is a noticeable most impressing difference in the male-female ratio. Neurologic deficit due to spinal cord compression is somewhat more common in meningiomas whereas radicular symptoms and signs predominate in neurofibromas (LEVY et al. 1986).

1.3.3
Leptomeningeal Metastases

Leptomeningeal metastases are rare in comparison to brain metastases or epidural metastases, although their frequency seems to be increasing (YAP et al. 1978; WAGGERSTROM et al. 1982). This increase is probably due to prolonged survival of patients with malignant disease and to increased awareness of this serious complication.

BOOGERD and co-workers (1991) found that pretreatment characteristics (age, presence of lung metastases, cranial nerve involvement, CSF glucose and CSF protein content) are more important for the prediction of the survival time than the intensity or the mode of treatment. Others found that the prognosis in patients with spinal cord involvement is better than the prognosis in patients with brain involvement (CLAMON and DOEBBELING 1987).

The most common primary solid tumors that give rise to leptomeningeal spread are breast carcinoma, lung carcinoma and melanoma. Leukemia and lymphoma may also metastasize to the lepto-meninges.

A number of clinical symptoms and signs can be caused by leptomeningeal metastases, depending on their location. Spinal symptoms and signs are present in the majority of patients (CLAMON and DOEBBELING 1987). However, radicular symptoms, giving rise to segmental deficits, may be overshadowed by more prominent cerebral disorders such as confusion, lowering of consciousness, seizures and headache (KAPLAN et al. 1990). The most important spinal symptoms are weakness and paresthesias, followed by radicular pain, back and neck pain and bladder or bowel dysfunction. Reflex abnormalities are found in most patients. Weakness and sensory loss also appear to be common signs. Nuchal rigidity is only an incidental finding. In the same series a cauda equina syndrome was found in one third of patients (KAPLAN et al. 1990).

The most important diagnostic test for leptomeningeal involvement is cytologic examination of the cerebrospinal fluid. In some cases repeated examinations of the CSF are necessary before the diagnosis is established. Apart from malignant cells, the CSF may contain an elevated number of white blood cells, probably reactive to the presence of tumor in the leptomeninges.

1.3.4
Other Intradural Tumors, Arising from the Cauda Equina

One case of an intradural, entirely extraosseous cervical chordoma has been described (VAZ et al. 1995).

Tumors from the cauda equina are usually neurofibromas or ependymomas. Ependymomas may become very large, but this is usually not the case with neurofibromas. There are, however, exceptions: in rare instances lumbosacral nerve sheath tumors may attain huge proportions, resulting in extensive changes of the vertebrae (BHATIA et al. 1992). The tumors are not encapsulated and may extend into the retroperitoneal space. Pain is an important feature in these patients. Neurological deficit in these patients may be of variable severity.

Primitive neuroectodermal tumors of the cauda equina are usually secondary to subarachnoid spread of cerebellar tumors (medulloblastomas or neuroblastomas). Primary malignant tumors of the cauda equina are extremely rare, especially in adults. KEPES and co-workers (1985) described three cases of primitive neuroectodermal tumors with neuro-blastic differentiation, that were located intradurally and that involved the cauda equina. Apparently these were primary tumors.

1.3.5
Other Intradural Abnormalities

Spinal meningeal cysts can be located intradurally as well as extradurally. NABORS and co-workers (1988) proposed a classification of spinal meningeal cysts. Three categories were distinguished. Type I cysts are located extradurally and do not contain spinal nerve root fibers. Type II cysts are also located extradurally and contain spinal nerve root fibers. Type III cysts are located intradurally.

Thoracic type I cysts occur mainly in adolescents, whereas sacral type I cysts are mostly seen in adult patients. Thoracic cysts may present with signs of myelopathy. Sacral cysts cause low back pain and radicular symptoms. Type II cysts appear as dilatations of spinal nerve root sleeves and are often multiple. They occur mostly in adults and as a rule are asymptomatic. Sacral type II cysts may cause sciatica. The intradural type III cysts are located along the posterior spinal subarachnoid space and are usually asymptomatic.

Spinal arachnoiditis is usually secondary to infection, hemorrhage or operation. Idiopathic cases are rare (VLOEBERGHS et al. 1992). The clinical symptoms and signs are usually confined to radicular pain syndromes. Myelopathy, caused by compression of dense fibrous tissue, is rare.

1.4
Tumors from the Intramedullary Space

Primary tumors of the spinal cord are rare and comprise 2%-4% of all central nervous system tumors (COOPER and EPSTEIN 1992; SLOOFF et al. 1964). Only in the first year of life is this percentage higher. There are a great variety of primary spinal cord tumors, mostly with similar clinical pictures.

1.4.1
Clinical Symptoms and Signs of Intramedullary Tumors

Patients with intramedullary tumors often complain initially of radicular pain at the level of the lesion. This pain may be aggravated by coughing or sneezing. Back pain is also frequently mentioned. This local back pain may become worse when the patient lies down. The patient often spends a part of the night sitting upright in a chair.

Most spinal cord tumors tend to grow slowly and therefore the clinical picture will develop slowly. When the neurological picture develops or deteriorates acutely, bleeding into the tumor must be suspected.

Various neurological syndromes may develop due to spinal cord tumors. Usually these neurological symptoms and signs are not specific for an intramedullary lesion, and in most cases it will not be possible to differentiate an intramedullary tumor from an extramedullary tumor on the basis of clinical symptomatology. If weakness in the arms is more serious than weakness in the legs, an intramedullary lesion will be more likely than an extramedullary tumor. Urinary incontinence and impotence may be early symptoms. If the tumor is located on one side of the spinal cord a (partial) Brown-Séquard syndrome may develop, with dissociation of sensory modalities below the level of the tumor. In intramedullary tumors sensory functions may be relatively spared in the perianal and perineal region. Motor dysfunction usually follows sensory dysfunction.

Intramedullary tumors may also rise in children. As in adults, spinal neoplasms in children are far less common than intracranial tumors, the ratio being 1:6.7; of these spinal tumors, less than 50% are intramedullary (DI LORENZO et al. 1982).

Ependymomas are the most common intramedullary tumors in adults, but astrocytomas predominate in children (STEINBOK et al. 1992). Intramedullary tumors in children occur most frequently in the rostral part of the cord. Typically in children, tumors (almost always astrocytomas) occur that involve the entire spinal cord (EPSTEIN and EPSTEIN 1982).

The diagnosis in children may be difficult: often it takes more than a year before the tumor is diagnosed (ROBERTSON et al. 1994). The most common initial symptoms are back pain and disturbance of gait. Scoliosis and torticollis are frequent symptoms at the time that the diagnosis is established. Especially in young children, presentation of complaints may be atypical: recurrent abdominal pain or pain in the limbs may for a long time not be recognized as symptoms from a spinal cord tumor (ROBERTSON 1992).

As many as 15% of children with an intramedullary spinal tumor suffer from associated hydrocephalus, resulting in increased intracranial pressure. The cause of the hydrocephalus may be the elevated cerebrospinal fluid protein, although

RIFKINSON-MANN et al. (1990) suggested two other mechanisms: in children with benign tumors rostral extension of the tumor into the medulla may block CSF pathways, while in children with malignant tumors subarachnoid metastases are the main cause for obstruction of CSF flow.

Magnetic resonance imaging is the method of choice in the visualization and evaluation of spinal cord tumors. Details on this procedure are discussed in Chap. 2.

Median and posterior somatosensory evoked potentials (SSEPs) show a good correlation with magnetic resonance imaging in patients with spinal cord tumors (JABBARI et al. 1990) and reflect the functions of the spinal cord. Recording of SSEPs may be an important means of peroperative monitoring of spinal cord function (FISCHER and BROTCH 1994).

1.4.2
Ependymomas

Ependymomas are the most common intramedullary tumors in adult patients. The majority of true intramedullary ependymomas are present in the cervical or upper thoracic region, but ependymomas may also involve the conus. A number of ependymomas arise from the cauda equina and filum terminale (SCHWEITZER and BATZDORF 1992). Pain is the most prominent presenting symptom in this latter group of patients.

Ependymomas are slowly growing tumors and may reach a considerable size before they become clinically manifest. In some cases the tumor extends over several vertebral spaces. In most cases the tumors are histologically benign and, although unencapsulated, rarely show local infiltration.

EPSTEIN et al. (1993) observed that initial symptoms were almost always sensory and consisted of dysesthesias which could be present in the arms, the chest wall or the legs, depending on the site of the tumor. The exclusive initial occurrence of sensory symptoms might be due to the origin of the tumor, being around the central canal. Crossing spinothalamic fibers may thus be compressed or interrupted. It is interesting that ependymomas differ from astrocytomas in this respect (EPSTEIN et al. 1993).

Isolated cases of intradural, extramedullary ependymoma have been reported. These tumors may have originated from ectopic ependymal cells (KATOH et al. 1995).

1.4.3
Astrocytomas

In children astrocytomas occur more frequently than ependymomas, but in adults the reverse is true.

The majority of astrocytomas in adult patients are low-grade tumors that appear as elongated swellings of the spinal cord. These tumors have a long natural history and it may take several years before the diagnosis is made. The prognosis of patients with low-grade astrocytomas after operation may be good, in contrast to anaplastic astrocytomas and glioblastomas (SANDLER et al. 1992; EPSTEIN et al. 1992).

Patients with pilocytic astrocytomas have a better prognosis than patients with diffuse fibrillary astrocytomas: the 10-year survival rate of these tumor types is 81% and 15%, respectively (MINEHAN et al. 1995).

The so-called "holocord tumors" that may be found in children have already been mentioned (EPSTEIN and EPSTEIN 1992).

Low-grade intramedullary gliomas may be associated with hydrocephalus in children, and in most cases the diagnosis of hydrocephalus is made prior to that of the spinal tumor (CINALLI et al. 1995).

1.4.4
Other Gliomas

Oligodendrogliomas of the spinal cord are extremely rare: the incidence as reported in the literature ranges from 0.8% to 4.7% of all tumors of the cord (FORTUNA et al. 1980). Symptoms and signs do not differ significantly from those of astrocytomas.

Gangliogliomas are rare central nervous system tumors that are composed of neuronal and glial elements. The glial cells are usually astrocytic, but may also have an oligodendroglial morphology. Usually the tumors behave relatively benignly, but several cases with a more malignant course have been described. About half of the gangliogliomas are intramedullary (MILLER et al. 1993). The majority of gangliogliomas occur during childhood with a median age at diagnosis of 8.5 years. The majority of children with spinal cord gangliogliomas present with back pain and associated weakness of the legs (LANG et al. 1993).

Intramedullary gliofibromas are extremely rare and are thought to be of mixed glial and mesenchymal origin (WINDISCH et al. 1995).

1.4.5
Hemangioblastomas

Spinal hemangioblastomas account for 1.5%-5.8% of all spinal cord neoplasms (RENGACHARY 1985; MUROTA and SYMON 1989). Hemangioblastomas may either occur sporadically or as a manifestation of Von Hippel-Lindau syndrome, an autosomally dominant inherited disorder characterized by tumors that develop in several organs. The majority of hemangioblastomas are found in the cerebellum. Spinal hemangioblastomas occur only in a minority of cases: in a series of 47 hemangioblastomas in 44 patients, only six patients had a spinal tumor (NEUMANN et al. 1989). These tumors may become manifest in the same way as other spinal tumors, with back pain or sensory or motor deficit as the initial symptom; alternatively the first symptom is a subarachnoid hemorrhage. In the same series it was found that 23% of patients with a hemangioblastoma suffered from Von Hippel-Lindau syndrome and the need for careful screening was stressed.

The onset of spinal symptoms is usually before the age of of 40.

1.4.6
Cavernous Hemangiomas

Cavernous malformations are composed of lobulated sinusoidal vascular channels, without a clear arterial supply or venous drainage. Cavernous hemangiomas of the central nervous system are usually found in the cerebral hemispheres. Intramedullary cavernous hemangiomas are extremely rare. OGILVY and co-workers (1992) reviewed the literature and added six patients to the 30 cases that had been described already. They distinguished four types of clinical presentation: (1) discrete episodes of neurological deterioration; (2) slow progression of neurological dysfunction; (3) acute onset of neurological symptoms with rapid deterioration; (4) acute onset of mild symptoms with gradual decline. Sudden onset or worsening of the neurological symptoms may be caused by minute hemorrhages from the lesions. They found that the peak age of presentation was in the fourth decade and that women were more affected than men. The six tumors all surgically removed, were described as well-demarcated, dark red or purple, soft, spongy masses of blood-filled minute vessels. At microscopic examination the vessel walls varied from thin and capillary-sized to extremely thickened and hyalinized.

Cavernous angiomas may be wholly intramedullary in location, but intradural extramedullary angiomas and intramedullary lesions with exophytic extramedullary extension have also been described (STONE et al. 1995).

1.4.7
Lipomas and Angiolipomas

There are three types of spinal lipomas: (1) intramedullary lipomas, (2) lipomyelo(meningo)celes and (3) lipomas of the filum terminale (McLONE and NAIDICH 1986). It is supposed that congenital spinal lipomas become clinically manifest during periods of rapid gain in height or in weight. Symptoms of intramedullary lipomas do not differ significantly from symptoms of other intramedullary tumors. Types 2 and 3 above may tether the spinal cord and cause symptoms through cord stretching and ischemia. McLONE and NAIDICH (1986) observed that only two of 50 consecutive pediatric patients had purely intramedullary lipomas. In 42 of these patients lipomas of the conus medullaris extended, in continuity, into the posterior subcutaneous plane via a posterior spina bifida. In six patients the tumor was more or less confined to the filum terminale.

In true intramedullary spinal cord lipomas presenting symptoms include spinal pain, dysesthetic sensory changes, gait difficulties, weakness, and incontinence. These intramedullary tumors may be located in the cervical as well as in the thoracic cord (LEE et al. 1995).

LUNARDI and co-workers (1990) divided spinal lipomas into congenital and (true) tumoral lipomas. They stated on the basis of their own observations that there is no difference in biological behavior between the two types.

Spinal angiolipomas accounted for 24% of spinal lipomas in the review by PREUL and co-workers (1993). Only two of 36 patients suffered from an intramedullary angiolipoma. In the other cases the tumor was located in the extradural space. These tumors are composed of adipocytes and abnormal blood vessels that vary widely in size. They show features of both lipomas and hemangiomas. The clinical presentation of these tumors does not differ from the presentation in lipomas.

One case of multiple intraspinal mixed tumors made up of astrocytes mingled with adipose cells has been described; the authors referred to this tumor type as "astrolipoma" (RODIA and GUTTIERET-MOLINA 1995).

1.4.8
Intramedullary Epidermoid and Dermoid Cysts

Spinal dermoid and epidermoid cysts are rare. Most intraspinal epidermoid cysts are subdural and extramedullary. Intramedullary epidermoid cysts are extremely rare. The cysts are lined by squamous epithelium. Progressive breakdown of tissue produces a soft waxy material that gradually increases in amount. Two types of epidermoid cysts can be distinguished: congenital and acquired (MANNO et al. 1962). Acquired cysts may occur after single or multiple lumbar punctures and result from outgrowth of penetrated skin fragments. ROUX et al. (1992) reviewed the data of 47 patients with intramedullary epidermoid cysts from the literature and found that the age ranged from 3 to 71 years with a mean age of 34 years. Symptoms and signs broadly resemble those of other intramedullary tumors. Epidermoid cysts tend to grow very slowly and often reach a considerable size (occupying two or more segments) before they become manifest. The mid-thoracic region is the most frequent site of these cysts.

Rupture of a dermoid cyst may result in the migration of free fat drops, eventually leading to obstructive hydrocephalus. The finding of intracranial fat should prompt one to look for an intraspinal dermoid or epidermoid cyst (CAVAZZANI et al. 1995).

1.4.9
Intramedullary Metastases

Spinal cord metastases are very rare compared with brain metastases and epidural metastases: the series that have appeared in the literature are mostly small (COSTIGAN and WINKELMAN 1985; GREM et al. 1985; WINKELMAN et al. 1987). Clinical manifestations do not differ significantly from those in other cases of myelopathy. Local back pain in combination with radicular pain is usually the first symptom. Neurological dysfunction develops soon afterwards. The most important differential diagnosis is epidural spinal cord compression and leptomeningeal carcinomatosis. Other rare causes of spinal dysfunction in cancer patients are radiation myelopathy and paraneoplastic necrotizing myelopathy. In these cases pain is usually not present. The prognosis of neurological dysfunction in patients with spinal cord metastasis is poor.

1.4.10
Other Intramedullary Tumors

Only a few isolated cases of *primary spinal intramedullary lymphoma* have been described (FISHER 1979; HAUTZER et al. 1983; SCHILD et al. 1995). The cerebrospinal fluid may be abnormal and MRI may reveal thickening of the cord. The prognosis is poor: patients will develop other lesions in the central nervous system and eventually die.

Primary spinal melanoma may be diagnosed after histological confirmation and when no lesions outside the spinal cord can be detected (HAYWARD 1976). The tumor probably arises from melanoblasts accompanying the pial sheaths of vascular bundles or from neuroectodermal congenital rests. Duration of symptoms before the diagnosis is made may be remarkably long (mean 29 months in a small series of five patients) (LARSON et al. 1987). The same authors suggest that spinal melanoma is more indolent than melanoma metastatic to the central nervous system: an average survival time of more than 6 years was noted.

Schwannomas (or neurilemmomas) are usually extramedullary. This is not surprising since these tumors originate from Schwann cells, which are not present in the spinal cord. HERREGODTS et al. (1991) found 35 cases of intramedullary schwannoma in the literature. Males are more often affected than females (ratio 2:1), and the median age of the patients is 40 years. In 63% of the cases the tumor was in the cervical cord. The tumors are located posteriorly or posteriolaterally.

Intramedullary germinomas are extremely rare and only a few isolated cases have been reported (MIYAUCHI et al. 1996; ITOH et al. 1996; MATSUYANA et al. 1995).

Intramedullary *meningiomas* are extremely rare. Salvati et al. reported a case in 1992 and mentioned that only three cases had been described previously. In all four cases the tumors were in the cervical spinal cord. Symptoms may be present for years before the diagnosis is made.

1.4.11
Other Intramedullary Abnormalities That May Mimic Intramedullary Tumors

Classical syringomyelia is defined as a slowly progressive, degenerative disorder of the spinal cord in which cavitation of the central parts of the spinal cord exists. The condition is usually associated with type 1 Chiari malformation. Symptoms usually begin in the fourth or fifth decade and depend on the location of the syrinx. Segmental paresis and atrophy of hand muscles in combination with segmental sensory loss of the dissociated type are more or less fundamental parts of the clinical picture. Involvement of ascending and descending tracts may cause sensory ataxia and spastic paresis of the legs. Kyphoscoliosis is commonly associated with neurological deficit. Pain may be present in or at the border of the area in which sensory disturbances exist.

Syringomyelia may be congenital or secondary to intramedullary tumor. SAMII et al. (1994) stated that "any cystic process in the spinal cord should be considered to be associated with an intramedullary tumor until proven otherwise". They used the term "syringomyelia" for cystic, fluid-containing cavities within the spinal cord that were not tumor cysts, in which tumor tissue makes up the wall of the cavity. In their series of 100 intramedullary tumors, 45 presented with associated syringes. Syringes could be present above tumor level, below tumor level or above and below tumor level. Syringes were especially found in ependymomas, hemangioblastomas and cavernomas and were less often present in astrocytomas. Especially tumors at the upper levels of the spinal cord were associated with a syrinx. Resection of a tumor appeared easier when an associated syrinx was present. Transudation and secretion by the intramedullary tumor may play a role in syrinx formation but are certainly not the only causative factors. Obstruction of CSF flow by an intramedullary tumor is related to obstruction of extracellular fluid flow in the spinal cord and is likely to contribute to syrinx formation.

Another cause of secondary syringomyelia is trauma of the spinal cord.

Radiation injury as a cause of spinal cord affection must be considered in those patients who have been treated with radiotherapy in the past. The latent period between irradiation and the manifestation of myelopathy is usually more than 1 year and may exceed 5 years.

Multiple sclerosis may cause neurological symptoms and signs mimicking intramedullary tumors, although pain will usually not be reported. MRI of the spine will easily differentiate between demyelination and neoplasm as a cause of neurological dysfunction.

A number of *viral infections* may lead to *myelitis.* Poliomyelitis causes anterior horn disease with motor deficit. Herpes zoster has an affinity for the dorsal root ganglia and causes sensory deficit with a dermatomere distribution. In HTLV virus infections affection of the white matter occurs with subsequent motor and sensory deficit below the level of the lesion.

Postinfectious and postvaccinal myelitis may develop within a few days in relation to a viral infection or a vaccination.

Paraneoplastic necrotic myelitis may develop in cancer patients, but may also be the first manifestation of malignant disease.

Intramedullary *spinal tuberculoma* is very rare in Europe and North America but may be more common in other areas of the world. MRI makes it possible to differentiate this abnormality from intradural, extramedullary lesions and from vertebral osteomyelitis in tuberculous patients (RHOTON et al. 1988).

Infarction of the spinal cord usually occurs in the territory of the anterior spinal artery. Symptoms develop acutely or within hours and consist of paralysis and dissociated sensory loss below the level of the infarction. Usually myelomalacia is associated with generalized vascular disease.

Vascular malformations of the spinal cord may mimic spinal neoplasms (Montine et al. 1995). CT and MR findings in these disorders may be falsely interpreted as spinal tumors.

Hematomyelia usually occurs secondary to a vascular malformation of the spinal cord and may be associated with anticoagulant therapy.

Hereditary spastic paraparesis is a degenerative disorder of the spinal cord which is characterized by slowly developing of spastic paresis of the legs.

Subacute combined degeneration of the spinal cord due to vitamin B12 deficiency usually begins with symptoms of posterior column involvement. Corticospinal tracts are affected later.

References

Algra PR, Heimans JJ, Valk J, Nauta JJ, Lachniet M, Van Kooten B (1992) Do metastases in vertebrae begin in the body or the pedicles ? Am J Radiol 158: 1275-1280

Bhatia S, Khosla A, Dhir R, Bhatia R, Banerij AK (1992) Giant lumbosacral nerve sheath tumors. Surg Neurol 37: 118-122

Boogerd W, Hart AAM, Van der Sande JJ, Engelsman E (1991) Meningeal carcinomatosis in breast cancer. Prognostic factors and influence of treatment. Cancer 67: 1685-1695

Boogerd W, Van der Sande JJ (1993) Diagnosis and treatment of spinal cord compression in malignant disease. Cancer Treat Rev 19: 129-150

Byrne TN, Waxman SG (1990) Spinal cord compression: diagnosis and principles of treatment. Contemporary neurology series, vol 33. Davis, Philadelphia

Cavazzani P, Ruelle A, Michelozzi G, Andrioli G (1995) Spinal dermoid cysts originating intracranial fat drops causing obstructive hydrocephalus: case report. Surg Neurol ; 43: 466-469

Chaparro MJ, Young RF, Smith M, Shen V, Choi BH(1993) Multiple spinal meningiomas: a case of 47 distinct lesions in the absence of neurofibromatosis or identified chromosomal abnormality. Neurosurgery 32:298-301

Ciapetta P, Domenicucci M, Raco A (1988) Spinal meningiomas: prognosis and recovery factors in 22 cases with severe motor deficits. Acta Neurol Scand 77:27-30

Cinalli G, Sainte-Rose C, Lellouch-Tubiana A, Sebag G, Renier D, Pierre-Kahn A (1995) Hydrocephalus associated with intramedullary low-grade glioma. J Neurosurg 83: 480-485

Clamon G, Doebbeling B(1987) Meningeal carcinomatosis from breast cancer: spinal cord vs. brain involvement. Breast Cancer Res and Treat 9:213-217

Cooper PR, Epstein FJ (1992) Intramedullary tumours. In: Findlay G, Owen T (eds). Surgery of the spine. A combined orthopaedic and neurosurgical approach. Blackwell, Oxford, pp 587-600

Costigan DA, Winkelman MD (1985) Intramedullary spinal cord metastasis. A clinicopathological study of 13 cases. J Neurosurg 62: 227-233

Dagi TF, Schmidek HH (1990) Vascular tumors of the spine. In: Sundaresan N, Schmidek HH, Schiller AL et al (eds) Tumors of the spine: diagnosis and clinical management. Saunders, Philadelphia, pp.181-191

Di Lorenzo N, Giuffre R, Fortuna A (1982) Primary spinal neoplasms in childhood: analysis of 1234 published cases (including 56 personal cases) by pathology, sex, age and site. Differences from the situation in adults. Neurochirurgia (Stuttg.) 25: 153-164

Dickinson LD, Farhat SM (1991) Eosinophilic granuloma of the cervical spine. Surg Neurol 35:57-63

Epstein FJ, Epstein N (1982) Surgical treatment of spinal cord astrocytomas of childhood. J Neurosurg; 57: 685-689

Epstein FJ, Farmer JP, Freed D (1993) Adult intramedullary spinal cord ependymomas: the result of surgery in 38 patients. J Neurosurg 79: 204-209

Epstein FJ, Farmer JP, Freed D(1992) Adult intramedullary astrocytomas of the spinal cord. J Neurosurg 77: 355-359.

Fischer G, Brotchi J (1994) Les tumeurs intramedullaires. Neurochirurgie; Suppl. 1

Fisher RG (1979) Intramedullary lymphoma of the spinal cord. Neurosurgery 5: 270-272

Fortuna A, Celli P, Palma L (1980) Oligodendroglioma of the spinal cord. Acta Neurochir (Wien) 52: 305-329

Fox MW, Onofrio BM (1993) The natural history and management of symptomatic and asymptomatic vertebral hemangiomas. J Neurosurg;78:36-45

Gaetani P, Tancioni F, Merlo P, Villani L, Spanu G, Baena RRY (1996) Spinal chondroma of the lumbar tract. Surg Neurol 46: 534-539

Gilbert RW, Kim JH, Posner JB (1978) Epidural spinal cord compression from metastatic tumor: diagnosis and treatment. Ann Neurol 3:40-51

Green NE, Robertson WW, Kilroy AW (1980) Eosinophilic granuloma of the spine with associated neural deficit. J Bone Joint Surg [Am] 62:1198-1202

Grem JL, Burgess J, Trump DL (1985) Clinical features and natural history of intramedullary spinal cord metastasis. Cancer 56: 2305-2314.

Hainline B, Tuszynski MH, Posner JB (1992) Ataxia in epidural spinal cord compression. Neurology 42:2193-2195

Hautzer NW, Aiyesimoju A, Robitaille Y (1983) "Primary" spinal intramedullary lymphomas: a review. Ann Neurol 14: 62-66

Hay MC, Paterson D, Yaylor TKF (1978) Aneurysmal bone cysts of the spine. J Bone Joint Surg [Br] 60:406-411

Hayward RD (1976)Malignant melanoma and the central nervous system. A guide for classification based on the clinical findings. J Neurol Neurosurg Psychiatry 39: 526-530

Helweg-Larsen S, Sørensen PS (1994) Symptoms and signs in metastatic spinal cord compression: a study of progression from first symptom until diagnosis in 153 patients. Eur J Cancer 30a:396-398

Herregodts P, Vloerberghs M, Schmedding E, Goossens A, Stadnik T, D'Haens J (1991) Solitary dorsal intramedullary schwannoma. J Neurosurg 74: 816-820

Itoh Y, Mineura K, Sasajima H, Kowada M (1996) Intramedullary spinal cord germinoma: case report and review of the literature. Neurosurgery 38: 187-190

Jabbari B, Geyer C, Schlatter M, Scherokman B, Mitchell M, McBurney JW, Elbrecht C, Gunderson CH (1990) Somatosensory evoked potentials and magnetic resonance imaging in intraspinal neoplasms. Electroencephalogr Clin Neurophysiol 77:101-111

Kandel E, Sungurov E, Morgunov V (1989) Cerebral and two spinal meningiomas removed from the same patient: case report. Neurosurgery 25:447-450

Kaplan JG, Portenoy RK, Pack DR, DeSouza T (1990) Polyradiculopathy in leptomeningeal metastasis: the role of EMG and late response studies. J Neuro-oncol 9:219-224

Katoh S, Ikata T, Inoue A, Takahashi M (1995) Intradural extramedullary ependymoma. A case report. Spine 20: 2036-2038

Kepes JJ, Belton K, Roessmann U, Ketcherside WJ (1985) Primitive neuroectodermal tumors of the cauda equina in adults with no detectable primary intracranial neoplasm - three case studies. Clin Neuropathol 4:1-11

Lang FF, Epstein FJ, Ransohoff J, Allen JC, Wisoff J, Abbott IR, Miller DC (1993) Central nervous system gangliogliomas. II. Clinical outcome. J Neurosurg 79: 867-873

Larson TC, Houser OW, Onofrio BM, Piepgras DG (1987) Primary spinal melanoma. J Neurosurg 66: 47-49

Lee M, Rezal AR, Abbott R, Coelho DH, Epstein FJ (1995) Intramedullary spinal cord lipomas. J Neurosurg 82: 394-400

Levy WJ, Bay J, Dohn D (1982) Spinal cord meningioma. J Neurosurg 57:804-812

Levy WJ, Latchaw J, Hahn JF, Sawhny B, Bay J, Dohn DF (1986) Spinal neurofibromas: a report of 66 cases and a comparison with meningiomas. Neurosurgery 18:331-334

Lunardi P, Missori P, Ferrante L, Fortuna A (1990) Long-term results of surgical treatment of spinal lipomas. Acta Neurochir (Wien) 104: 64-68

Lunardi P, Missori P, Franco C, Delfini R, Fortuna A (1992) Hard-rock spinal meningioma. J Neurosurg Sci 136:243-246

Manno NJ, Uihlein A, Kernohan JW (1962) Intraspinal epidermoids. J Neurosurg 19: 754-765

Matsuyama Y, Nagasaka T, Mimatsu K, Inoue K, Mii K, Iwata H (1995) Intramedullary spinal cord germinoma. Spine 20: 2338-2340

McLone DG, Naidich TP (1986) Laser resection of fifty spinal lipomas. Neurosurgery 18: 611-615

Miller DC, Lang FF, Epstein FJ (1993) Central nervous system gangliogliomas. J Neurosurg 79: 859-866

Minehan KJ, Shaw EG, Scheithauer BW, Davis DL, Onofrio BM (1995) Spinal cord astrocytoma: pathological and treatment considerations. J Neurosurg 83: 590-595

Miyauchi A, Matsumoto K, Kohmura E, Doi T (1996) Primary intramedullary spinal cord germinoma. J Neurosurg 84: 1060-1061

Montine TJ, O'Keane JC, Eskin TA, Giangaspero F, Gray L, Friedman AH, Burger PC (1995) Vascular malformations presenting as spinal cord neoplasm: case report. Neurosurgery 36: 194-197

Murota T, Symon L (1989) Surgical management of hemangioblastoma of the spinal cord: a report of 18 cases. Neurosurgery 25: 699-707

Nabors MW, Patt TG, Byrd EB, Karim NO, Davis DO, Kobrine AI, Rizzoli HV (1988) Updated assessment and current classification of spinal meningeal cysts. J Neurosurg 68:366-377

Namer IJ, Pamir MN, Benli K, Saglam S, Erbengi A (1987) Spinal meningiomas. Neurochirurgia (Stuttgart) 30:11-15

Neumann HPH, Eggert HR, Weigel K, Friedburg H, Wiestler OD, Schollmeyer P (1989) Hemangioblastomas of the central nervous system. A 10-year study with special reference to Von Hippel Lindau syndrome. J Neurosurg 70: 24-30

Ogilvy CS, Louis DN, Ojemann RG (1992) Intramedullary cavernous angiomas of the spinal cord: clinical presentation, pathological features, and surgical management. Neurosurgery 31: 219-230.

Pagni CA, Canavero S, Cento A (1990) Multiple spinal meningiomas: case report and review of the literature. Zentralbl Neurochir 51:225-228

Pettine KE, Klassen RA (1986) Osteoid-osteoma and osteoblastoma of the spine. J Bone Joint Surg [Am] 68 A:354-361

Pilepich MV, Vietti TJ, Nesbit ME, Tefft M, Kissane J, Burgert O, Pritchard D, Gehan EA (1981) Ewing's sarcoma of the vertebral column. Int J Radiat Oncol Biol Phys 1981 7:27-31

Preul MC, Leblanc R, Tampieri D, Robitaille Y, Pokrupa R (1993) Spinal angiolipomas. J Neurosurg 78:280-286

Rengachary SS (1985) Hemangioblastomas. In: Wilkins RH, Rengachary SS (eds) Neurosurgery. McGraw-Hill, New York, pp 772-782

Rhoton EL, Ballinger WE, Quisling R, Sypert GW (1988) Intramedullary spinal tuberculoma. Neurosurgery 22:733-736

Rifkinson-Mann S, Wisoff JH, Epstein F (1990) The association of hydrocephalus with intramedullary spinal cord tumors: A series of 25 patients. Neurosurgery 27: 749-754

Robertson PL (1992) Atypical presentation of spinal cord tumors in children. J Child Neurol 7: 360-363

Robertson PL, Allen JC, Abbott IR, Miller DC, Fidel J, Epstein FJ (1994) Cervicomedullary tumors in children: a distinct subset of brainstem gliomas. Neurology 44: 1798-1803

Roda JM, Guttierrez-Molina M (1995) Multiple intraspinal low-grade astrocytomas mixed with lipoma (astrolipoma). J Neurosurg 82: 891-894

Roux A, Mercier C, Larbrisseau A, Dube L-J, Dupuis C, Del Carpio R (1992) Intramedullary epidermoid cysts of the spinal cord. J Neurosurg 76: 528-533

Rubinstein AB, Kuritzky A (1990) Paroxysmal sensory-motor attack as the only manifestation of thoracic spinal meningioma. Neurology 40:722

Salvati M, Artico M, Lunardi P, Gagliardi FM (1992) Intramedullary meningioma: case report and review of the literature. Surg Neurol 37:42-45

Samii M, Klekamp J (1994) Surgical results of 100 intramedullary tumors in relation to accompanying syringomyelia. Neurosurgery 35: 865-873

Sandler HM, Papadopoulos SM, Thornton AF, Ross DA (1992) Spinal cord asrocytomas: results of therapy. Neurosurgery 30: 490-493

Sanjay BKS, Sim FH, Unni KK, McLeod RA, Klassen RA (1993) Giant-cell tumours of the spine. J Bone Joint Surg [Br] 75b:148-154

Schild SE, Wharen RE Jr, Menke DM, Folger WN, Colon-Otero G (1995). Primary lymphoma of the spinal cord. Mayo Clin Proc 70: 256-260

Schweitzer JS, Batzdorf U (1992) Ependymoma of the cauda equina region: diagnosis, treatment and outcome in 15 patients. Neurosurgery 30: 202-207

Seppala MT, Haltia MJ, Sankila RJ, Jaaskelainen JE, Heiskanen O (1995) Long-term outcome after removal of spinal Schwannoma: a clinicopathological study of 187 cases. J Neurosurg 83: 621-626

Sharafuddin MJA, Haddad FS, Hitchon PW, Haddad SF, El-Khoury GY (1992) Treatment options in primary Ewing's sarcoma of the spine: report of seven cases and review of the literature. Neurosurgery 30:610-618

Shives TC, Dahlin DC, Sim FH, Pritchard DJ, Earle JD (1986) Osteosarcomas of the spine. J Bone Joint Surg [Am]68 a:660-668

Shives TC, McLeod RA, Unni KK, Schray MF (1989) Chondrosarcoma of the spine. J Bone Joint Surg [Am]71 a:1158-1165

Slooff JL, Kernohan JW, McCarty CS (1964) Primary intramedullary tumors of the spinal cord and filum terminale. Philadelphia, Saunders: 1-255

Solero CL, Fornari M, Giombini S, Lasio G, Oliveri G, Cimino C, Pluchino F (1989) Spinal meningiomas: review of 174 operated cases. Neurosurgery 25: 153-160

Souweidane MM, Benjamin V (1994) Spinal cord meningiomas. Neurosurg Clin North Am 5:283-291

Stechison MT, Tasker RR, Wortzman G (1987) Spinal meningioma en plaque. Neurosurgery 67:452-455

Steinbok P, Cochrane D, Poskitt K (1992) Intramedullary spinal cord tumors in children.Neurosurg Clin North Am. 3: 931-945

Stone JL, Lichtor T, Ruge JR (1995) Cavernous angioma of the upper cervical spinal cord. A case report. Spine 20: 1205-1207

Sundaresan N (1986) Chordomas. Clin Orthop 204:135-142.

Sundaresan N, Galicich JH, Chu FC, Huvos AG (1979) Spinal chordomas. J Neurosurg 50:312

Tönnis W, Krenkel W, Nittner K (1963) Ein als Bandscheibenvorfall imponierendes Kauda-Neurinom. Zentralbl Chir 88:1293-1297

Vaz RM, Pereira JC, Ramos U, Cruz CR (1995) Intradural cervical chordoma without bone involvement. J Neurosurg 82: 650-653

Vloeberghs M, Herregodts P, Stadnik T, Goossens A, D'Haens J (1992) Surg Neurol 37:211-215

Wasserstrom WR, Glass JP, Posner JB (1982) Diagnosis and treatment of leptomeningeal metastases from solid tumors: experience with 90 patients. Cancer 49:759-772

Weil SM, Gewirtz RJ, Tew JM (1990) Concurrent intradural and extradural meningiomas of the cervical spine. Neurosurgery 27:629-631

Windisch TR, Naul LG, Bauserman SC (1995) Intramedullary gliofibroma: MR, ultrasound, and pathologic correlation. J Comput Assist Tomogr 19: 646-648

Winkelman MD, Adelstein DJ, Karlins NL (1987) Intramedullary spinal cord metastasis. Diagnostic and therapeutic considerations. Arch Neurol 44: 526-531

Yap HY, Yap BS, Tashima CK, DiStefano A, Blumenschein GR (1978) Meningeal carcinomatosis in breast cancer. Cancer 42:283-286

2 Imaging of the Spine: Techniques and Indications

P.M. PARIZEL and J.T. WILMINK

CONTENTS

2.1 Introduction

In 1995 the radiological community commemorated the 100th anniversary of Wilhelm Conrad Röntgen's discovery of a type of radiation with extraordinary powers of penetration which he named X-rays. This remarkable modality has formed the mainstay of medical imaging during the past century, and is only recently in the process of being superseded by the even more versatile technique of magnetic resonance imaging.

P.M. PARIZEL, MD, PhD, Department of Radiology, Universitair Ziekenhuis Antwerpen (University of Antwerp), Wilrijkstraat 10, B-2650 Edegem, Belgium
J.T. WILMINK, MD,PhD, Department of Radiology, Academisch Ziekenhuis Maastricht, P. Debeyelaan 25, P.B. 5800, 6202 AZ Maastricht, The Netherlands

Early X-ray technology was adequate for the depiction of dense skeletal structures and air-containing organs, but resolution was insufficient for imaging of soft tissue structures and abnormalities. The development of tomography improved spatial resolution. Better contrast resolution could only be achieved by introducing into the body radiological contrast media. These were either "negative" (air) or "positive" (high-density fluids or semi-fluids containing iodine or barium). In neuroradiology this led to the development of encephalography and cisternography, cerebral and spinal angiography, myelography and radiculography. These imaging techniques, though often invasive and unpleasant for the patient, did however produce diagnostic images of the cerebrospinal fluid (CSF) spaces within and around the central nervous system as well as normal and abnormal blood vessels. Unfortunately, the substance of the brain and spinal cord itself was not directly visualised.

Computed tomography (CT) revolutionised X-ray imaging by its greatly improved contrast resolution coupled to a superior tomographic capability and the advantage of digital data manipulation. In the cranium, this resulted in the elimination of the dreaded air study, as the brain could now easily be distinguished from the adjacent CSF by CT. Moreover, thanks to the improved contrast resolution in the brain substance, even the grey matter could be distinguished from the white matter. In spinal diagnosis, however, the situation was different. Due to the dense bony vertebral structures surrounding the relatively small spinal canal, the spinal cord could not be discerned sufficiently well for diagnostic purposes. CT is capable of demonstrating degenerative, neoplastic or traumatic lesions of the spinal skeleton and even some soft tissue encroachments such as caused by lumbar disc herniation. In the cervical and thoracic spine especially, opacification of the CSF by a radiological contrast medium is often necessary to assess the presence of soft tissue masses within the spinal canal and their effects upon the spinal cord and nerve roots. In patients with spinal tumours, a

CT-myelographic procedure can be painful and time-consuming and involves the risk of neurological deterioration due to disturbed spinal CSF hydrodynamics.

The introduction of *magnetic resonance (MR) imaging* has proved to be a significant stride forward beyond X-ray based imaging techniques. The first effects of this new revolution have been perhaps even more profound in spinal diagnosis than in brain imaging. MR imaging provides yet again improved contrast resolution in soft tissue structures. The shape and structure of the spinal cord can easily be ascertained due to the lack of the bone artefacts that are so troublesome in X-ray CT imaging. In all X-ray techniques, image contrast is basically determined by a single tissue variable: electron density. Conversely, in MR imaging of the spine, several tissue variables (proton density, longitudinal and transverse magnetisation characteristics) can be utilised to optimise image contrast for various types of pathology. In addition, diagnostic information can be increased by making use of flow phenomena in moving fluids (blood, CSF) and also, as in X-ray imaging, by intravenous injection of contrast media that selectively increase signal intensity in specific structures and lesions.

Although MR imaging utilises a computed tomographic image reconstruction technique as X-ray CT does, the tomographic sections are acquired in multi-slice sets unlike the sequential images acquired by X-ray CT. Examination speed and diagnostic quality are improved by the multiplanar imaging capability of the MR technique. X-ray CT sections of the spine are virtually limited to the axial imaging plane, with time-consuming reformatting procedures providing less than optimal sagittal and coronal views.

In summary it can be said that the introduction of digital imaging techniques has brought great benefits to patients with spinal tumours. X-ray CT literally added a new dimension to contrast myelography with its axial views and greatly improved spinal cord definition. MR imaging has further improved the picture of the spinal cord and spinal canal, but its greatest benefit has been the provision of rapid, reliable and non-invasive spinal imaging. This allows for earlier and thus more effective diagnosis of potentially invalidating and even life-threatening spinal tumours. For these reasons, MR imaging, when available, is the modality of choice for imaging of spinal tumours in all but exceptional cases.

2.2
Conventional X-Ray Imaging

2.2.1
General Principles

Conventional X-ray imaging of the spine is an easy and inexpensive technique, but the diagnostic yield in patients with spinal tumours is rather low. The main advantage is that, with only a few films (AP and lateral view), a good overview of a large section of the spine can be obtained. The main disadvantage is the intrinsically low soft tissue resolution of conventional X-ray imaging. Another problem is the superimposition of other soft tissue structures over the spine, which renders interpretation of images difficult. In AP views, soft tissue structures of the mediastinum and heart are superimposed over the thoracic spine. In the lumbar spine, there may be superimposition by bowel contents, aortic calcifications etc. In the lateral projection, the cervico-thoracic junction is difficult to evaluate because of superimposition of the shoulders. This can be avoided by using the so-called swimmers position requiring a cooperative patient, however. Due to superimposition of the diaphragm, the thoraco-lumbar junction may be difficult to visualise in the lateral projection. Superimposition of other structures can be avoided by using conventional tomography, but this technique also suffers from poor contrast resolution.

2.2.2
Specific Findings on Conventional X-Rays in Spinal Tumours

Slowly growing mass lesions within the spinal canal erode osseous structures of the spine. Signs of *chronic bony compression (pressure erosion)* on plain X-ray films include: enlargement of the spinal canal, scalloping of the posterior surface of the vertebrae, thinning of vertebral pedicles, widening of the interpedicular distance or widening of neural foramina (MITCHELL et al 1967). Widening of the spinal canal with thinning of pedicles may be observed in ependymomas (e.g. the slowly growing myxopapillary ependymomas of the conus medullaris). Dumbbell shaped neurogenic tumours typically cause enlargement of a neural foramen and pedicle erosion. In patients with neurofibromatosis, paraspinal extension of a tumour may cause erosion of ribs ("ribbon ribs") and kyphoscoliosis. Bone erosion can also be caused by non-tumoural conditions, such as meningocoeles, which are dural develop-

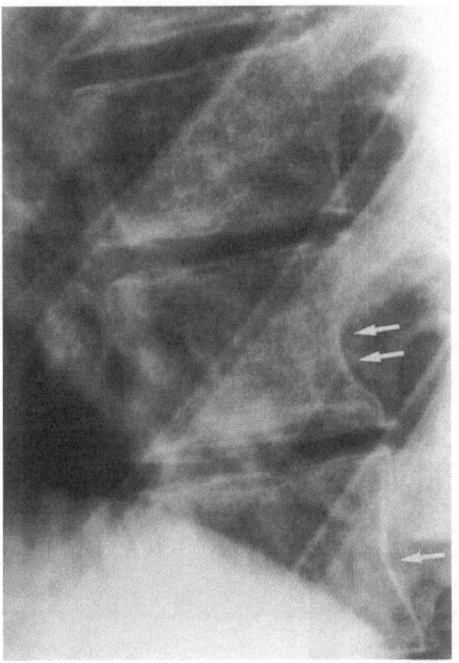

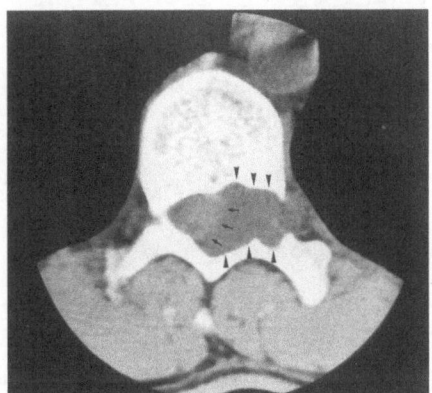

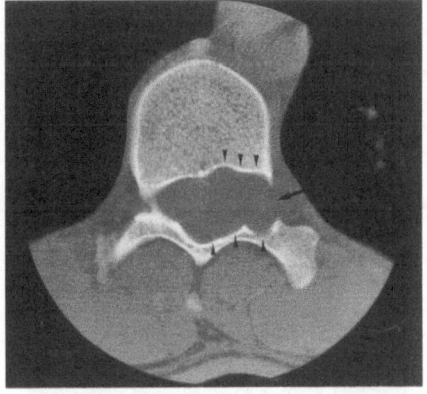

Fig. 2.1a-c. Posterior vertebral scalloping by dural ectasia and lateral thoracic meningocoeles in a patient with neurofibromatosis type 1. a Lateral plain X-ray shows scalloping of the posterior wall of T9 and T10 (*arrows*). b. Axial CT scan through T9 with soft tissue window setting. There is a sharply marginated hypodense lesion (*arrowheads*) in the left lateral half of the spinal canal extending into the left neural foramen. The density of the lesion is 0 H.U., indicating fluid contents. The spinal cord is pushed over to the right (*small arrows*). c Axial CT scan through the same level with bone window setting. There is smooth expansion of the spinal canal (*arrowheads*) and left neural foramen (*arrow*).

mental malformations. These CSF-filled outpouchings erode bone through transmitted cerebrospinal fluid pulsations (Fig. 2.1). They can occur as an isolated defect or may be associated with mesenchymal disorders such as neurofibromatosis type 1 and Marfan syndrome (OSBORN 1994)

Osteolytic spinal metastases are a frequent cause of focal areas of abnormality on plain X-ray films. The most common plain radiographic finding is destruction of a pedicle (ALGRA et al 1991c) This results in the "one-eyed vertebra" sign on AP films. This sign is, however, not pathognomonic for metastasis and can be observed in other osteolytic lesions involving the pedicle (Fig. 2.2). Other frequent abnormalities include: multifocal lytic vertebral body lesions, pathologic compression fracture, paraspinal

soft tissue mass and destruction of the cortical lining of vertebrae. An indistinct posterior vertebral body margin may be a subtle sign of metastatic involvement of the extradural space (OLCOTT and DILLON 1993). Fig. 2.3 illustrates the degree of vertebral destruction that can take place with only minimal findings on plain X-ray films. Most osteolytic metastases develop first in the posterior half of the vertebrae due to the proximity of the basivertebral vein, which is the entry-route for haematogenic dissemination of metastatic cells deposited in the intravertebral venous system (ALGRA et al 1991b,c; ALGRA 1995).

Dense osteoblastic or sclerotic metastatic lesions are encountered much less frequently, mainly in patients with metastasised prostate carcinoma

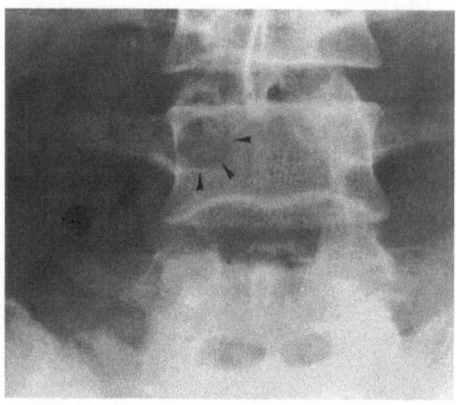
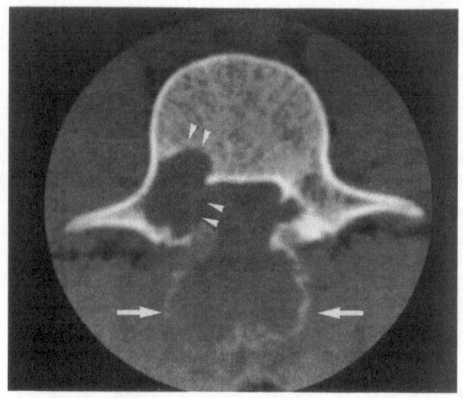

a   b

Fig. 2. 2a,b. One eyed vertebra due to pedicle destruction. a AP plain radiograph shows destruction of the right pedicle of L4 (*arrowheads*). This results in the "one-eyed vertebra" sign. Note that the spinous process of L4 is also missing. b Axial CT scan through L4, bone window, shows a lytic, expansile mass that involves the right L4 vertebral pedicle (*paired arrowheads*) as well as the neural arch and spinous process (*arrows*). Aneurysmal bone cyst was found at surgery

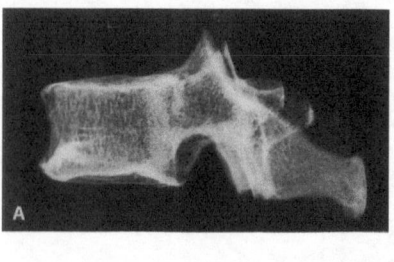
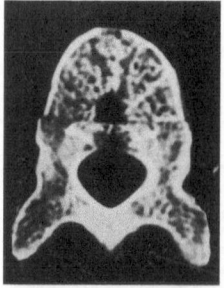

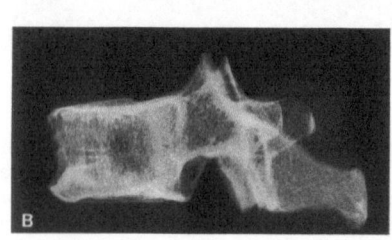
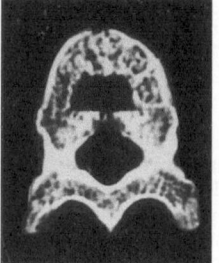

Fig. 2.3a,b. Preparations of a thoracic vertebra with artificial defects in the spongiosa of the vertebral body show the difficulty of recognising osteolytic lesions on plain X-ray films. a An 8-mm defect is not visualised. b A 16-mm defect is seen as a faint osteolytic lesion. (Courtesy of H. van der Zwaag)

(Fig. 2.4). Mixed osteolytic-osteoblastic metastases often originate from breast and lung carcinoma.

Pathological compression fractures in patients with vertebral metastasis are well seen on plain X-rays of the spine. Lateral views show anteriorly flattened, wedge-shaped vertebral bodies. Wafer-like compression of vertebral bodies can be observed in AP and lateral projections. Compression fractures may cause the posterior wall of the vertebral body to be displaced posteriorly, with compression of the thecal sac and its contents (spinal cord, conus or cauda equina). Collapse of a vertebral body can also be observed in other vertebral tumours such as eosinophilic granuloma; this results in the so-called vertebra plana appearance (DE SCHEPPER et al. 1993). Preservation of intervertebral disc spaces is characteristic of tumours involving the vertebral body and constitutes a differential diagnostic criterion for distinguishing such a tumour from an infectious process (GREENFIELD 1980).

2.3
Myelography

2.3.1
General Principles and Technique

Myelography is an imaging technique performed by the injection of contrast medium into the subarachnoid space to opacify the cerebrospinal fluid and thereby produce the radiological contrast necessary for the visualisation of the spinal cord, cauda equina, nerve roots and the surrounding subarachnoid space. The contrast agent used can be negative (air, CO_2 or O_2) or positive (iodinated oil or water-soluble iodinated contrast medium). Myelography with water-soluble iodinated contrast agents is the preferred technique. In addition to being safer for the patient (little risk of delayed arachnoiditis), these contrast agents provide greatly improved anatomical detail. The myelographic contrast can be administered via lumbar puncture or lateral C1-C2 puncture. The lumbar puncture technique is preferred for myelography of the lumbar and thoracic spine and is preferably performed at the L3-L4 intervertebral

disc space (the L4 vertebra is usually at the level of the iliac crest).

2.3.2
Indications

Until a decade ago, suspicion of a space-occupying lesion of the spinal cord, nerve roots, meninges or spinal canal was an indication for myelography. MR imaging has taken over most of the indications for myelography because of its obvious advantages over myelography: no X-ray irradiation, painless procedure performed on out-patients, no need for a lumbar puncture, multiplanar imaging capability and superior soft tissue contrast resolution. Moreover, because MR imaging is a non-invasive technique it prevents the risk of myelographic complications (WILMINK et al. 1984; VAN DE KELFT et al. 1991) Therefore, there must be a firm clinical indication for myelography, a technique which is always uncomfortable for the patient and may be followed by mild to severe headache in up to 50% of patients. The frequency and severity of headache after lumbar myelography can be reduced by using a 25-gauge pencil point (Whitacre) spinal needle instead

a

b

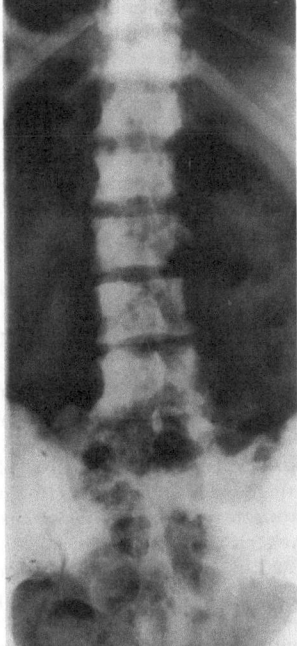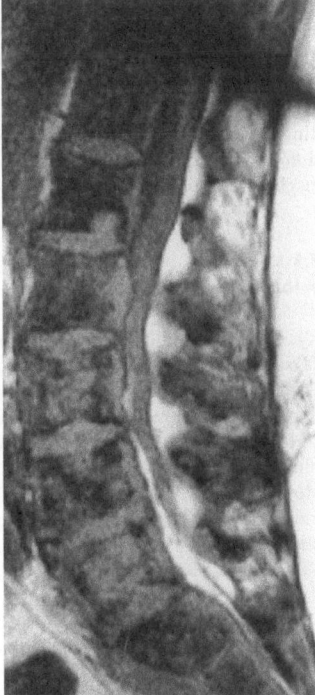

Fig. 2.4a,b. Osteoblastic vertebral metastasis in a patient with prostate carcinoma. **a** AP plain radiograph shows numerous osteoblastic or sclerotic lesions in the spine, sacrum and pelvis. **b** Sagittal SE T1-W MR image through the lumbar spine shows extensive multifocal metastatic lesions in the vertebral bodies, with replacement of fatty marrow. There is involvement of the anterior epidural space as well.

of the usual 20 to 22-gauge Quinke-point spinal needle (QUAYNOR et al. 1995). An essential consideration should be that the outcome of the myelographic
examination will affect the subsequent management
of the patient. At present, only a few indications for
myelography in patients with suspected tumour remain:

1 Absence (or unavailability) of MR imaging
2 Contra-indication for the patient`s being posi-
   tioned in a strong magnetic field (e.g. patients
   with pacemakers or ferromagnetic aneurysm
   clips in the brain)
3 Severely claustrophobic patients.

In all other instances, MR imaging has superseded myelography for the diagnosis of spinal
space-occupying lesions.

Patients referred for emergency myelography
usually have neurological abnormalities and/or evidence of severe vertebral destruction (>50% loss of
vertebral body height). If the neurological level is
not clinically evident, the myelogram should ideally
depict the entire spinal canal. It must be remembered that 10%-20% of patients in whom extradural
metastatic disease is shown have asymptomatic (extradural) metastases at another level. In approximately 15% of patients, extradural tumours extend
over more than one vertebral segment.

Finally, myelography has the advantage of providing a CSF sample that should be examined for:
cell count, cell differentiation, cytology, total protein, glucose and micro-organisms.

2.3.3
Myelographic Findings

Myelographic semiology can best be understood by
analysing the location of the lesion and its relationship to the contrast-filled subarachnoid space. Traditionally, spinal tumours are classified by location
as: intramedullary, intradural extramedullary, or extradural (synonym: epidural). This classification
represents somewhat of an oversimplification. Some
tumours may in fact reside in two compartments simultaneously, e.g. a dumbbell shaped neurogenic tumour extends into both the extradural and intradural extramedullary spaces.

Intramedullary neoplasms cause fusiform enlargement of the spinal cord. The surrounding subarachnoid space, which is opacified by contrast medium, is flattened by the thickened cord. Unless they

are very large or produce a complete myelographic
block, myelographic recognition of intramedullary
lesions is difficult. Moreover, enlargement of the spinal cord is not pathognomonic of tumour, but is also
observed in non-tumoral conditions such as syringomyelia or myelitis. Magnetic resonance imaging
has completely replaced myelography in the diagnostic work-up of patients with suspected intramedullary disease.

Myelography is a sensitive technique for showing
intradural extramedullary lesions. These lesions lie
within the subarachnoid space and consequently
produce sharply defined rounded filling defects at
the interface between the tumour and the contrast
medium (SHAPIRO 1984). When an intradural tumour produces a complete myelographic obstruction, the margin of the tumour abutting the contrast
is outlined as a "cap" defect. Intradural tumours include, among others, leptomeningeal metastatic deposits, schwannomas and meningiomas. They are illustrated in Fig. 2.5a,b.

Extradural lesions lie outside the subarachnoid
space and produce an extrinsic compression upon
the thecal sac. Benign extradural tumours (e.g. disc
herniation) indent the side of the contrast column;
the filling defect is usually limited to one or two vertebral segments (WILMINK et al. 1984; WILMINK
1988). Large extradural tumours may produce a
complete myelographic block. Extradural metastasis often produces a circumferential cuff of tumour
invasion around the thecal sac, resulting in a complete myelographic block. In the lumbar spine, an
extradural lesion can be suspected by its feathered,
serrated interface due to the fact that the opacified
subarachnoid space over the nerve roots is not in direct contact with the extradural lesion (Fig. 2.5c).
There is a generally accepted risk of neurological
deterioration after removal of CSF below the level of
a complete spinal subarachnoid block (SHAPIRO
1984; HOLLIS et al. 1986). Worsening of the clinical
condition following lumbar puncture is due to
changes in CSF hydrodynamics that may result in
downward spinal coning (HOLLIS et al. 1986). When
a total myelographic block is found, it is recommended to also demonstrate the other limit of the
obstruction, either by CT myelography (see Section
2.4.4) or by injecting contrast medium into the subarachnoid space on the other side of the block, e.g.
via lateral C1-C2 puncture. The degree of myelographic block and the neurological loss of function
are not directly related.

When a complete myelographic block is present,
it may not be possible to determine the exact loca-

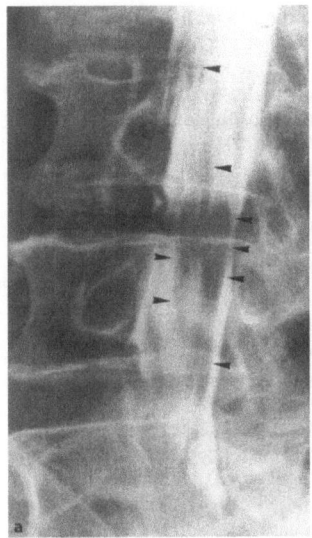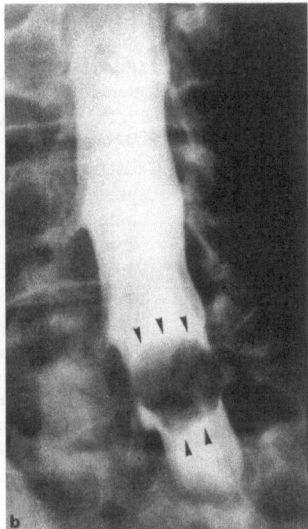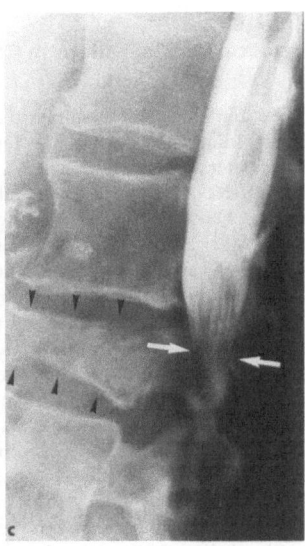

Fig. 2.3a–c. Myelographic findings in intradural and epidural lesions. **a** Lumbar myelogram (*oblique view*) in a patient with poorly differentiated bronchgenic carcinoma. Intradural metastatic nodules adhere to the thickened cauda equina nerve roots. They are shown as multiple filling defects of varying size (*arrowheads*). **b** Lumbar myelogram (*oblique view*) in a patient with a intradural schwannoma. The tumor is seen as a smooth, sharply marginated filling defect at L5-S1 (*arrowheads*). **c** Lumbar myelogram in a patient with breast carcinoma (*lateral projection*). Metastatic invasion of the anterior extradural space produces a complete myelographic block at L3 (*white arrows*). The feathered appearance at the head of the contrast column indicates an extradural lesion with block. There is a pathologic compression fracture of L3 (*black arrowheads*). Contrast from previous lymphography remains in lymph nodes which project over the anterior margin of L2

tion of a spinal tumour from its myelographic appearance (SHAPIRO 1984). A complete myelographic block can be produced by intramedullary, intradural, extramedullary or extradural tumours.

2.4
X-Ray Computed Tomography

2.4.1
General Principles

Since its introduction in the 1970s, computed tomography (CT) has become established as one of the most effective radiological techniques for the examination of the spine in a wide range of clinical situations. A detailed overview of the basic physics and instrumentation of CT is beyond the scope of this chapter. The reader is referred to more basic textbooks. Essentially, the reader should keep in mind that, as in conventional radiography, CT provides images which are grey-scale representations of the tissues' X-Ray density (attenuation values).

The attenuation value of a tissue is related to its electron density, and is expressed in CT imaging as Hounsfield units (HU). In other words, the Hounsfield value of tissue is determined by the degree to which it attenuates or weakens the X-ray beam. By convention, the attenuation value of air is –1000 HU, that of water 0 (zero) HU and that of bone +1000 HU In order to improve assessment of dense bony structures, most scanners feature an extended Hounsfield scale of up to + 4000 HU

Because in CT the X-ray tube moves around the patient in a plane perpendicular to the patient's long axis, it provides cross-sectional cuts. Each image is built up of a matrix of small squares (known as pixels, from picture elements) each representing the attenuation values of the tissues at that point. CT is superior to conventional X-ray imaging because the cross-sectional display implies that there is no superimposition of anatomic structures. A drawback is that, because of the cross-sectional nature of the images, each 'slice' represents only a relatively small volume of tissue, and imaging a large segment of the spine can be time-consuming and involves a large radiation dose to the patient. State-of-the-art spiral or helical CT scanners have greatly reduced the imaging time needed to examine longer segments of the spine.

2.4.2
Technical Considerations in CT of the Spine

CT examinations of the spine usually start with a digital radiograph known as the 'localiser' or 'scout' image (lateral or AP view or both). It is used to define the area of interest, to plan and record the level of the sections, and to determine the degree of angulation of the gantry. The choice of slice thickness depends on the area of examination and the suspected pathology. Thin sections can be obtained if the examination is specifically directed towards a small area of interest. When a larger anatomical region needs to be covered, the slice thickness (and/or) increment (interslice gap) will be increased to limit the number of scans and the radiation dose to the patient. In conventional CT scanning, it is not feasible to scan the entire spine, because this would involve a prohibitively lengthy examination time. This is changing to some extent with the introduction of spiral or helical CT scanning, but the impact of this technique in evaluating tumours of the spine still needs to be established.

Because the information contained in a CT image is digital, it can be viewed with different window and level settings. The window level is usually best set between the Hounsfield values for normal and abnormal tissues. For example, when the objective of the CT examination is to determine the soft tissue extension of a spinal lesion, soft tissue window settings with a window width of 300-500 HU will be used (Fig. 2.1b). Conversely, the vertebral bony structures, which include a wide range of attenuation values, should be viewed at window widths of 1500 to 4000 Hounsfield units (Fig. 2.1c; Fig. 2.2b). In looking for spinal lesions, in many cases the images will be studied with two different window/level settings, one for soft tissues and one for bony structures. There are software algorithms available for reprocessing data to give high-resolution images by applying specific convolution filters. A major advantage of CT over plain X-ray imaging lies in its ability to define subcortical and trabecular destruction (ALGRA 1995).

2.4.3
Contrast Enhancement

The use of intravenously injected, iodine-based contrast agents is the most important modification of the CT technique. Accumulation of the contrast agent causes a local increase in attenuation values known as 'enhancement'. In examinations of the spine, CT will be performed without or with intravenous contrast injection, depending on the indication for the study and the clinical status of the patient.

Non-contrast CT (NCCT) provides excellent visualisation of soft tissue structures adjacent to the spine, intervertebral discs and bony elements of the spine. Unfortunately, contrast resolution of structures within the bony spinal canal is not as good (except, perhaps, at the cranio-cervical junction and in the upper cervical spine). This is due to the fact that the spinal canal is relatively small, and surrounded by very dense osseous structures that attenuate the X-ray beam and cause beam hardening artefacts.

Contrast-enhanced CT (CECT) can occasionally be useful for visualising spinal lesions that possess increased vascularity (e.g. highly vascular tumours or vascular malformations). Normal enhancing structures in the spinal canal include the epidural veins and, in some cases, the anterior spinal artery. Dilatation of epidural veins is an indirect sign of an extradural lesion blocking the flow in the epidural venous channels and leading to venous congestion (Fig. 2.6). The epidural venous plexus is connected to the external vertebral plexus via intervertebral veins that accompany spinal nerves within the neural foramina. The external vertebral plexus is a network of veins along the vertebral body, laminae, and spinous, transverse and articular processes. CECT can also be used for showing vascular intradural extramedullary tumours such as schwannomas or meningiomas. Nevertheless, even with optimal technique, the performance of CT in the diagnosis of intramedullary lesions remains disappointing compared to MR imaging.

2.4.4
CT Myelography

CT myelography (CTM) is an adjunct to conventional myelography. This method provides information about intraspinal soft tissue masses and their effects upon the cord and nerve roots. Purely intramedullary lesions are often overlooked unless they are accompanied by gross swelling of the cord. Conversely, intradural extramedullary tumours are easily recognised as filling defects within the subarachnoid space that is opacified by the contrast agent (Fig. 2.7a,b). The use of sagittal, coronal or oblique reformatted images helps to gain insight into the morphology and spatial relationships of the tumour

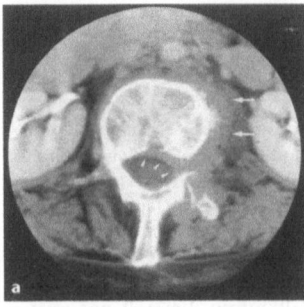
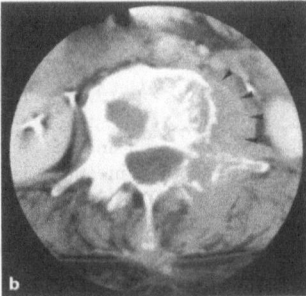
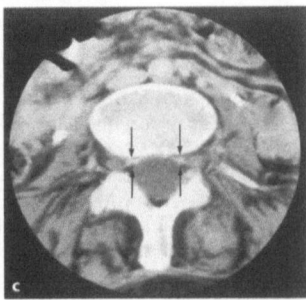

Fig. 2.6a-c. Contrast-enhanced CT in a 33-year-old woman with metastatic breast carcinoma showing invasion of the epidural space and congestion of the epidural veins. **a** Metastatic tumour extends from the paravertebral region (*arrows*) through the left neural foramen L2-L3 into the extradural space around the thecal sac (*arrowheads*). The soft tissue component of the metastasis enhances with intravenous contrast. **b** Section through L3 shows a large paravertebral soft tissue mass (*arrowheads*) with associated bone destruction involving the vertebral body, lamina, spinous and transverse processes. **c** Section through L4 reveals dilatation and congestion of the anterior epidural veins (*arrows*) due to tumour obstruction at a higher segment

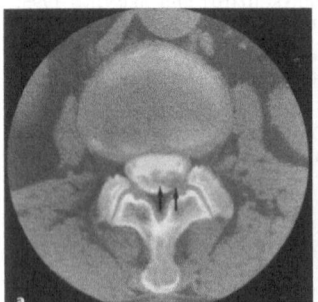
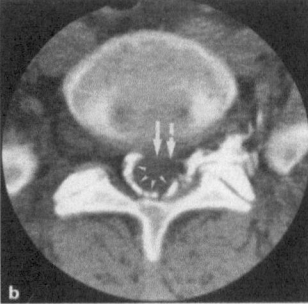
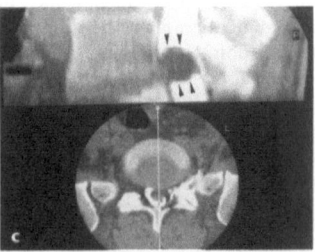
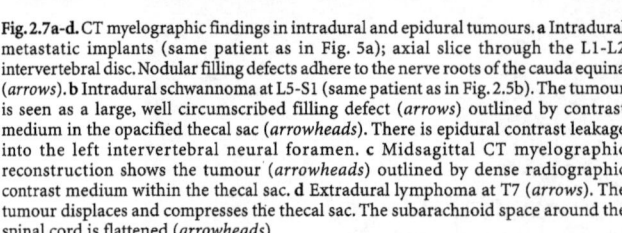
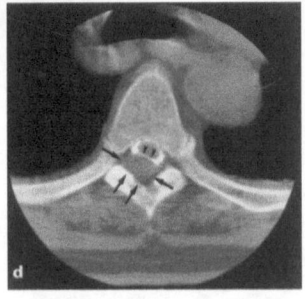

Fig. 2.7a-d. CT myelographic findings in intradural and epidural tumours. **a** Intradural metastatic implants (same patient as in Fig. 5a); axial slice through the L1-L2 intervertebral disc. Nodular filling defects adhere to the nerve roots of the cauda equina (*arrows*). **b** Intradural schwannoma at L5-S1 (same patient as in Fig. 2.5b). The tumour is seen as a large, well circumscribed filling defect (*arrows*) outlined by contrast medium in the opacified thecal sac (*arrowheads*). There is epidural contrast leakage into the left intervertebral neural foramen. **c** Midsagittal CT myelographic reconstruction shows the tumour (*arrowheads*) outlined by dense radiographic contrast medium within the thecal sac. **d** Extradural lymphoma at T7 (*arrows*). The tumour displaces and compresses the thecal sac. The subarachnoid space around the spinal cord is flattened (*arrowheads*)

(Fig. 2.7c). Extradural tumour invasion is seen as extrinsic compression of the contrast-filled thecal sac (Fig. 2.7d).

When the conventional myelographic examination shows a total block, CTM may help to depict the other margin of the block due to the intrinsically greater contrast resolution and the delay between the myelographic procedure and the CTM examination (Fig. 2.8). Similarly, when the quality of the conventional myelogram is inadequate due to dilution of the intradural contrast medium, CTM with its superior contrast resolution may save the examination.

A disadvantage with all CT techniques is that the location and extent of the lesion must be anticipated before starting the examination, so that the CT technique can be optimised with regard to slice thickness, interval or overlap, starting and ending location.

2.4.5
CT-Guided Biopsy

CT has proved to be a useful method of guiding per-cutaneous biopsy for diagnosing spinal or para-spinal tumours (KATTAPURAM and ROSENTHAL, 1987; KATTAPURAM et al. 1992; FREYSCHMIDT and BERNING, 1995; ALGRA 1995). The procedure is gen-erally performed under local anaesthesia. Thoracic and lumbar vertebrae are reached from a posterior lateral approach with the patient in prone position (Fig. 2.9). From a diagnostic CT scan series, a slice is selected that shows both the lesion and an approach route. A suitable point on the body surface is chosen to begin the procedure. The position is confirmed by placing a marker on the skin (e.g. a hypodermic nee-dle or a catheter segment) across the plane of the CT scan. A new CT image is then acquired and the bi-opsy route is determined by measuring the distance and angulation from the skin marker to the lesion (target point). Ideally the needle should follow the shortest possible path, but in case of a planned sur-gical excision it is important that the needle track should be excised completely to avoid tumour seed-ing. Vessels must be avoided in mapping the ap-proach. When in doubt regarding certain structures,

a new CT section after bolus enhancement of vessels should be obtained. After the approach has thus been determined, the skin is infiltrated with local anaesthetic and the biopsy needle is inserted. Pref-erably this is carried out with suspended respira-tion and it is important that the patient should hold his breath in the same phase of respiration for the imaging guidance to be accurate. Depth and angle of the needle are confirmed by one or more CT sections with the needle in place. The angle is approximately 30°-45° from the sagittal plane (FREYSCHMIDT and BERNING, 1995). If necessary, adjustments are made. A CT image is always made with the tip of the needle situated at the desired tar-get point (Fig 2.9)

Several types of needle can be used: needles for cytological diagnosis (aspiration needles) and needles for histological diagnosis (cutting and tre-phine needles) (FREYSCHMIDT and BERNING 1995; HAUENSTEIN et al. 1988). The choice of needle de-pends on several factors: tissue to be biopsied, depth of the target point, previous experience with a par-ticular type of needle and personal preference of the radiologist. Ideally a needle must be chosen that is easy to manipulate, reliable and safe and that pro-

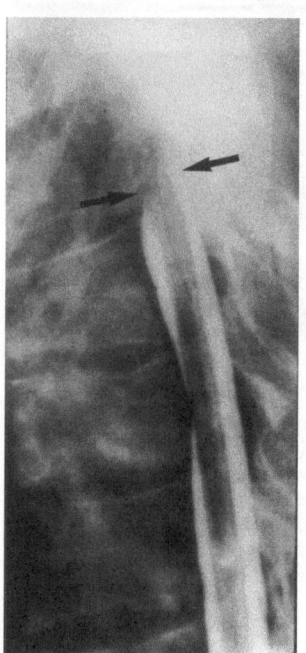

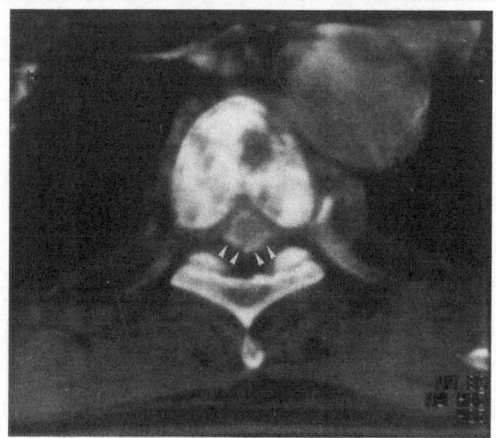

Fig. 2.8a,b. Myelography and CT myelography in a 75-year-old woman with metastatic breast carcinoma. **a** Thoracic myelogram, lateral view, shows a complete myelographic block (*arrows*). **b** Axial CT myelographic image obtained 2 cm above the level of the block shows faint opacification of the subarachnoid spaces around the cord (*arrowheads*). This illustrates the superior contrast resolution of CT. Note the osteolytic and osteoblastic metastatic lesions in the vertebral body

a
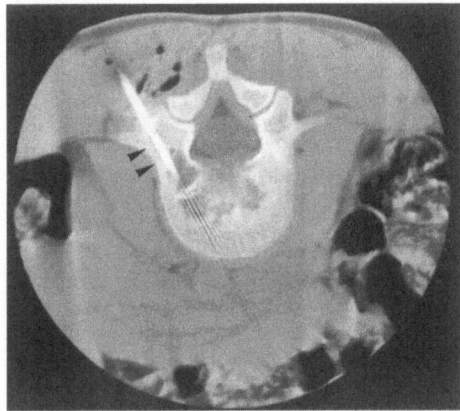

b
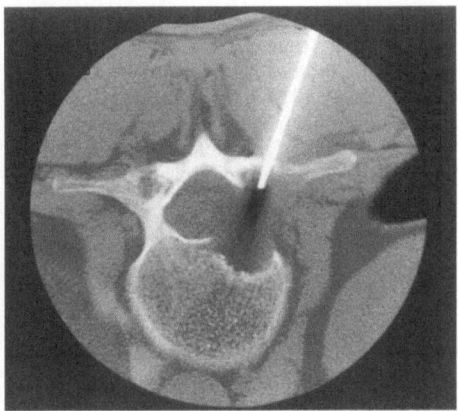

Fig. 2.9a,b. CT-guided needle biopsy. **a** CT-guided biopsy of L3 in a 10-year-old boy. Axial CT scan with the patient in prone position. The CT image shows the course of the needle, which enters through the right pedicle (*arrowheads*). Histology demonstrated a non-specific granulomatous disorder; no malignancy was found. **b** CT-guided biopsy in a 46-year-old man with an osteolytic mass in the left pedicle of L1. The needle tip is positioned in the lesion with the patient in prone position. Histological diagnosis: metastasis from adenocarcinoma

vides a cylinder of bone or tissue for histological examination.

2.5
Magnetic Resonance Imaging

2.5.1
General Principles

In this section we do not intend to provide an in-depth explanation of the basic physical principles, instrumentation aspects and image formation theory pertaining to MR imaging. This is clearly beyond the scope of this chapter. Rather, it is our aim to provide an expanded and annotated glossary of terms and concepts that the reader is likely to encounter in the daily practice of spinal MR imaging. Interested readers are referred to more basic works and textbooks (ATLAS 1996; KETT and PRÜLL 1990; RUNGE 1996; STARK and BRADLEY 1992; WEHRLI and McGOWAN 1996; RINCK 1993).

When an object consisting largely of water such as the human body is placed in a magnetic field, its protons and other nuclei possessing a magnetic moment will become aligned parallel or anti-parallel to the external magnetic field with a slight excess of the parallel orientation. In effect the body becomes slightly magnetised with its magnetic vector parallel to the longitudinal axis of the external field. If an ex-

ternal radiofrequency (RF) signal is now applied, several processes ensue which result in the magnetic vector in effect being tipped out of the longitudinal direction and rotating in the direction transverse to the external field. This rotating vector is the sum of the vectors of the individual protons spinning or precessing in phase and produces an RF signal of the same frequency as the external RF pulse and related to the field strength of the magnet. This process of magnetic resonance is called *excitation*. It can be compared to the resonance of a tuning fork, which starts to oscillate when exposed to sound waves of appropriate frequency.

An RF pulse with sufficient power and duration to flip the magnetisation vector from the longitudinal to the fully transverse direction is called a 90° pulse. After such a pulse has been applied, the protons are said to be saturated.

When the external RF source is switched off, the original conditions are restored. Longitudinal magnetisation is regained and transverse magnetisation decays, a process which is called *relaxation*. Longitudinal and transverse relaxation occur at different rates and are influenced by different tissue factors. The RF signal from the protons fades with the decay in transverse magnetisation. Regrowth of longitudinal magnetisation is characterised by the longitudinal relaxation time T1 and decay of transverse magnetisation by the transverse relaxation time T2.

By employing repetitive RF pulses at varying intervals (repetition time or TR) and recording the RF signal from the protons at varying times after excitation (echo time or TE), information can be elicited regarding longitudinal and transverse magnetisation characteristics of the protons in various tissue compositions within the body. Thus an MR image can be "*T1-weighted*" (T1-W), "*proton-density weighted*" (PD-W) "*T2-weighted*" (T2-W) (Fig. 2.10). These three basic types of image contrast reflect tissue differences and variations in T1 relaxation time, density of protons, and T2 relaxation time of the anatomic region being imaged (PLEWES 1994).

The capability for sampling several tissue characteristics is one of the factors that makes MR imaging superior to other radiographic techniques, including X-ray CT imaging in which contrast is determined by only a single variable, X-ray attenuation, through variations in electron density. Conversely, in MR imaging, contrast between a suspected lesion and surrounding tissues can be optimised by appropriate T1, PD or T2 weighting or by the use of an intravenously injected contrast medium (see Section 2.5.7). Although PD-W images are useful in diagnosing inflammatory intramedullary lesions (e.g. multiple sclerosis), they are of little use in imaging spinal tumours, because the intrinsic contrast resolution is poor.

Apart from excitation, RF pulses are also used for other purposes in MR imaging. One of these is the 180° refocusing pulse used to counteract dephasing of the precessing protons and premature loss of the RF signal by magnetic field inhomogeneity. The spin echo sequence, which is produced in this way, is the most universally applied technique in MR imaging. In order to produce tomographic cuts of the body (MR imaging is also a form of computed tomography), the signals from groups of protons must be spatially encoded to permit localisation in three dimensions. This is done by the use of weaker accessory magnetic fields that induce variations in strength or gradients in the main magnetic field. The RF frequency needed to excite the protons as well as the frequency of the signal emitted by these protons depends on the strength of the magnetic field influencing the protons in question.

In gradient echo imaging, refocusing of the protons is not achieved by a 180° pulse as with the spin echo technique. Instead, the gradients are briefly applied in opposing directions (gradient reversal). Using this technique, images can be produced with T1- and T2 weighting. More correctly, the symbol T2* should be used, because this value is not independent of magnetic field inhomogeneities as T2 is. Therefore, T2* is shorter than T2, especially at high field strengths.

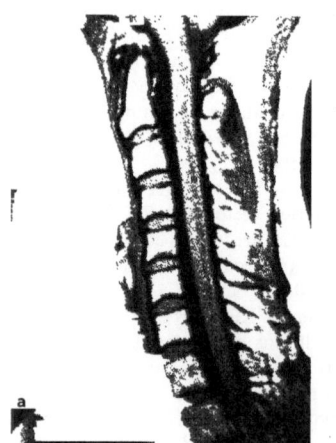 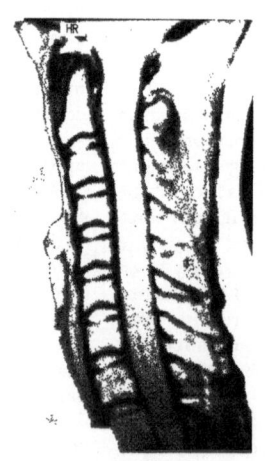 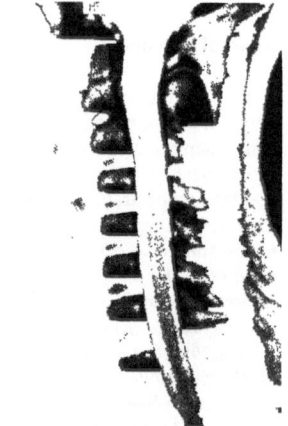

Fig. 2.10a-c. Midsagittal spin echo T1-W, PD-W and T2-W images of the cervical spine. **a** T1-W image is obtained with short TR (500 ms) and short TE (15 ms). This provides an 'anatomical' image in which fat is hyperintense ('bright') and CSF is hypointense ('dark'). Intervertebral discs are hypointense relative to bone marrow in the vertebral bodies. **b** PD-W image is obtained with long TR (2500 ms) and short TE (20 ms). Contrast resolution of tissues within the spinal canal is poor: the spinal cord cannot be distinguished from the surrounding CSF. PD-W images are not often used in the evaluation of spinal mass lesions. **c** T2-W image is obtained with long TR (2500 ms) and long TE (80 ms). This image provides a 'myelographic' effect: the spinal cord is silhouetted by high signal intensity CSF. Normal intervertebral discs are hyperintense relative to the vertebral bodies

Let us consider a transverse cut through the body. A gradient is applied longitudinal to the body along the so-called z-axis, and an RF frequency is selected to excite only that section of protons at the appropriate level of the gradient (and body). The *slice selection gradient* thus provides localisation along the long axis of the body. Spatial encoding in the other two axes (x and y) is accomplished by manipulating the emitted RF signal. The *frequency encoding gradient* is switched on, and along this gradient the precession frequency of protons changes. As field strength increases along the gradient, the protons precess more rapidly and the frequency of the emitted RF signal increases. The third spatial dimension is defined by the use of the *phase encoding* gradient. This gradient is briefly switched on, and along the gradient phase changes occur in precessing protons and their emitted RF signals.

By using a Fourier transform, groups of protons from a stimulated slice of the body are now assigned spatial co-ordinates based on the frequency and phase of their RF signals. Signal strength, as determined among others by PD, T1 and T2, is expressed as grey scale values of the pixels making up the image.

2.5.2
Practical Considerations

The diagnostic principle of MR imaging, as with all other imaging techniques, lies in its ability to convert anatomical shapes or tissue characteristics within the body into linear contours and grey-scale values in an image on a TV monitor or a hard copy. The sharpness with which contours are defined is expressed as *spatial resolution* and the accuracy with which low-contrast objects can be distinguished from the background as *contrast resolution*. Contrast resolution is adversely affected by an increase in the level of background noise or statistical fluctuations in grey-scale values. Noise is inherent to the imaging system and is also generated within the patient. Signal-to-noise ratio (SNR) and contrast-to-noise (CNR) ratio are important parameters influencing image quality. Depending on the clinical query, trade-offs have to be made between spatial resolution and contrast resolution. Each can be improved at the expense of the other, with *imaging time (or temporal resolution)* constituting a third variable.

Now the trade-off can begin. Spatial resolution or image sharpness can be improved by acquiring thinner slices, reducing the field of view (FOV) or using a finer image matrix. All these measures result in smaller tissue volumes, or voxels, being sampled. Besides increasing spatial resolution this results in less precise measurements of tissue characteristics or increase in statistical noise which can be countered by increasing the number of measurements (syn. excitations or averages) at the cost of increasing the acquisition time. Unfortunately, SNR increases not in direct proportion to the number of excitations, but in proportion to their square root (Fig. 2.11).

Spatial resolution can be improved by increasing the matrix size. This can be achieved in two ways. When the number of phase encoding steps is increased, the acquisition time increases accordingly (Fig. 2.12a,b). Conversely the number of frequency encoding steps can be increased without incurring a time penalty (Fig. 2.12c). For spinal imaging, most current MR scanners employ a rectangular FOV (recFOV). With a recFOV the number of phase encoding steps can be reduced and acquisition time can be shortened while maintaining the same spatial resolution (Fig. 2.12d). Conversely, when it is necessary to limit the examination time and the number of excitations is reduced, this results in a decrease in SNR, which can accordingly be compensated by sacrificing spatial resolution (selecting a larger FOV, greater slice thickness or coarser matrix).

Background noise is reduced by the selection of an appropriate coil or RF antenna (the smaller a coil, the less noise is picked up from the patient, but also the smaller the volume imaged). A difficult trade-off in imaging spinal tumours is between the length of the spine to be examined, image quality and imaging time. If it is not possible to establish a reliable level by clinical examination, a large segment of the spine needs to be imaged. Here a choice must be made between multiple acquisitions at several levels versus a single acquisition sequence with a large whole-body coil and a large FOV. In the first case, with dedicated surface or saddle coils, the imaging volume is limited, and typically only the cervical, thoracic or lumbar spine can be covered in any one scan acquisition. Thus, if the entire spine must be examined, the examination time is greatly prolonged, but in each section, the SNR will be high due to the close proximity of the examined anatomical spine segment to the coil. Conversely, if a whole body volume coil is used (RF transmission and reception), image quality will suffer (poor SNR when compared to a surface coil, decreased spatial resolution due to the large FOV). This dilemma is being alleviated by improved surface coil technology (phased array coils), but a good

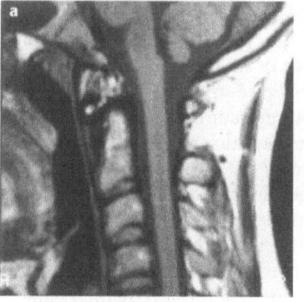 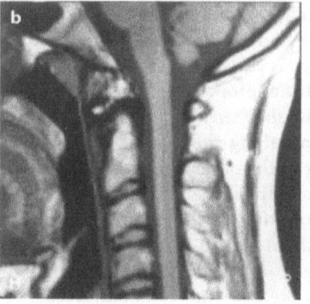 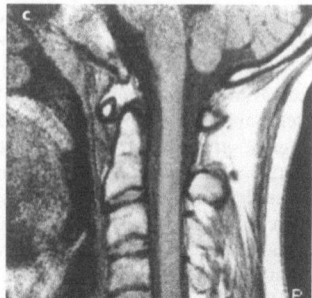

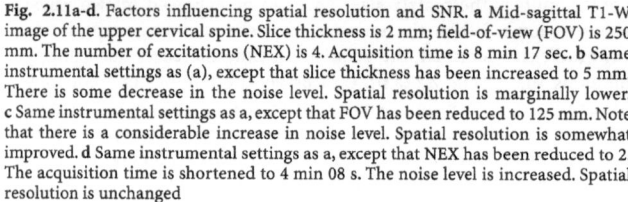 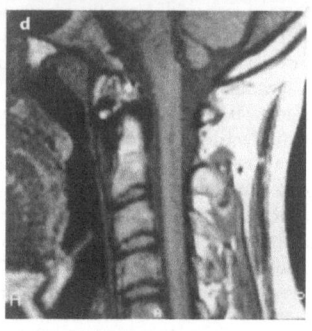

Fig. 2.11a-d. Factors influencing spatial resolution and SNR. **a** Mid-sagittal T1-W image of the upper cervical spine. Slice thickness is 2 mm; field-of-view (FOV) is 250 mm. The number of excitations (NEX) is 4. Acquisition time is 8 min 17 sec. **b** Same instrumental settings as (a), except that slice thickness has been increased to 5 mm. There is some decrease in the noise level. Spatial resolution is marginally lower. **c** Same instrumental settings as a, except that FOV has been reduced to 125 mm. Note that there is a considerable increase in noise level. Spatial resolution is somewhat improved. **d** Same instrumental settings as a, except that NEX has been reduced to 2. The acquisition time is shortened to 4 min 08 s. The noise level is increased. Spatial resolution is unchanged

clinical examination is still of paramount importance in limiting, where possible, the length of the spine to be examined.

2.5.3
Spin Echo T1-Weighted MR Imaging

An MR image is called "T1-weighted" (T1-W) when image contrast is based upon tissue differences in T1, i.e. the longitudinal relaxation time. The time constant T1 of a biological tissue characterises the rate at which spin-lattice relaxation occurs (the speed with which the protons reorient themselves parallel to the main magnetic field) and longitudinal magnetisation is restored.

Traditionally, T1-W images have been produced by using a *spin echo (SE) sequence* with a short repetition time (TR: 300-700 ms, depending on field strength) and a short echo time (TE: 30 ms or less). The sequence derives its name from the 180° SE pulse that is used to refocus the protons. After the 90° excitation pulse the precessing protons undergo dephasing due to magnetic field inhomogeneities, and the RF signal is progressively lost. The SE pulse inverts the rotational axis of the precessing protons, so rephasing occurs and at the appropriate moment an SE signal can be registered.

When an SE technique is used with a short TR, spins with a long T1 relaxation time cannot completely relax or regain magnetisation between excitations and therefore do not contribute to the signal. It follows that the corresponding biological tissues (e.g. cerebrospinal fluid) are seen as low-intensity (dark or black) structures in the resulting MR image. Conversely, biological tissues with a short T1 relaxation time relax completely between successive excitations, are fully magnetised and contribute strongly to the signal. These are hyperintense (bright) in T1-W MR images, e.g. fat (Fig. 2.13). Parameter settings for a T1-W sequence are chosen in such a way that most biological tissues have intermediate relaxation times and are seen as shades of grey. The use of a short TE value makes the signal (and the resulting image) independent of T2 because the T2 decay process is just beginning.

T1 W images provide excellent anatomical information on the spine; the spinal cord is outlined by hypointense cerebrospinal fluid (CSF), and the thecal sac is outlined by hyperintense epidural fat.

2.5.4
Spin Echo and Fast Spin Echo T2-Weighted MR Imaging

An MR image is called "T2-weighted" (T2-W), when image contrast is based upon tissue differences in T2, i.e. the transverse relaxation time. In *SE sequences*, T2 weighting is achieved by combining a long repetition time TR (usually 2000-3000 ms) with a long echo time TE (80-120 ms or more). Long TR reduces T1-contrast, while long TE produces strong T2 contrast. A disadvantage of conventional SE imaging lies in the lengthy acquisition time imposed by long TR.

Conversely, in *fast spin echo (FSE) sequences*, also known as turbo spin echo (TSE) sequences, multiple phase-encoding steps are acquired per excitation instead of a single step as in conventional SE imaging (LISTERUD et al. 1992; ATLAS et al. 1993). Acquisition times for FSE T2-W "myelographic" images are typically reduced to one third or one quarter of the time necessary for conventional SE imaging. This has proved to be very useful in spinal imaging. Due to shorter imaging times, patient motion is reduced, throughput is increased and per-patient examination costs can be reduced (PETERSEIN and SAINI 1995). Alternatively, the implementation of faster sequences can be utilised to perform one or more supplementary sequences. In this way, the potential reduction in imaging time is traded for an improved, more complete MR examination. Due to

the repetitive 180° pulses, FSE sequences are less sensitive to susceptibility and metallic artefacts. This constitutes an advantage when imaging postoperative patients (TARTAGLINO et al. 1994). Conversely, the decreased sensitivity to susceptibility artefacts is a drawback when searching for old haemorrhagic foci.

Image characteristics of T2-W FSE images are comparable to those acquired with conventional SE sequences with equal effective TE (CHAPPELL et al. 1995). However, fat (including vertebral fatty bone marrow) is imaged with a higher signal intensity on FSE than on SE images (HENKELMAN et al. 1992). The brighter signal intensity of bone marrow fat on T2-W FSE images may mask vertebral metastases which are already difficult to detect on conventional SE T2-W images. In these instances, fat suppression is useful (see also Section 2.5.8).

The hallmark of T2-W images is the high signal from CSF, which creates a 'myelographic' effect. When short TEs and short echo trains are used, the visibility of subtle spinal cord lesions such as multiple sclerosis plaques is improved (HITTMAIR et al. 1996). Long TE values and long echo trains are ben-

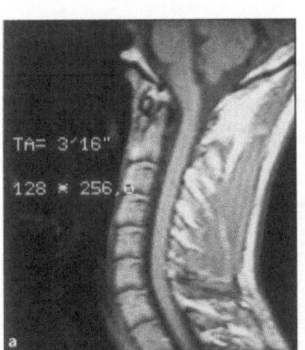
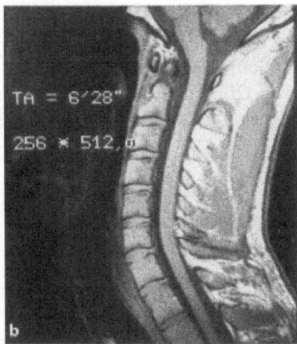
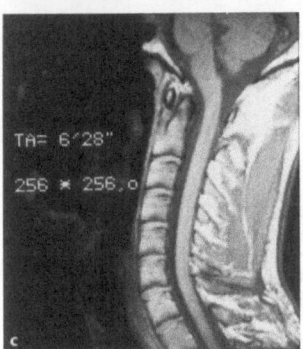
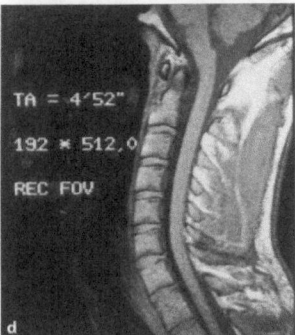

Fig. 2.12a-d. Influence of matrix size on acquisition time. a Midsagittal T1-W MR image (SE 500/15) obtained with a matrix of 128 phase encoding steps and 256 frequency encoding steps (matrix 128 · 256). Acquisition time is 3 min 16 s. b When the number of phase-encoding steps is increased to 256 (matrix 256·256), spatial resolution improves and the acquisition time is doubled to 6 min 28 s. c The number of frequency encoding steps can be increased from 256 to 512 (matrix 256 · 512) with no increase in the acquisition time (6 min 28 secs). Spatial resolution is improved. d When a rectangular field-of-view (rec FOV) of 6/8 (75%) is used, the number of phase encoding steps can be decreased to 192 (matrix 192 · 512) while maintaining the same spatial resolution. Imaging time decreases to 4 min 52 s.

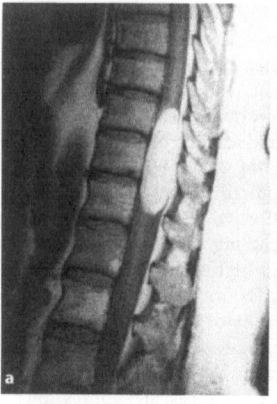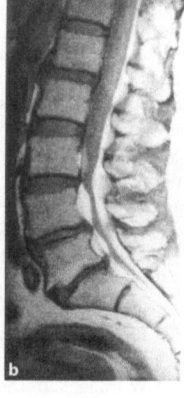

Fig. 2.13a,b. Fat produces high signal intensity in T1-W images. **a** Midsagittal SE T1-W image shows a uniformly hyperintense intradural mass in the lower thoracic spine. The findings are pathognomonic for lipoma (see also Fig. 2.28). **b** Midsagittal SE T1-W in a patient with severe epidural lipomatosis, seen as widespread high signal intensity around the thecal sac. The epidural fat impinges upon the thecal sac in the lower lumbar spine

ing nerve roots. A maximum intensity projection (MIP) algorithm, such as that utilized in MR angiography, can be used to create a 3D representation from multiple FSE T2-W images (see also Section 2.5.6). This generates a so-called "MR myelogram" (KRUDY 1992; HOFMAN and WILMINK 1996) (Fig. 2.14). Extrinsic impressions upon the dural sac by vertebral or extradural lesions are well imaged; T2-W images have supplanted myelography in these cases. Intradural lesions, such as leptomeningeal metastases, are also well demonstrated especially when heavily T2-W FSE sequences are employed (SCHUKNECHT et al. 1992). (Fig. 2.14b, Fig. 2. 15). These images provide anatomical detail comparable to T1-W images after contrast injection. Artefacts resulting from pulsatile CSF flow in the perimedullary subarachnoid spaces can provide misleading images, especially in the thoracic region. A method of suppressing these artefacts is 3D imaging (see Section 5.6.).

eficial for showing extramedullary and extradural disease (HITTMAIR et al. 1996). Sagittal FSE T2-W images provide an excellent depiction of the spinal canal and its contents, i.e. outlines of the thecal sac as well as the spinal cord and nerve roots contained within. Slice thickness is generally 3-5 mm. Oblique coronal views can be useful for depicting the emerg-

2.5.5
Gradient Echo Imaging

2.5.5.1
Principle

In gradient echo (GRE) sequences, the echo is a gradient echo (also known as field echo, as opposed to

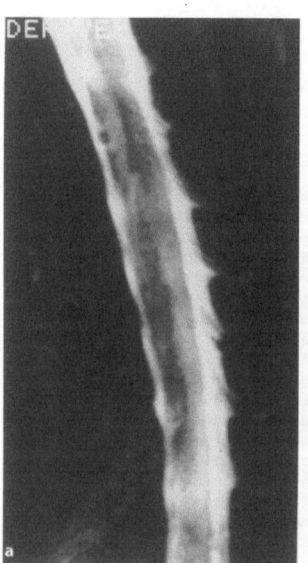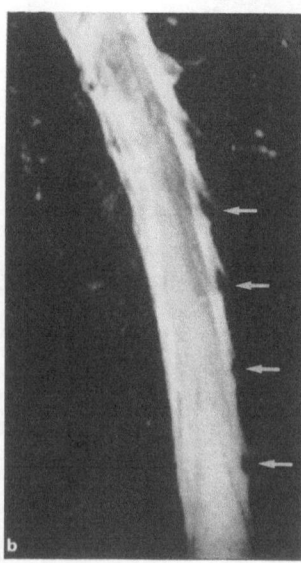

Fig. 2.14a,b Maximum intensity projection (MIP) reformats of oblique coronal heavily T2-W slice set can be used to produce an MR myelogram. **a** Normal individual. **b** Patient with lymphomatous deposits on several cervical nerve roots, seen as 'filling defects' (*arrows*)

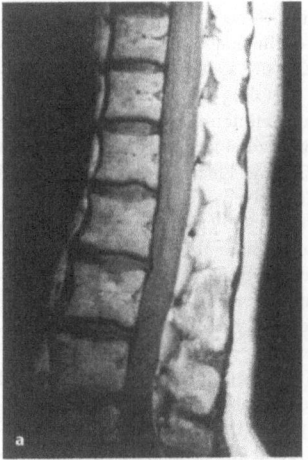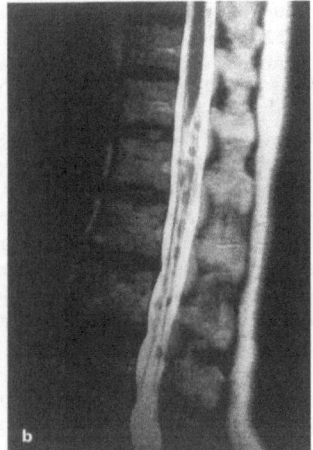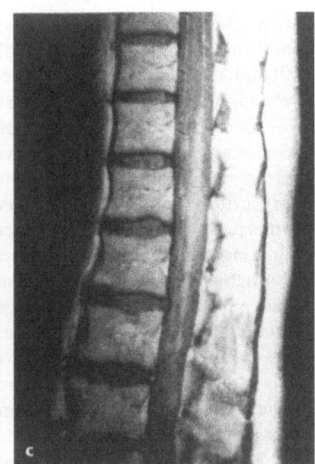

Fig. 2.15a-c. Myelographic effect in FSE T2-W images outlines small metastatic deposits. **a** Sagittal SE T1-W image shows thickening of cauda equina nerve roots, but contrast resolution between nerve roots and surrounding CSF is poor. **b** Midsagittal FSE T2-W image silhouettes the small metastatic nodules adherent to the nerve roots of the cauda equina. The lesions appear as "beads on a string". **c** Midsagittal SE T1-W image after intravenous contrast medium administration shows enhancement of the neoplastic coating along the cauda equina nerve roots and on the surface of the conus medullaris

spin echo) generated by applying a pair of balanced gradients of opposite signs (HAASE et al. 1986). GRE sequences use a single RF pulse, usually with a flip angle of less than 90°. If the flip angle is less than 90°, 180° can not be used. Therefore, in GRE imaging the echo must be created by gradient refocusing instead of RF refocusing. GRE sequences come in a wide variety of types, most of which are identified by their acronyms. Several different types of GRE sequences are currently used in clinical practice. These methods all rely on a reduced flip angle to enhance signal with short TR, but differ in the architecture of the pulse sequence. The modifications, however, significantly influence image contrast. Signal and contrast behaviour in GRE sequences are more complex than in conventional SE sequences (PRICE RR 1995). Tissue contrast is governed not only by TR and TE, but can also be varied by changing the flip angle (in SE sequences, the flip angle is 90°). In fact, in GRE sequences, the flip angle is the main determinant of contrast.

Two major 'families' of GRE sequences are used in clinical practice: spoiled GRE and rephased GRE (NITZ 1995). GRE images can be obtained in 2D or 3D data sets.

2.5.5.2
Spoiled GRE

In *"spoiled" GRE*, an RF spoiler is used to destroy coherency of transverse magnetisation (NITZ 1995). Therefore, transverse magnetisation does not contribute to the signal. Longitudinal magnetisation is allowed to recover and reach steady-state condition. Spoiled GRE imaging is known by the acronyms of FLASH (fast low angle shot; Siemens), SPGR (spoiled gradient recalled acquisition in the steady state; General Electric) or CE-FFE-T1 (contrast-enhanced fast field echo with T1 weighting; Philips).

When spoiled GRE imaging with a long TR (e.g. 500 ms) and a *large flip angle* (90°) is used, as in 2 D FLASH sequences, T1 contrast similar to that of spin echo imaging can be obtained. Short TE intervals (≤ 10 ms) minimise T2* weighting. The tendency towards T1 weighting occurs at higher flip angles at lower field strength (PARIZEL 1994). When a spoiled GRE sequence with short TR (e.g. 40 ms) is chosen, as in a 3 D FLASH sequence, there are less T2 effects at low flip angles. Therefore T1 contrast is achieved more rapidly, even with relatively small flip angles (30° at high field strengths; 60° at lower field strengths).

GRE techniques with small flip angle (e.g. 20-30°) can be used to provide images with bright CSF signals of the spine (T2*-W images). They resemble conventional SE or FSE 'myelographic' T2-W images with high CSF signals, low signal vertebrae, and relatively high signal of the intervertebral discs (Fig. 2.16). Blood flow produces high signal intensity in these images (Fig. 2.16b). A disadvantage is that the contrast resolution of GRE sequences for intramedullary lesions is not as good as that of their SE or FSE counterparts. Thus, GRE sequences are useful for evaluating degenerative or disc pathology, but are less sensitive in detecting of intramedullary lesions. An advantage of GRE T2*-W images over their conventional SE T2-W counterparts is that imaging times are shorter, since when a flip angle of less than 90° is used, relaxation occurs more quickly and TR can be reduced. For the same reason, however, SNR is lower in small flip angle GRE images. In terms of SNR, FSE images are presently proving superior.

2.5.5.3
Rephased GRE

"*Rephased*" or "*steady-state*" GRE sequences operate with a steady state for both longitudinal and trans-verse magnetisation (NITZ 1995). Thus, the transverse component of the magnetisation vector is preserved. Steady-state GRE sequences with free induction decay (FID) sampling are known by the acronyms of FISP (free induction in the steady state; Siemens), GRASS (gradient recalled acquisition in the steady state; General Electric) or FFE (fast field echo; Philips). Alternatively, steady-state GRE can be used with SE or stimulated echo sampling, in which case they are known under the acronyms PSIF (reversed FISP; Siemens), SSFP (steady-state free precession technique; General Electric) or CE-FFE-T2 (contrast-enhanced fast field echo with T2 weighting; Philips).

Steady-state GRE imaging differs from spoiled GRE imaging in that the steady-state free precession echo contributes to the signal, an effect that increases at short TR and large flip angle. Because the greatest signal contribution to this sequence is from tissues with a long T2 relaxation time, the signal intensity from CSF is higher, especially when short TR values (e.g. 50 ms) and large flip angles are used. Therefore, these sequences are less useful for achieving true T1 contrast, because the CSF retains high to very high signal intensity, especially with short TR

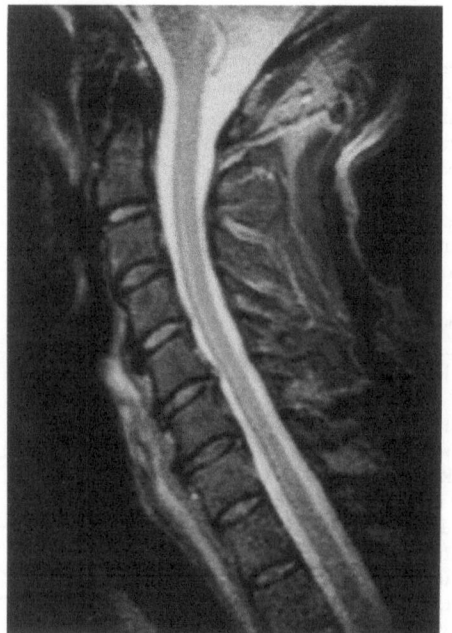

a

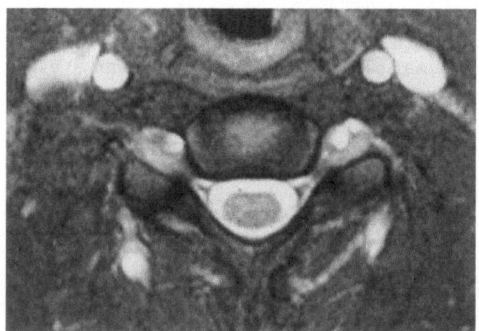

b

Fig. 2.16a,b. Spoiled gradient echo T2*-W images of the cervical spine obtained at low field strength (0.2 T) with a collar-shaped solenoidal coil. a Sagittal T2*-W 2D FLASH sequence (TR/TE/flip angle: 518/45/25°) provides excellent myelographic effect, and is therefore particularly useful for evaluating extradural disease. Within the spinal cord differentiation between grey and white matter is seen. b Axial T2*-W 2D-FLASH image (TR/TE/flip angle: 435/45/25°) through the C5-C6 intervertebral disc. Note the butterfly shape of the intramedullary grey matter.

values (e.g. 50 ms). With 'long' TR values (≥ 500 ms), spoiled and rephased GRE sequences can be considered equivalent in terms of contrast behaviour, though CSF generally displays a higher SI in the rephased GRE sequences.

2.5.5.4
Susceptibility

Magnetic-susceptibility-induced misregistration along the frequency-encoding axis occurs in all pulse sequence types (CZERVIONKE et al. 1988). However, susceptibility induced artefactual tissue loss is negligible in SE imaging; in FSE sequences, suceptibility effects are even less than in conventional SE imaging. This is because in SE and FSE sequences, the phenomenon of spin dephasing is corrected by one or more 180° refocusing RF pulses. Due to the absence of a 180° refocusing pulse in GRE sequences, local field inhomogeneities caused by differences in magnetic susceptibility (bone/air tissue interfaces, calcium and iron deposits, metallic fixation devices) cause loss of signal (POSSE and AUE 1990). This is observed as artefactual dark areas in the image. These artefacts can severely degrade image quality, but can also be used as an aid in diagnosis (e.g. detection of haemosiderin in old haemorrhagic foci). Foreign *ferromagnetic objects*, such as spinal fixation devices, cause severe local magnetic field distortion (PARIZEL et al. 1996). If the material is ferromagnetic (e.g. stainless steel), a large distortion of the magnetic field deforms the MR image, and may render interpretation of anatomical structures completely impossible. Even *nonferromagnetic materials* (e.g. titanium or tantalum) can cause image artefacts because eddy currents are generated in these objects by gradient magnetic fields that disrupt the local magnetic field (BELLON et al. 1986; SHELLOCK and CRUES 1988). In clinical practice, the presence of large metallic spinal fixation devices renders MRI of the involved region of the spine virtually impossible (PARIZEL et al. 1996).

2.5.6
Three-Dimensional Imaging

Three-dimensional (3D) imaging or volume scanning is a method of acquiring thinner slices without a concomitant penalty in terms of reduced SNR or increased imaging time. In 3D imaging, the slice selection z-gradient used in 2D imaging is omitted,

and signal is acquired from the entire volume scanned rather than a single slice. Slice selection in 3D imaging is achieved by application of a second set of phase-encoding pulses along the z-axis.

Two pulse sequence techniques can be used to obtain 3D data sets: GRE (T1-W or T2*-W) and FSE (HOFMAN and WILMINK 1995) imaging. When 3D volume imaging is performed with GRE, a sequence with short TR is preferred because of the large number of phase-encoding pulses required (ROSS 1992) (Fig. 17). This sequence type is vulnerable to motion induced phase shifts across the image. At high field, interference of both echoes causes dark interference bands ; in order to overcome this problem, the sequence must be applied twice, once with 180° phase-alternated RF and once with non-phase alternated RF (ROSS 1992; ROSS et al. 1993).

Alternatively, a transverse FSE sequence with thin, high resolution sections (1-2 mm) can be used to cover a segment of the spine (Fig. 2.18). In the lumbar spine, excellent visualisation of intradural nerve roots has been reported with a heavy T2-W FSE sequence; the slices obtained with this technique can be reformatted with an MIP protocol to obtain 'MR radiculography' images (HOFMAN and WILMINK 1996). An advantage of 3D FSE volume scanning is that CSF flow void artefacts, often troublesome in the thoracic and cervical regions in 2D FSE pulse sequences, are not present.

The 3D data sets with thin slices are very suitable for post-processing into other image planes by using multiplanar reformatting (MPR) (Fig. 2.17, Fig. 2.18) algorithms. In conclusion, 3D volume scanning is useful for acquiring large sets of contiguous or overlapping thin sections with acceptable SNR.

2.5.7
Contrast-Enhanced T1-Weighted MR Imaging

2.5.7.1
General Principles

Contrast agents for spinal MR imaging contain ions with a high electron spin. In a magnetic field, this causes shortening of the relaxation time of adjacent molecules. The result is known as a paramagnetic effect. Paramagnetic contrast agents for intravenous injection are gadolinium chelates. In these products, the paramagnetic metal ion gadolinium (Gd3+) is the active ingredient. The chelate tightly binds the Gd ion and assures complete elimination by the kidneys. There are a variety of such agents. The first

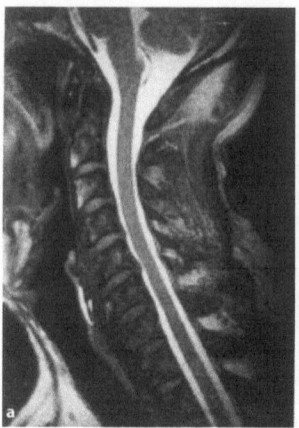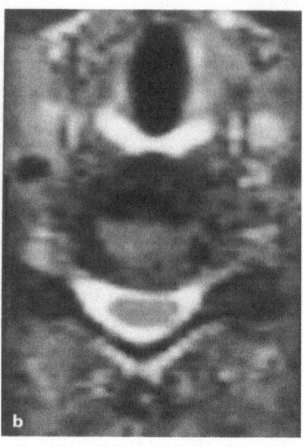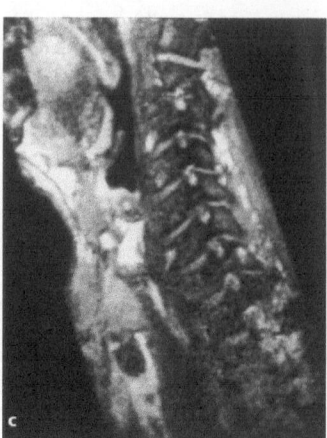

Fig. 2.17a-c. 3D volume acquisition with multiplanar reformatting using a GRE sequence. a Midsagittal slice of GRE 'true' FISP 3D data acquisition obtained at 0.2 T (TR/TE/flip angle: 17/7/3/50°). In this steady-state volume acquisition, 32 slices with an effective thickness of 2 mm are obtained. These thin slices can be reconstructed in other imaging planes. b Axial reformatted image through the C5-C6 intervertebral disc space (2 mm slice thickness) shows mild disc protrusion. c Left oblique reformatted image (1 mm slice thickness) shows narrowing of several neural foramina. Note the anatomical detail of the exiting nerve root ganglia and the facet joints

generation of paramagnetic compounds was introduced in the late 1980s and includes products such as gadopentate dimeglumine (Gd-DTPA, Magnevist, Schering AG) and gadoterate meglumine (Gd-DOTA, Dotarem, Laboratoires Guerbet; RUNGE et al. 1988; PARIZEL et al. 1989b; MEYER et al. 1988). Recently, non-ionic paramagnetic agents such as gadodiamide (Gd-DTPA-BMA, Omniscan, Nycomed) have complemented the older ionic agents (CHANG 1993; ASLANIAN et al. 1996). However, the differences in systemic toxicity between ionic and non-ionic paramagnetic agents are substantially less than those of iodinated compounds. The standard dose for intravenously injected paramagnetic contrast media is 0.1 mmol/kg body weight. Gadolinium-based paramagnetic contrast agents are relatively safe: contrast media reactions are rare and usually mild (BRUGIÈRES et al. 1994; ASLANIAN et al. 1996). Nevertheless, one should always keep in mind that there is a small risk of anaphylactic shock.

The effect of paramagnetic contrast agents is best visualized on T1-W images. It should be kept in mind, however, that Gd chelates not only shorten T1, but also T2. Enhancement is observed as an increase in signal intensity. For definitive identification of enhancement, pre- and post-contrast images are recommended; otherwise other high signal intensity materials such as blood or fat could be mistaken for

contrast agent (RUNGE 1996). An alternative is to use spectral fat suppression techniques. After contrast injection, it is advisable to use SE T1-W sequences, since GRE T1-W images are less sensitive to enhancement. Normal enhancing structures in the spine include the basivertebral and epidural veins along the posterior longitudinal ligament. Disappearance of the basivertebral vein can be an early sign of metastatic bone marrow disease (ALGRA et al. 1991b).

The application of intravenously injected paramagnetic contrast agents has greatly improved the sensitivity and specificity of MR imaging in certain processes. The mechanism of enhancement is different in intra- and extra-axial lesions. In intra-axial lesions enhancement is seen with disruption of the blood-cord barrier; in extra-axial lesions enhancement is due to intrinsic vascularity. In *intramedullary neoplasms,* Gd chelates improve visualisation of tumour extent, provide differentiation of enhancing viable tumour components from surrounding cysts, and may contribute to differential diagnosis (VALK 1988; SZE et al. 1988b; PARIZEL et al. 1989a) (Fig. 2.19). In *intradural extramedullary* tumours, paramagnetic contrast agents dramatically improve lesion conspicuity, especially when the tumour is isointense to CSF in the thecal sac in pre-contrast images (SZE et al. 1988a; PARIZEL et al. 1989a) (Fig.

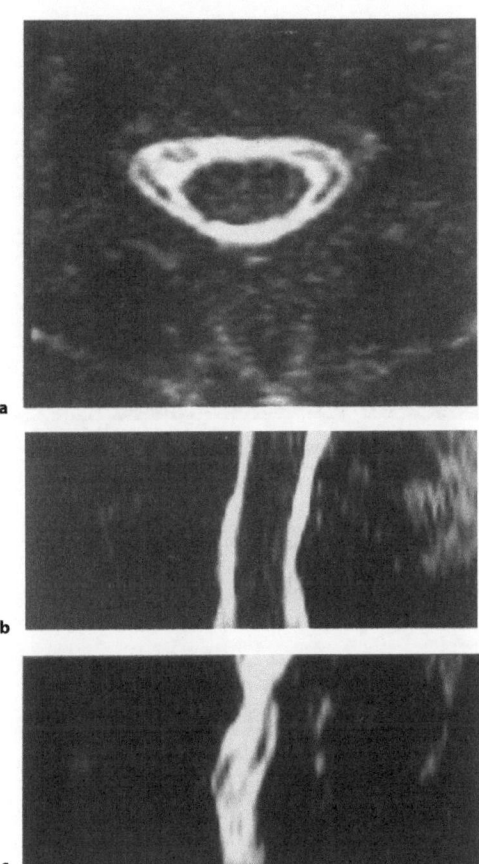

a

b

c

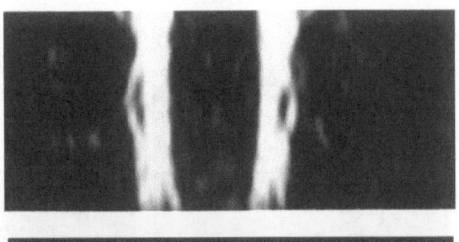

d

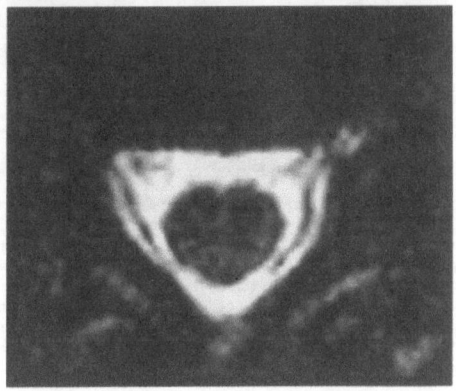

e

Fig. 2.18a-e. 3D volume acquisition with multiplanar reformatting using a FSE sequence. **a** Heavily T2-W FSE sequence produces multiple thin-section (2 mm) transverse cervical images. From this 3D dataset **b** midsagittal, **c** parasagittal and **d** coronal images can be reconstructed. Note the excellent depiction of nerve roots in lateral regions. **e** Oblique coronal reformatted images can be constructed to follow the course of nerve roots from the spinal cord to the neural foramina

2.20). Enhancing lesions stand against a background of dark CSF and are readily detected. In the *extra-dural space*, contrast-enhanced imaging is generally not required for the detection of metastatic invasion. However, paramagnetic contrast agents are of great value in post-operative patients for differentiating recurrent disc herniation from epidural scar formation (VAN GOETHEM et al. 1996).

2.5.7.2.
Use of Contrast Media in Spinal Metastases

On T1-W SE images, normal vertebral bone marrow does not enhance appreciably after intravenous administration of paramagnetic contrast agents. However, vertebral metastases are vascularised and do enhance. Therefore, in cases of *osteolytic vertebral*

metastases, which are hypointense on T1-W images, Gd enhancement may actually obscure the lesions, because the enhancing vertebral metastases become isointense with normal bone marrow (Fig. 2.21). Therefore, in cases of suspected vertebral metastases, pre-contrast T1-W images must always be obtained unless sequences with spectral fat suppression are employed (see Section 2.5.8.2). Gd-enhanced sequences are useful in outlining the soft-tissue tumour components in the paravertebral region.

In the *extradural space* contrast administration is generally not very useful in detecting metastasis. This is because the epidural fat acts as a natural contrast agent on non-enhanced T1-W images and the CSF-filled dural sac provides bright contrast on T2-W images (Fig. 2.22).

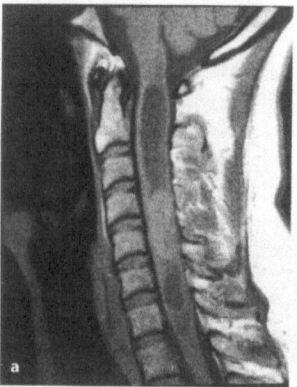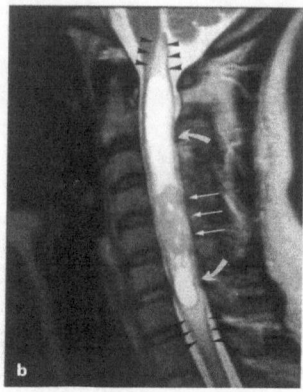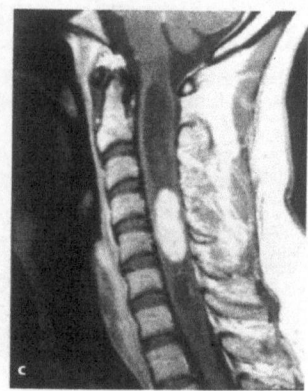

Fig. 2.19a-c. Value of paramagnetic contrast in intramedullary tumour in a 41-year-old woman. a Midsagittal T1-W image (SE 500/15). The cervical spinal cord is expanded by an intramedullary mass with heterogeneous signal characteristics. The central portion of the tumour at C4-C5, which is almost isointense to the normal cord segments, is flanked proximally and distally by hypointense areas. b Midsagittal T2-W image (TSE 4600/91). Tumour architecture is now better delineated. The central portion of the tumour is heterogeneous (*arrows*). It is flanked on either side by high signal intensity intramedullary cysts (*curved arrows*) and by areas of intramedullary oedema triangular in appearance which extend to the obex proximally and the thoracic cord distally (*arrowheads*). c Midsagittal T1-W image (SE 500/15) after Gd administration. Intense contrast enhancement is seen in the central, solid tumour nodule. Conversely, there is no enhancement in the cystic and oedematous regions

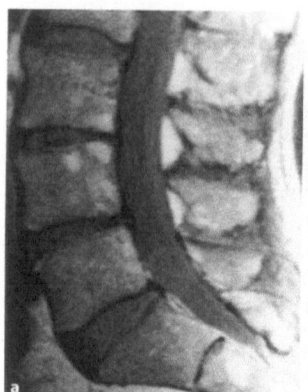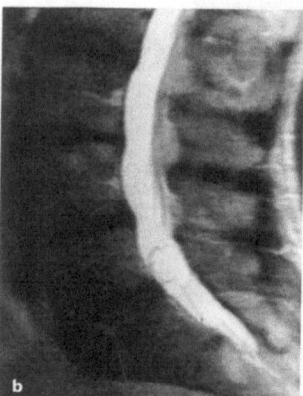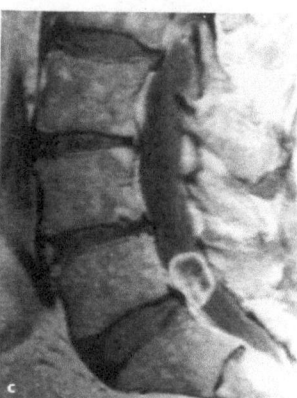

Fig. 2.20a-c. Value of paramagnetic contrast in intradural extramedullary tumour. The patient is a 69-year old man with a schwannoma at L5-S1 (same patient as in Fig. 2.5,b and Fig. 2.7b, c). a Sagittal T1-W MR image (SE 630/15). The intradural mass is almost isointense to the surrounding CSF in the dural sac. b Sagittal T2-W MR image (TSE 5500/91). The tumour is outlined by a hypointense peripheral rim or capsule, whereas the central portion of the tumour is isointense to CSF. c Sagittal T1-W MR image (SE 630/15) after contrast injection. The tumour enhances inhomogeneously; nonenhancing portions presumably reflect cyst formation or necrosis

In *leptomeningeal metastasis,* intravenously administered contrast agents show the enhancing lesions brightly (RODESCH et al. 1990; SCHUKNECHT et al. 1992) (Fig.2. 23). High- resolution T2-W images can provide similar information. Leptomeningeal metastatic deposits along nerve roots can appear as 'beads on a string' (Fig. 2.15). However, when thin-section transverse sets of images are acquired, the spinal segment that can be covered is rather small.

In *intramedullary metastases* the use of contrast agents is of great benefit in detection and classification.

2.5.8
Fat Suppression Techniques

MR imaging of neoplastic spinal lesions depends on its ability to distinguish tumour from bone marrow in the case of vertebral metastases, from CSF in the case of extradural and leptomeningeal involvement and from the spinal cord in the case of intramedullary location.

Metastasis to the vertebral body is the most common form of spinal neoplastic disease, occurring in 10% of cancer patients (MEHTA et al. 1995). MRI is considerably more sensitive than bone scintigraphy in detecting neoplastic infiltration of bone marrow (FRANK et al. 1990; ALGRA et al. 1991a; KATTAPURAM et al. 1990). The high fat content of vertebral bone marrow (25%-50%) in young adults, increasing with age (MEHTA et al. 1995; DE

BISSCHOP et al. 1993) presents a bright contrast to low-signal- intensity metastases on T1-W images. In T2-W images the same lesions are characterised by a higher signal intensity than the surrounding bone marrow, since they have a higher water content. This is, however, not always the case. In FSE sequences, fat retains a relatively high signal intensity and fatty bone marrow can remain isointense to the metastatic lesion. Acquisition of T2-W images in suspected neoplastic spinal disease is desirable, however, as intramedullary lesions are much better defined on T2-W than on non-contrast T1-W images, and the same applies to extradural lesions and lesions of the posterior vertebral elements (JONES et al. 1994). In order to improve conspicuity of vertebral lesions, various fat suppression techniques can be applied (TIEN 1992).

2.5.8.1
Short Tau Inversion Recovery

The inversion recovery (IR) sequence uses a 180° RF pulse to invert the longitudinal magnetisation from the parallel to the anti-parallel direction. After cessation of the pulse, spins are allowed to relax for a short time (TI). During this time, the magnetisation vector returns to the parallel direction at a rate depending on the T1 value of the tissue. When the magnetisation vector of fat is crossing from anti-parallel to parallel (crosses the null point), a 90° RF pulse is applied. This affects all tissues except for fat,

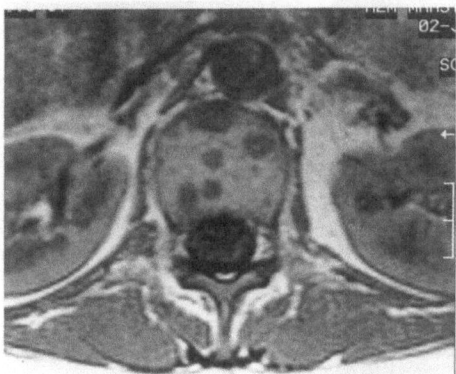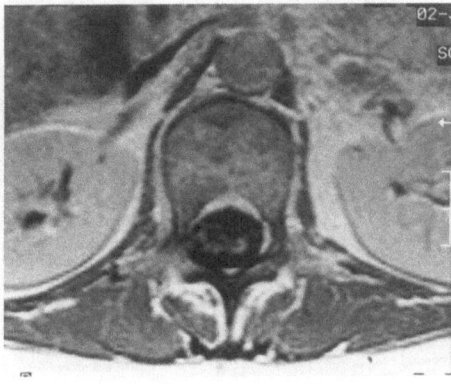

a   b

Fig. 2.21a,b. Influence of paramagnetic contrast agents on vertebral and leptomeningeal metastases of breast carcinoma. **a** Axial T-W MR image through L2 vertebral body. Osteolytic metastases are easily recognised as hypointense lesions within the vertebral body. **b** After intravenous Gd injection, there is filling in of the vertebral lesions, which become isointense to normal bone marrow. Conversely, the cauda equina deposits enhance and become more conspicuous

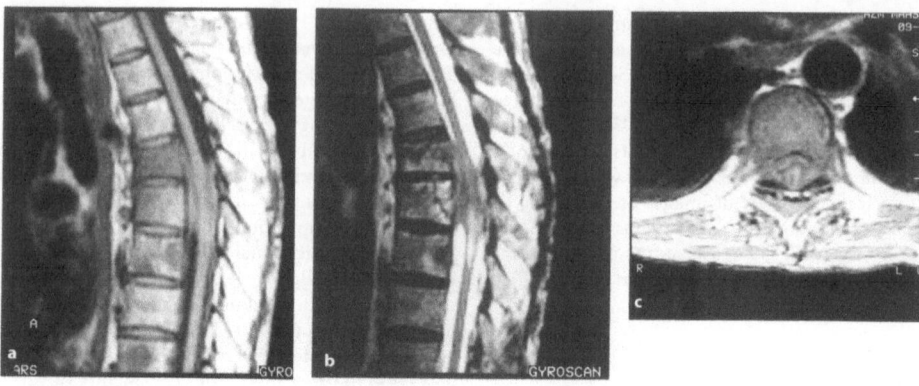

Fig. 2.22a-c. Mid-thoracic metastases of lung carcinoma with marked epidural extension and concentric compression of the thecal sac. **a** Sagittal SE T1-W image shows multiple low signal intensity lesions replacing vertebral bone narrow. There is epidural tumour extension around the thecal sac. **b** The vertebral lesions are less visible when a sagittal FSE T2-W sequence is used. However, cord oedema is much better seen as an intramedullary region of high signal intensity. Epidural spread is well visualised. **c** Transverse SE T1-W image demonstrates cuff-like concentric spread of epidural tumour and deformation of cord

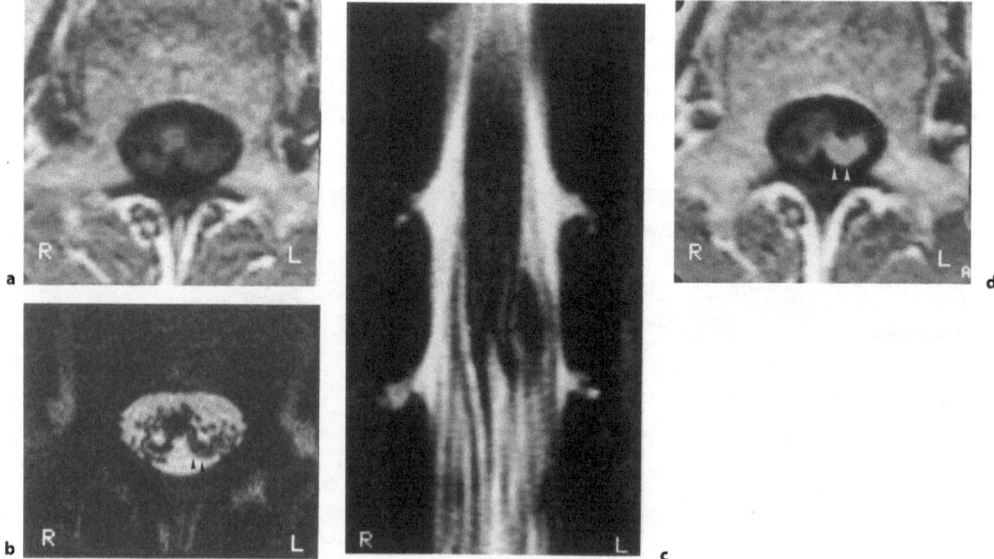

Fig. 2.23a-d. Imaging characteristics of leptomeningeal metastasis (adenocarcinoma of lung) adjacent to conus medullaris in various pulse sequences. **a** Pre-contrast transverse T1-W image. **b** Transverse thin-section 3D T2-W FSE image. Nerve roots of the cauda equina are thickened by adherent tumour nodules (*arrowheads*).**c** Coronal T2-W FSE image. **d** Post-contrast transverse T1-W image shows enhancement of the metastatic deposits (*arrowheads*).

which therefore does not contribute to the MR signal. Short tau inversion recovery effectively suppresses fat signals with the correct choice of TI, which is field -strength- dependent (usually 100-150 ms). The sequence is also extremely sensitive to differences in water content of tissues. Disadvantages of STIR are: long scanning times, suboptimal spatial resolution and motion and flow artefacts, particularly in the thoracic spine (JONES et al. 1992). A major disadvantage is that the signal from methaemoglobin in haematomas and from Gd -enhancing structures is also suppressed. Therefore, unlike the frequency selective techniques discussed in Section 2.5.8.2, STIR should not be used in conjunction with paramagnetic contrast agents.

Compared to T1-W SE images, STIR provides an improved conspicuity of lesions in vertebral red haematopoietic bone marrow, where there is less fat to provide contrast in T1-W images (JONES et al. 1992; MEHTA et al. 1995). The sensitivity of STIR towards water content provides bright lesion contrast against a dark background. In fatty bone marrow (peripheral bones, elderly patients, post-radiation therapy), lesion contrast of T1-W images is improved, and there is little difference in lesion conspicuity (JONES et al. 1992). Compared to FSE T2-W images, STIR is clearly superior in terms of lesion detection with 14 of 65 lesions missed on FSE T2-W images demonstrated by STIR (Mehta et al. 1995) (Fig. 2.24). Moreover, STIR images have been shown to be effective in MR imaging of intramedullary spinal lesions (MASCALCHI et al. 1993).

The relatively long acquisition time of STIR can be reduced without loss of lesion conspicuity or contrast-to-noise ratio when FSE STIR is implemented

(MEHTA et al. 1995). This sequence is excellent for detecting intramedullary lesions such as multiple sclerosis plaques (HITTMAIR et al. 1996).

When a long TI value (e.g. 2000 ms) is chosen instead of a short one , the signal of the CSF can be suppressed. This technique is known as fluid-attenuated inversion recovery (FLAIR) and it has been applied for imaging spinal cord lesions (WHITE et al. 1993). This method can also be combined with an FSE technique, and is then known as fast FLAIR or FSE-FLAIR. It has been found to contribute little to the detection of spinal multiple sclerosis plaques (HITTMAIR et al. 1996).

2.5.8.2
Spectral Fat Saturation (Frequency Selective)

Spectral fat saturation distinguishes water and fat protons on the basis of differences in their resonance frequencies (Larmor frequencies). The frequency difference between water and fat protons is approximately 3.5 parts per million (ppm). This corresponds with $\pm$ 220 Hz at 1.5 Tesla (T), $\pm$ 150 Hz at 1 T, $\pm$ 70 Hz at 0.5 T and $\pm$ 30 Hz at 0.2 T. Prior to the actual imaging pulses, fat is saturated selectively by the application of a frequency selective saturation pulse. The method is known as 'fat sat' imaging or as CHESS (chemical shift selective saturation) and can be combined with any imaging technique, which is an advantage over STIR. Thus it is possible to acquire fat-saturated T1-W, PD-W and T2-W images with SE, FSE or GRE sequences. An important advantage over STIR is that spectral fat saturation can be used in combination with paramagnetic contrast agents.

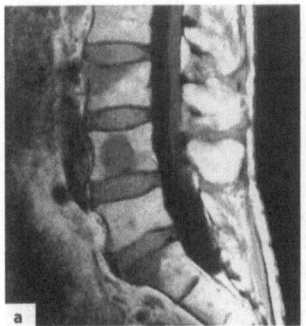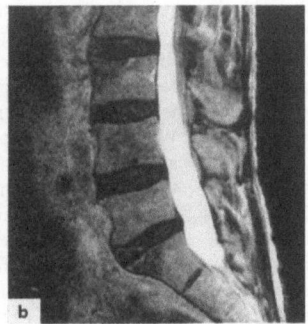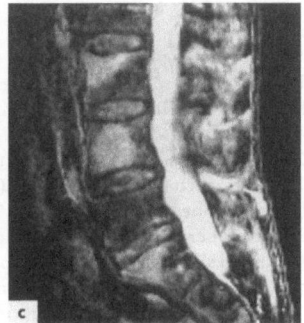

Fig. 2.24a-c. Choice of pulse sequence in diagnosing lumbar vertebral metastases of oesophageal adenocarcinoma. a On a SE T1-W image, vertebral metastases in the lumbar spine are seen as hypo-intense lesions outlined by high signal intensity bone marrow in L3, L4, and S1. b Heavily T2-W FSE image does not show the lesions. c Fat-suppressed STIR image confirms the metastatic lesions, which are seen here as high intensity areas against a dark background

Disadvantages lie in the degradation of fat suppression by magnetic field inhomogeneities and in the fact that less slices can be acquired in a multi-slice SE set.

An alternative frequency-selective fat suppression method is SPIR (selective presaturation inversion recovery or selective partial inversion recovery). In SPIR fat protons are selectively exposed to a 180° inversion pulse and nulled as in STIR. Because only the signal of fat protons is suppressed and water protons are not affected, SPIR can also be used in combination with intravenous contrast agents.

The use of fat saturation in conjunction with Gd-enhanced MR imaging is a sensitive method of imaging spinal diseases (TIEN et al. 1992). Advantages of this technique include: increased conspicuity of pathological lesions, improved detection of subtle enhancement, and the ability to show more lesions compared to contrast-enhanced images without fat saturation (GEORGY et al. 1995). The greater sensitivity and increased contrast are attributed to the elimination of chemical shift artefacts and the surrounding high signal from fat as well as the expanded grey scale of the images (GEORGY et al. 1995). Gd-enhanced fat saturated imaging is useful in postoperative patients (MIROWITZ and SHADY 1992).

Metastatic disease, but also focal fatty infiltration can result in a mixed appearance of areas with higher and lower SI on T1-W images. When the fat signal is selectively suppressed, malignant bone marrow lesions will be seen with relatively high SI (UCHIDA et al. 1993). Areas with fatty infiltration have a homogeneous, low SI appearance.

In contrast-enhanced T1-W studies, as we have shown before, leptomeningeal and intramedullary lesions are seen more clearly. Hypointense vertebral lesions, however, may enhance to isointensity with the normal fatty marrow and be obscured. Pre-enhancement studies are mandatory unless fat suppression is applied, in which case the enhancing lesions show up brightly against the dark fat-suppressed bone marrow and epidural fat (TIEN et al. 1992).

T2-W sequences have not proved useful for the detection of vertebral metastases (JONES et al. 1994). This applies especially to FSE T2-W images with their higher bone marrow fat signal masking the high SI lesions. Selective fat suppression improves the conspicuity of vertebral metastases in FSE T2-W images (CHRYSIKOPOULOS et al. 1996). Fat suppression is considerably better when STIR is employed, however, anatomical detail is better in the FSE T2-W images (JONES et al. 1994) (Figs. 2.24, 2.25).

At present, therefore it appears, that spectral fat saturation techniques are especially useful in post-contrast T1-W images, to reduce the signal of fat and increase the effect of enhancement. T2-W fat-suppressed images are less sensitive than STIR in detecting bone marrow lesions.

2.5.8.3
GRE Imaging in Opposed Phase

With the aim to improve the visualisation of abnormal tissues, DIXON, (1984) first described a chemical-shift SE technique that consisted of generating opposed-phase images in which the magnetisation vectors of water and fat protons are 180° out of phase during sampling. By subtraction, water-only or fat-only images can be produced. The opposed phase images are very sensitive to changes in the ratio of fat and water protons in the imaged tissue. Bone marrow imaging with the Dixon method was introduced in the mid 1980s (WISMER et al. 1985).

Opposed-phase images can also be generated by using GRE sequences (WEHRLI et al. 1987; TILLING et al. 1988). Due to the absence of a 180° refocusing pulse, GRE sequences are sensitive to field variations caused by magnetic field inhomogeneities, susceptibility effects and chemical shift differences (WEHRLI et al. 1987). This has implications for the signal amplitude in MR images obtained with gradient refocusing, especially if the tissue to be imaged contains more than one spectral component (such as bone marrow). It follows that signal decay in GRE sequences is not only governed by $T2^*$ decay, but also by in-phase/out-of-phase oscillations (phase cycling; PARIZEL et al. 1995). The amplitude modulation of signal decay is due to chemical shift effects (WEHRLI et al. 1987). Hydrogen nuclei in different types of tissue (e.g. water and fat) possess slightly different resonance frequencies. The difference in resonance frequency between fat and water protons is ± 3.5 ppm (WISMER et al. 1987; WEHRLI 1991). When the two spectral components are in-phase, the signal intensity contributions of water and fat protons are added to one another; in opposed-phase orientation they are subtracted from one another. The relative phase shift between fat and water protons thus results in a frequency modulation, which is superimposed on the $T2^*$ exponential signal decay (PARIZEL et al. 1995). The signal intensity of structures containing both fat and water protons (e.g. vertebral bone marrow) depends on the chosen TE (WEHRLI 1991; PARIZEL et al. 1995). It also depends on the magnetic field strength B_0, that determines

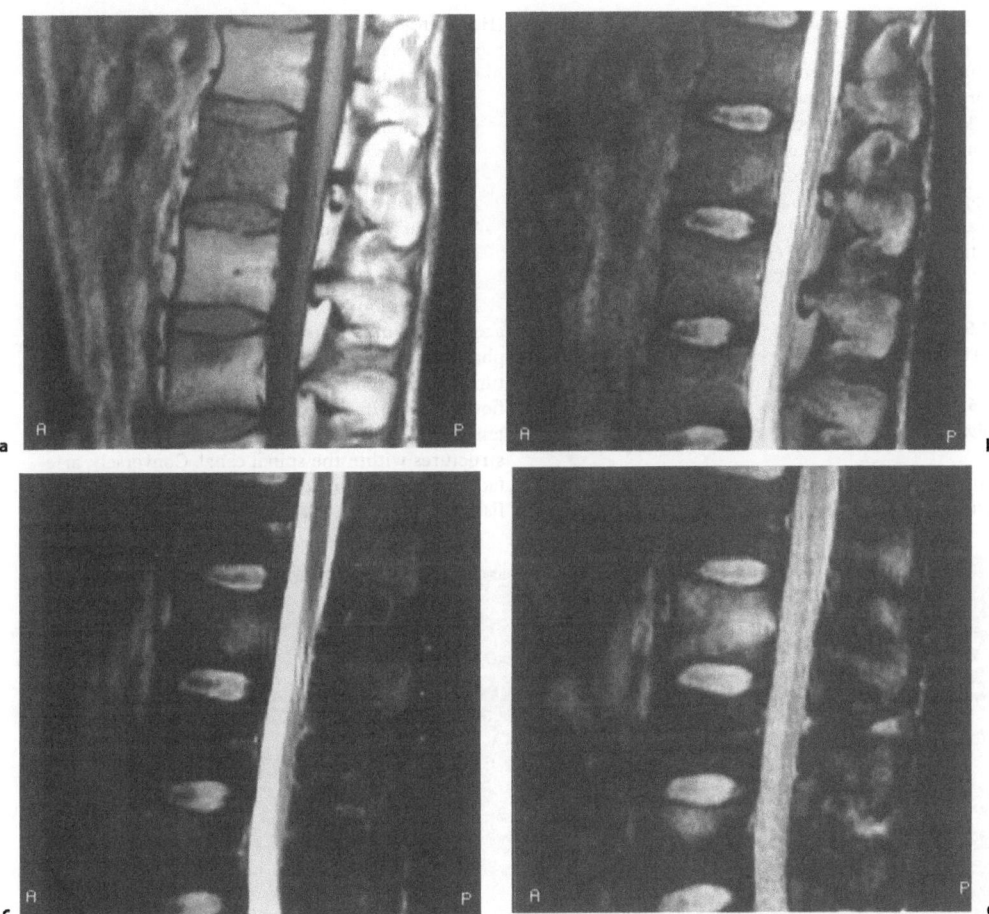

Fig. 2.25a-d. Influence of sequence type on the visualisation of lumbar vertebral metastases (Ewing sarcoma). a Sagittal SE T1-W MR image shows multifocal vertebral metastases as hypointense lesions replacing high signal intensity fatty bone marrow. b The lesions are poorly demonstrated on a sagittal FSE T2-W MR image. c With FSE T2 SPIR MR imaging technique, there is only marginal improvement in visibility of the metastatic lesions. d A sagittal STIR image shows the metastatic deposits as well as the T1-W image. However, contrast is reversed: lesions are now of high signal intensity against a dark background because signal from fatty vertebral bone marrow is suppressed

the chemical shift-induced frequency difference (PARIZEL et al. 1995).

When GRE sequences are used, bone marrow should be considered of as consisting of two separate compartments. Signal intensity in the first compartment is generated by water-bound protons; in the second compartment signal intensity is generated by fat-bound protons. The overall signal intensity of the bone marrow space is determined by the sum of signal intensities of these two compartments. By

appropiately choosing the TE value, an in-phase or opposed-phase image can be generated. Normal red bone marrow is dark on out-of-phase images because fat and water signals cancel each other out (NEUMANN et al. 1995; PARIZEL et al. 1995). When the bone marrow is replaced by a cellular infiltrate (e.g. leukaemic infiltration, metastatic disease), the increased water content of the bone marrow is reflected as increased signal intensity on opposed-phase GRE images. This technique can disclose vertebral metastases earlier than bone scintigraphy (NEUMANN et al. 1995). With the body coil, opposed-phase GRE images can be successfully applied to screen for vertebral metastases (NEUMANN et al. 1995) (Fig. 2.26). However, the technique is not specific: benign conditions (diffuse osteoporosis, vertebral haemangiomas) can also display an increased signal intensity on opposed-phase GRE images. Conversely, purely osteoblastic metastases may be overlooked due to susceptibility effects (NEUMANN et al. 1995).

2.5.9
Artefacts

2.5.9.1.
Motion and Flow Artefacts

An important source of artefacts is motion of or within the object being studied (the patient)

(HENDRICK et al. 1993). Five different sources of motion artefacts are distinguished:
- Cardiac pulsations
- Pulsatile flow (arterial blood flow, CSF pulsations in the subarachnoid space; Fig. 2.27)
- Respiration
- Involuntary motion (peristalsis, deglutition, eye movement)
- Voluntary motion in non-co-operative patients (e.g. an unsedated child)

Motion and/or flow in any direction during image acquisition manifests itself as an artefact in the phase-encoding direction of the image. Most disturbing are the artefacts produced by pulsatile CSF flow on T2-W images (when CSF is of high signal intensity). These artefacts can obscure visualisation of structures within the spinal canal. Conversely, artefacts may mimic disease (e.g. dural arteriovenous fistula) and lead to false-positive interpretations.

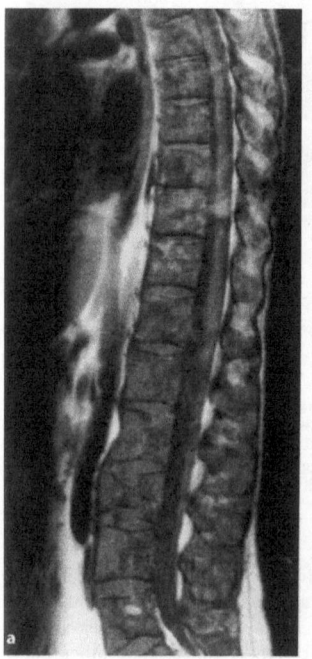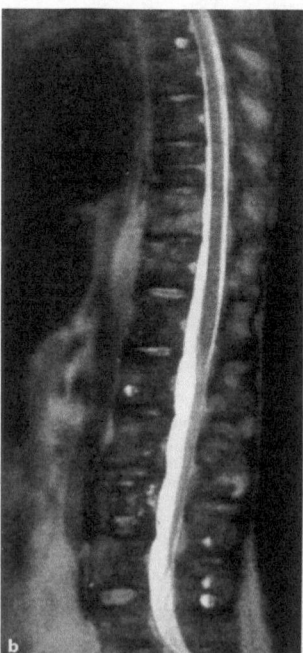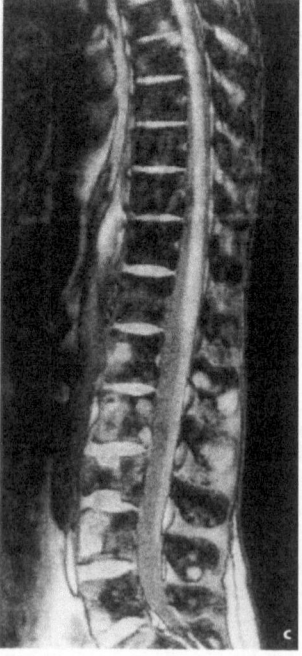

Fig. 2.26a-c. Opposed phase gradient echo in diagnosing vertebral metastases in a patient with metastatic breast carcinoma to the spine. Images obtained with body coil at 1.5 T. a Midsagittal T1-weighted image (SE 660/15) shows diffuse metastatic involvement of the thoracic and lumbar spine. The multifocal confluent vertebral lesions are hypointense and have almost completely replaced fatty bone marrow. b Midsagittal T2-weighted image (FSE 4500/90) provides excellent myelographic contrast with bright CSF outlining the spinal cord. However, this sequence is less sensitive to vertebral metastases. c Gradient echo image in opposed phase conditions (FLASH 350/7/90°) outlines multiple metastatic lesions especially in the lumbar spine. Note improved visualisation of metastatic involvement of the spinous processes. At 1.5 T, a TE of 7 ms corresponds to an opposed phase condition

There are several ways of reducing motion artefacts (although they cannot be completely eliminated). Some remedies are given here:

• Use of sequences with gradient moment nulling (also known as flow compensation, motion artefact suppression technique or gradient moment rephasing). This method, which can be applied to most MR scan techniques, incorporates additional gradient pulses into the scanning sequence to eliminate phase-encoding errors. The contribution of motion occuring during the time interval TE is reduced. The correction can be for velocity (first order), acceleration (second order) or higher orders of motion. Most routinely applied techniques compensate only for velocity. The implementation of gradient moment nulling methods increases the minimum TE value of the sequence.

• Use of presaturation regions anterior to the spine. These presaturation or 'SAT pulses' can be applied perpendicular or parallel to the plane of acquisition. *Perpendicular* presaturation slabs are typically used to reduce bulk motion artefacts. When imaging is performed in the sagittal plane, coronal presaturation pulses are placed over the face and neck in the cervical spine, the heart and lungs in the thoracic spine and the anterior abdomen in the lumbar spine. Presaturation pulses parallel to the plane of acquisition are applied in axial images of the spine to prevent CSF flow artefacts. Presaturation pulses are repeated at each TR interval and prevent increase of longitudinal magnetisation in the applied area. They increase the specific absorption rate (SAR) and require time within a scan sequence (therefore the total number of slices that can be acquired is reduced unless TR is prolonged; RUNGE 1996).

• Use of physiological synchronisation (ECG triggering, pulse triggering, respiratory gating). The purpose of ECG or pulse triggering is to synchronise data collection with the cardiac cycle. This minimises the contribution of motion occuring between successive TR intervals. The implementation of these techniques restricts the free choice of TR for a given sequence.

• By interchanging the phase-and frequency - encoding directions of the image ('swapping'), the direction of the artefact can be changed. The orientation of encoding can be selected to reduce artefacts across the region of interest. However, the choice of axis may be restricted by 'wrap around': it is necessary to choose the frequency axis in such a way as to prevent image aliasing (see Section 2.5.9.2).

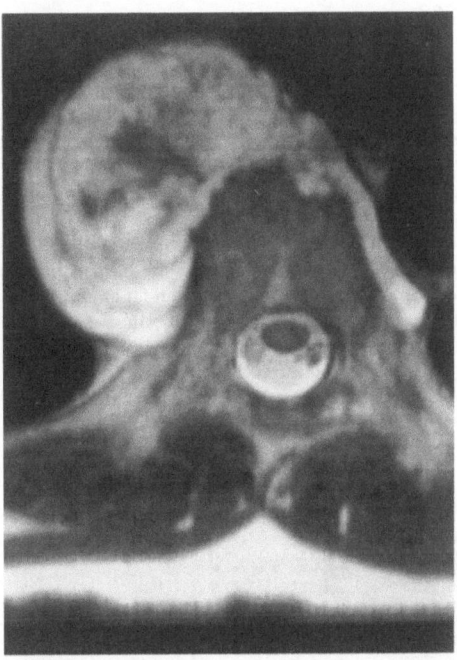

Fig. 2.27. Flow artefacts resulting from CSF pulsations may cause misleading images in the subarachnoid space in this patient with a large chordoma of the thoracic spine

2.5.9.2
Aliasing Artefact (syn. 'Wrap Around' Artefact)

The aliasing artefact occurs when the diametre of the object under study exceeds the FOV of the chosen imaging sequence. Signals generated outside the FOV are superimposed on the opposite side of the image. One the most typical examples of aliasing artefact is encountered in sagittal images of the cervical spine where the chin and nose of the patient, structures supposedly outside the FOV, are superimposed on the occiput. Another example is the quality loss that occurs in the outer images of 3 D volume acquisition. Aliasing artefacts can be encountered both in the frequency- and the phase-encoding direction of an image (JOSEPH and ATLAS 1996).

In order to avoid aliasing artefacts in the frequency encoding direction, a technique called 'oversampling' is recommended. Oversampling doubles the FOV in the frequency-encoding direction, while maintaining the same pixel size.

2.5.9.3
Chemical Shift Artefact

Chemical shift artefact (CSA) (Fig. 2.28) is due to spatial misregistration of the resonance frequency between protons in a 'watery' and 'fatty' environment (PARIZEL et al. 1994; JOSEPH and ATLAS 1996). The difference in resonance frequency between fat and water protons is 3.5 ppm (parts per million). In a magnetic field of 1.5 T, where the resonance frequency is 63 MHz, the chemical-shift-induced resonance frequency difference between fat and water is approximately 220 Hz. Conversely, in a magnetic field strength of 0.2 T, the difference is only 28 Hz. It is easily understood that the spatial misregistration generated by the resonance frequency difference between fat and water protons is directly proportional to the magnetic field strength. Furthermore, the artefact is inversely proportional to the receiver bandwidth: the narrower the bandwidth, the greater the CSA observed (PARIZEL et al. 1994).

Since frequency is equivalent to a position in 2 D Fourier transform imaging and fat protons resonate at a lower frequency, they appear shifted in position along the frequency -encoding axis to the lower frequency side of the image (WEINREB et al. 1985). The boundary artefact occurs only in the direction of the read or frequency-encoding gradient, as such, it is oriented within the plane of the phase-encoding and section-select directions. It causes the boundaries of some anatomical structures to appear asymmetric. In sagittal MR images of the spine, the frequency-encoding direction is usually cranio-caudad, while the phase encoding direction is antero-posterior. At high field strengths, artefactual white and dark bands can be seen at the upper and lower vertebral endplates (SMITH et al. 1991).

There are several ways to reduce chemical shift artefacts of the spine. One of the easiest is to use pulse sequences with a wide receiver bandwidth. Unfortunately, this decreases SNR, as bandwidth is inversely related to SNR. At high field strength this is generally not a problem, since SNR is high.

When performing MR imaging at low field strengths, CSA is reduced. Moreover, at low field strength it is possible to use sequences with a narrower receiver bandwidth in order to increase SNR, yet without incurring the penalty of unacceptably high CSA.

CSA occurs by definition in the frequency encoding direction of the image. By switching the read and phase directions of an image, CSA can be changed.

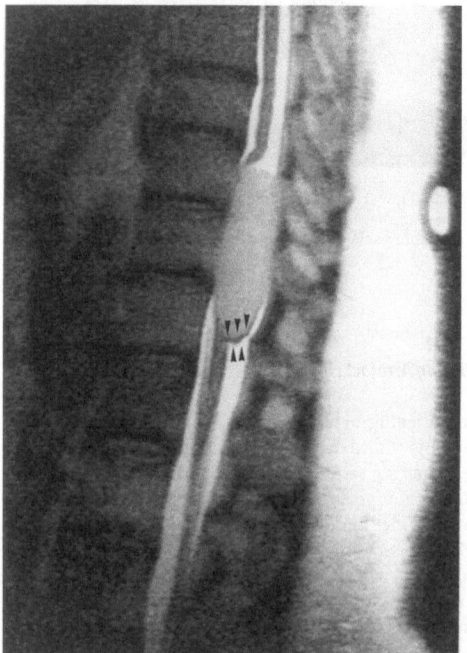

Fig. 2.28. Chemical shift misregistration artefact in a patient with an intradural lipoma in the lower thoracic spine (same patient as Fig. 2.13a). The artefact occurs in the frequency-encoding direction. The dark rim (*arrowheads*) of the chemical shift artefact at the lower pole of the tumour confirms the lipomatous nature of the tumour. The bright rim of the artefact of the upper pole of the tumour is not seen because of the bright CSF signal. Note that signal intensity of fat remains high in this TSE T2-W image

2.5.9.4
Truncation Artefact (Gibbs Phenomenon)

The trunctation artefact is due to imperfections in the Fourier transformation. It occurs at the boundary between two regions with markedly different signal intensity. Because the Fourier transformation used in image processing is limited to a finite number of terms, this can result in the formation of artefactual bands with alternating high and low intensity that are parallel to the interface of two tissues with markedly different signal intensity. This produces an image with ripples, the spacing of which is a direct reflection of the highest spatial frequency used (JOSEPH and ATLAS 1996). Truncation artefacts are potentiated when a small matrix is used (because the pixel size then becomes larger). They have been designated as a possible cause of overestimation of spinal canal stenosis on MR images (REUL et al. 1995).

Truncation artefacts can be diminished by increasing the matrix size (e.g. by increasing the number of phase-encoding steps). Actually, when the number of phase-encoding steps is increased, the truncation artefact becomes less obvious to the human eye because the frequency of the oscillating high-low- intensity bands increases.

2.5.9.5
Susceptibility Artefact

Magnetic susceptibility is a measure of the extent to which a tissue can be magnetised. Susceptibility artefacts occur at the boundary of two tissues with markedly different magnetic susceptibility. This artefact is especially obvious in GRE sequences, which do not compensate for field inhomogeneities (no refocusing 180° pulses in the XY-plane). The extent of sensitivity of the different pulse sequence families to susceptibility induced artefacts is as follows: echoplanar (EPI) > gradient echo (GRE) > spin echo (SE) > fast spin echo (FSE). It should also be kept in mind, that magnetic susceptibility effects are directly related to field strength (PARIZEL 1994).

Susceptibility artefacts can be useful in detecting haemosiderin in old haemorrhagic foci, calcifications, epidural gas or retained foreign bodies (Van GOETHEM et al. 1991). Conversely, susceptibility artefacts are detrimental to image quality and may obscure visualisation of spinal structures in patients with metallic implants (PARIZEL et al. 1996). In order to avoid susceptibility artefacts, it is advisable to use SE or, even better, FSE sequences and to avoid GRE and EPI sequences. Therefore FSE sequences should be preferred in the postoperative spine (TARTAGLINO et al. 1994). In GRE sequences susceptibility artefacts can be decreased by using a short TE, a small FOV and high bandwidth per pixel. Susceptibility artefacts are greatly reduced when MR imaging is performed at low field strengths (PARIZEL 1994).

2.6
Review of Imaging Options

The most common form of spinal neoplastic disease consists of metastasis from a primary tumour located elsewhere. Although tumour seeding may occur directly to the spinal cord, leptomeninges or epidural space, the most common sequence is the appearance of lesions in the vertebral bone marrow, followed by invasion of the epidural space within the spinal canal and compression of the dural sac and the nervous tissue within. In patients with a known malignancy, the manifestation of novel back pain carries with it a high degree of suspicion for vertebral metastasis (specificity 98%; DEYO and DIEHL 1988). When signs of radicular compression and/or neurologic deficit occur, this constitutes an emergency situation requiring urgent diagnosis and appropriate therapy. Once severe signs of motor deficit through cord compression have set in, they are usually irreversible.

Plain X-ray films are inadequate for detecting vertebral metastases by reason of their poor accuracy. When plain X-ray films demonstrate severe vertebral involvement, it is likely that there is epidural encroachment as well, although the latter cannot be visualised directly. Epidural and leptomeningeal metastasis is not visualised by plain films, and the same applies to most medullary tumours. Slowly expanding lesions such as neurinoma may produce bony erosive changes.

Computed tomography (CT) is superior to plain X-ray films in detecting vertebral metastases. CT allows visualisation of lesions that only cause trabecular disruption without cortical bony changes (ALGRA 1995). Invasion of the spinal canal can be detected by changes of the bony margins. Sometimes epidural involvement is better evaluated after intravenous contrast injection. However, even contrast-enhanced CT is unable to reliably diagnose leptomeningeal and intramedullary metastases. The same applies to intramedullary tumours, nerve roots and meninges, unless bony erosion is present or the lesions are highly vascular and show intense enhancement. Examination of long sections of the spine involves a high radiation dose to the patient.

Myelography suffers the same low accuracy as plain X-ray films in detecting vertebral metastases. Conversely, mass lesions that deform the thecal sac or are located within it are demonstrated with adequate sensitivity. The quality of myelographic diagnosis is highly dependent on the proficiency and experience of the examiner performing the study and reading the films. Patient cooperation is essential, especially when the entire spinal canal must be examined. In elderly patients and in patients with painful spinal metastases, myelographic examination can be problematic. CSF is obtained for cytological examination. It is important to remember that a lumbar puncture in a patient with a spinal block carries a risk of rapid neurological deterioration (HOLLIS et al. 1986).

CT myelography (CTM) is a technique that combines the advantages of CT and myelography. High resolution transverse images show vertebral lesions, epidural irregularities, leptomeningeal changes and abnormalities of the spinal cord and nerve roots more clearly than conventional myelography. CTM is less technically demanding in patients who are partially immobilised or unable to cooperate fully. However, CTM involves a high radiation dose to the patient when long stretches of the spine are imaged with thin sections. Moreover, this is time-consuming unless spiral CT scanning is performed. For these reasons, CTM is often used as an adjunct to conventional myelography, and the examination is focused on selected regions of the spine.

Magnetic resonance (MR) imaging is the method of choice in practically all cases of spinal neoplastic disease. It is the most sensitive method for detecting vertebral metastasis because areas with only bone marrow infiltration and no trabecular destruction can be visualised. Encroachment upon the extradural space and compression of the thecal sac are easily assessed. Intravenous injection of paramagnetic contrast media can improve detection of small lesions in the meninges, spinal cord and nerve roots. Contrast injection is generally not needed for detecting epidural encroachment. Low-intensity vertebral metastases on T1-W images may be masked by contrast injection, because the lesions enhance to isointensity with normal bone marrow. The sagittal imaging plane is preferred for screening sections of the spine, while transverse images provide a better view of possible encroachment upon the spinal canal. When no abnormalities are detected on T1-W images, it is unlikely that neoplastic infiltration of bone marrow is present. Low-signal intensity areas are not always attributable to metastasis, but can also be due to degenerative changes, which are typically located at the vertebral endplates. T2-W images are very useful in providing a 'myelographic' effect, in which high intensity CSF outlines the thecal sac and its contents. However, T2-W images have proved to be rather unreliable for detecting metastatic bone marrow changes, especially when FSE sequences are used. Fat-suppressed sequences such as STIR are much more sensitive for this purpose.

References

Algra PR (1995) Diagnostic imaging of vertebral metastases. Riv Neuroradiol Suppl 8 : 165-175

Algra PR, Bloem JL, Tissing H, Falke THM, Arndt JW, Verboom LJ (1991a) Detection of vertebral metastases: comparison between MR imaging and bone scintigraphy. Radiographics 11: 219-232

Algra PR, Bloem JL, Valk J (1991b) Disappearance of the basivertebral vein: a new MR imaging sign of bone marrow disease. AJR Am J Roentgenol 157: 1129-1130

Algra PR, Heimans JJ, Valk J, Nauta JJ, Lachniet M, Van Kooten B (1991c) Do metastases in vertebrae begin in the body or pedicles? Imaging study in 45 patients. AJR Am J Roentgenol 158: 1275-1279

Aslanian V, Lemaignen H, Bunouf P, Svaland MG, Borseth A, Lundby B (1996) Evaluation of the clinical safety of gadodiamide injection, a new nonionic MRI contrast medium for the central nervous system: a European perspective. Neuroradiology 38: 537-541

Atlas SW (1996) Magnetic resonance imaging of the brain and spine. Lippincott-Raven, Philadelphia

Atlas SW, Hackney DB, Listerud J (1993) Fast spin echo imaging of the brain and spine. Magn Reson Q 9: 61-83

Balériaux D, Parizel P, Rodesch et al.(1988) Magnetic resonance imaging (MRI) of the spinal cord and intracanalar lesions. J Belge Radiol 71: 79-90

Balériaux D, Parizel P, Bank WO (1992) Intraspinal and intramedullary pathology. In: Manelfe C (ed) Imaging of the spine and spinal cord. Raven, New York, pp 513-564

Bellon EM, Haacke EM, Coleman PE, Sacco DC, Steiger DA, Gangarosa RE (1986) MR artifacts: a review. AJR Am J Roentgenol 147: 1271-1281

Brugières P, Gaston A, Degryse HR et al. (1994) Randomised double blind trial of the safety and efficacy of two gadolinium complexes (Gd-DTPA and Gd-DOTA). Neuroradiology 36: 27-30

Chang CA (1993) Magnetic resonance imaging contrast agents. Design and physicochemical properties of gadodiamide. Invest Radiol 28: 21-27

Chappell PM, Glover GH, Enzman DR (1995) Contrast on T2-weighted images of the lumbar spine using fast spin-echo and gated conventional spin-echo sequences. Neuroradiology 37: 183-186

Chrysikopoulos H, Pappas J, Papanikolau N (1996) Bone marrow lesions: evaluation with fat-suppression turbo spin echo MR imaging at 0.5 T. Eur Radiol 6: 895-899

Czervionke LF, Daniels DL, Wehrli FW et al. (1988) Magnetic susceptibility artifacts in gradient-recalled echo MR imaging. AJNR 9: 1149-1155

De Bisschop E, Luypaert R, Louis O, Osteaux M (1993) Fat fraction of lumbar bone marrow using in vivo proton nuclear magnetic resonance spectroscopy. Bone 14:133-136

De Schepper AMA, Ramon F, Van Marck E (1993) MR imaging of eosinophilic granuloma: report of 11 cases. Skeletal Radiol 22: 163-166

Deyo RA, Diehl AK (1988) Cancer as a cause of low back pain. J Gen Intern Med 3: 230-238

Dixon WT (1984) Simple proton spectroscpic imaging. Radiology 153: 189-194

Frank JA, Ling A, Patronas NJ et al (1990). Detection of malignant bone tumours: MR imaging versus scintigraphy. AJR Am J Roentgenol 155: 1043-1048

Freyschmidt J, Berning W (1995) Musculoskeletal interventions. Part 2: Percutaneous bone biopsy. In: Baert AL, Grenier P, Willi UV, Bloem JL (eds) Musculoskeletal imaging: an update. Syllabus Categorical Course, European Congress of Radiology ECR 95, pp 19-23

Georgy BA, Hesselink JR, Middleton MS (1995) Fat-suppression contrast-enhanced MRI in the failed back surgery syndrome: a prospective study. Neuroradiology 37: 51-57

Greenfield GB (1980) Radiology of bone diseases, 3rd edn. Lippincott, Philadelphia; pp. 401-414

Haase A, Frahm J, Matthaei D, Hänicke W, Merboldt K-D (1986) FLASH imaging: rapid NMR imaging using low-flip angle pulses. J Magn Reson B 67: 258-266

Hauenstein KH, Wimmer B, Beck A (1988) Knochenbiopsie unklarer Knochenläsionen mit einer neuen 1.4 mm messenden Biopsiekanüle. Radiologe 28: 251-256

Hendrick RE, Russ PD, Simon JS (1993) MRI principles and artifacts. The Raven MRI teaching file. Raven, New York

Henkelman RM, Hardy PA, Bishop JE, Coons CS, Plewes DB (1992). Why fat is bright in RARE and fast spin-echo imaging. J Magn Reson Imaging 2: 533-540

Hittmair K, Mallek R, Prayer D, Schindler EG, Kolleger H (1996) Spinal cord lesions in patients with multiple sclerosis: comparison of MR pulse sequences. AJNR 17: 1555-1565

Hofman PAM, Wilmink JT (1995) 3-D volume scanning: a new technique for lumbar MR imaging. Acta Neurochir (Wien) 134: 108-112

Hofman PAM, Wilmink JT (1996) Optimising the image of the intradural nerve root: the value of MR radiculography. Neuroradiology 38: 654-657

Hollis PH, Malis LI, Zappulla RA (1986) Neurological deterioration after lumbar puncture below complete spinal subarachnoid block. J Neurosurg 64: 253-256

Jones KM, Unger EC, Granstrom P, et al (1992) Bone marrow imaging using STIR at 0.5 and 1.5 T. Magn Reson Imaging 10: 169-176

Jones KM, Schwartz RB, Mantello MT, et al. (1994). Fast spin-echo MR in the detection of vertebral metastases: comparison of three sequences. AJNR 15: 401-407

Joseph PM, Atlas SW (1996) Artifacts. In: Atlas SW (ed. Magnetic resonance imaging of the brain and spine. Lippincott-Raven, Philadelphia

Kattapuram SV, Rosenthal DI (1987) Percutaneous biopsy of the cervical spine using CT guidance. AJR Am J Roentgenol 149: 539-541

Kattapuram SV, Khurana JS, Scott JA, El-Khoury GY (1990) Negative scintigraphy with positive magnetic resonance imaging in bone metastases. Skeletal Radiol 19: 113-116

Kattapuram SV, Khurana JS, Rosenthal DI (1992) Percutaneous needle biopsy of the spine. Spine 17: 561-564

Kett H, Prüll C (1990) Physical principles and signal behaviour in magnetic resonance imaging. In: Breit A (ed) magnetic resonance in oncology. Springer, Berlin Heidelberg New York, pp 3-14

Krudy AG (1992) MR myelography using heavily T2-weighted fast spin echo pulse sequences with fat suppression. AJR Am J Roentgenol 159: 1315-1320

Listerud JL, Einstein S, Outwater E, Kressel HY (1992) First principles of fast spin echo. Magn Reson Q 8: 199-244

Mascalchi M, Dal Pozzo G, Bartolozzi C (1993) Effectiveness of the short TI inversion recovery (STIR) sequence in MR imaging of intramedullary spinal lesions. Magn Reson Imaging 11: 17-25

Mehta RC, Marks MP, Hinks RS, Glover GH, Enzmann DR (1995) MR evaluation of vertebral metastases: T1-weighted, STIR, FSE and IRFSE sequences. AJNR 16: 281-288

Meyer D, Schaefer M, Bonnemain B (1988) Gd-DOTA, a potential MRI contrast agent: current status of physicochemical knowledge. Invest Radiol 23 (1): 232-235

Mirowitz SA, Shady KL (1992) Gadopentate dimeglumine-enhanced MR imaging of the post-operative lumbar spine: comparison of fat-suppression and conventional T1-weighted images. AJR 159: 385-389

Mitchell GE, Louri H, Berne AS (1967) The various causes of scalloped vertebrae with notes on their pathogenesis. Radiology 89: 67-74

Neumann K, Hosten N, Venz S (1995) Screening for skeletal metastases of the spine and pelvis: gradient echo opposed-phase MRI compared with bone scintigraphy. Eur Radio 5: 276-284

Nitz WR (1995) Fast MR imaging techniques. In: Parizel PM, Van Goethem JW, van den Hauwe L, De Schepper AM, Balériaux D, David P (eds) Erasmus course on magnetic resonance imaging, syllabus 'Central Nervous System II'. University of Antwerp

Olcott EW, Dillon WP (1993) Plain film clues to the diagnosis of spinal epidural neoplasm and infection. Neuroradiology 35: 288-292

Osborn AG (1994) Diagnostic neuroradiology. Mosby, St. Louis

Parizel PM (1994) The influence of field strength on magnetic resonance imaging (a comparative study in physicochemical phantoms, isolated brain specimens and clinical applications). PhD thesis, University of Antwerp

Parizel PM, Balériaux D, Rodesch G, et al (1989a) Gd-DTPA-enhanced MR imaging of spinal tumors. AJR Am J Roentgenol 152: 1087-1096; AJNR 10: 249-258

Parizel PM, Degryse HR, Gheuens J et al. (1989b) Gadolinium DOTA enhanced MR of intracranial lesions. J Comput Assist Tomogr 13: 378-385

Parizel PM, van Hasselt BAAM, van den Hauwe L, Van Goethem JWM, De Schepper AMA (1994) Understanding chemical shift induced boundary artefacts as a function of field strength: influence of imaging parameters (bandwidth, field-of-view, and matrix size). Eur J Radiol 18: 158-164

Parizel PM, Van Riet B, van Hasselt BAAM et al.(1995) Influence of magnetic field strength on T2* decay and phase effects in gradient echo MRI of vertebral bone marrow. J Comput Assist Tomogr 19: 465-471

Parizel PM, Van Goethem JW, van den Hauwe L, Deckers F, Gunzburg R, De Schepper AM (1996) Imaging of spinal implants and radiologic assessment of fusion. In: Szpalski M, Gunzburg R, Spengler DM, Nachemson A (eds): Instrumented fusion of the degenerative lumbar spine: state of the art, questions, and controversies. Lippincott-Raven, Philadelphia, pp 25-33

Petersein J, Saini S (1995) Fast MR imaging: technical strategies. AJR Am J Roentgenol 165: 1105-1109

Plewes DB (1994) Contrast mechanisms in spin echo MR imaging. Radiographics 14: 1389-1404

Posse S, Aue WP (1990) Susceptibility artifacts in spin echo and gradient echo imaging. J Magn Res on B88: 473-492

Price RR (1995) Contrast mechanisms in gradient-echo imaging and an introduction to fast imaging. Radiographics 15: 165-178

Quaynor H, Tronstad A, Heldaas O (1995) Frequency and severity of headache after lumbar myelography using a 25-gauge pencil point (Whitacre) spinal needle. Neuroradiology 37: 553-556

Reul J, Gievers B, Weis J, Thron A (1995) Assessment of the narrow cervical spinal canal: a prospective comparison of MRI, myelography and CT-myelography. Neuroradiology 37: 187-191

Rinck PA (1993). Magnetic resonance in medicine (the basic textbook of the European magnetic resonance forum), 3rd edn. Balckwell, Oxford

Rodesch G, Van Bogaert P, Mavroudakis N et al. (1990) Neuroradiologic findings in leptomeningeal carcinomatosis: the value interest of gadolinium-enhanced MRI. Neuroradiology 32: 26-32

Ross JS (1992) MR Imaging of the cervical spine: techniques for two- and three-dimensional imaging. AJR Am J Roentgenol 159: 779-786

Ross JS, Ruggieri PM, Glicklich M et al. (1993) 3D MRI of the cervical spine: low flip angle FISP vs. Gd-DTPA turbo FLASH in degenerative disc disease. J Comput Assist Tomogr 17: 26-33

Runge VM (1996) Review of neuroradiology. Saunders, Philadelphia

Runge VM, Wood ML, Kaufman D, Price AC (1988) Gd-DTPA future applications with advanced imaging techniques. Radiographics 8: 161-179

Schuknecht B, Huber P, Büller B, Nadjmi M (1992) Spinal leptomeningeal neoplastic disease. Eur Neurol 32: 11-16

Shapiro R (1984) Myelography, 4th edn. Year Book, Chicago

Shellock FG, Crues JV (1988) High field-strength MR imaging and metallic biomedical implants: an ex vivo evaluation of deflection forces. AJR Am J Roentgenol 151: 389-392

Smith RC, Lange RC, McCarthy SM (1991) Chemical shift artifact: dependence on shape and orientation of the lipid-water interface. Radiology 181: 225-229

Stark DD, Bradley WG (1992) Magnetic resonance imaging. 2nd edn. Mosby Year Book, St. Louis

Sze G (1990) Magnetic resonance imaging of the spine in oncology. In: Breit A (ed) Magnetic resonance in oncology. Springer, Berlin Heidelberg New York, pp 41-54

Sze G, Abramson A, Krol G, et al (1988a) Gadolinium-DTPA/dimeglumine in the MR evaluation of intradural extramedullary spinal disease. AJNR 9: 153-163; AJR Am J Roentgenol 150: 911-921

Sze G, Krol G, Zimmerman RD, Deck MDF (1988b) Intramedullary disease of the spine: diagnosis using gadolinium-DTPA enhanced MR imaging. AJNR 9: 847-858; AJR Am J Roentgenol 151: 1193-1204

Tartaglino LM, Flanders AE, Vinitski S, Friedman DP (1994) Metallic artifacts on MR images of the postoperative spine: reduction with fast spin-echo techniques. Radiology 190: 565-569

Tien RD (1992) Fat-suppression MR imaging in neuroradiology: techniques and clinical application. Review article. AJR Am J Roentgenol 158: 369-379.

Tien RD, Olson EM, Zee CS (1992) Diseases of the lumbar spine: findings on fat-suppressed MR imaging. AJR Am J Roentgenol 159: 95-99.

Tilling R, Fink U, Deimling M, Bauer WM, Yousry T, Krauss B (1988) Klinische Anwendung von Gradientenecho-Sequenzen mit längeren Repetitionszeiten. Fortschr Röntgenstr 149: 303-309

Uchida N, Sugimara K, Kajitani A et al (1993). MR imaging of vertebral metastases: evaluation of fat-saturation imaging. Enr J Radiol 17: 91-94

Valk J (1988) Gadolinium-DTPA in MR of spinal lesions. AJNR 9: 345-350

Van de Kelft E, Bosmans J, Parizel PM, Van Vyve M, Selosse P (1991) Intracerebral hemorrhage after lumbar myelography with iohexol: report of a case and review of the literature. Neurosurgery 28(4): 570-574

Van Goethem JWM, Parizel PM, Perdieus D, Hermans P, de Moor J (1991) MR and CT imaging of paraspinal textiloma (gossybipoma). J Comput Assist Tomogr 15: 1000-1003

Van Goethem JWM, Van de Kelft E, Biltjes IGGM, van Hasselt BAAM, van den Hauwe L, Parizel PM, De Schepper AMA (1996) MRI after successful lumbar discectomy. Neuroradiology 38: 90-96

Wehrli FW (1991) Fast-scan magnetic resonance (principles and applications). Raven, New York

Wehrli FW, McGowan JC (1996). The basis of MR contrast. In: Atlas SW (ed) Magnetic resonance imaging of the brain and spine. Lippincott-Raven, Philadelphia

Wehrli FW, Perkins TG, Shimakawa A, Roberts F (1987) Chemical shift-induced amplitude modulations in images obtained with gradient refocusing. Magn Reson Imaging 5: 157-158

Weinreb JC, Brateman L, Babcock EE, Maravilla KR, Cohen JM, Horner SD (1985) Chemical shift artifact in clinical magnetic resonance images at 0.35 T. AJR Am J Roentgenol 145: 183-185

White SJ, Hajnal JV, Young IR, Bydder GM (1993) Use of fluid attenuated inversion recovery pulse sequences for imaging the spinal cord. Magn Reson Med 28: 153-162

Wilmink JT (1988) Radiology of sciatica. PhD thesis, University of Groningen, Van Denderen, Groningen

Wilmink JT, Lindeboom SF, Vencken LM, van den Burg W (1984) Relationship between contrast medium dose and adverse effects in lumbar myelography. Diagn Imaging Clin Med 53: 208-214

Wismer GL, Rosen BR, Buxton R, Stark DD, Brady TJ (1985) Chemical shift imaging of bone marrow: preliminary experience. AJR Am J Roentgenol 145: 1031-1037

3 Imaging Intradural Extra and Intramedullary Tumours

J. VALK and J. WEERTS

CONTENTS

3.1 Introduction

In the classic division, spinal tumours are differentiated as extradural and intradural, and the latter subdivided into intra- and extramedullary tumours. Though not all tumours are confined to the boundaries suggested by this division, it is nevertheless useful in describing location and extent of space-occupying lesions (BALÉRIAUX 1986; BALÉRIAUX et al. 1989, 1992). The relative incidence of tumours in the various spinal compartments is given in Table 3.1.

J.VALK, MD,PhD, Department of Radiology, Free University Hospital, Academisch Ziekenhuis, Postbus 7057, 1007 MB Amsterdam, The Netherlands
J.WEERTS, MD, Department of Radiology, Free University Hospital, Academisch Ziekenhuis, Postbus 7057, 1007 MB Amsterdam, The Netherlands

Table 3.1. Relative incidence of spinal canal tumours by compartment

	Overall	Adult	Child
Intramedullary	20%	1/3	1/2
Extramedullary	50%	2/3	1/2
Extradural	30%		

Of the primary intramedullary tumours, astrocytoma occurs most frequently, followed by ependymoma and finally haemangioblastoma. Less frequent are tumours of non-glial origin, dysembryogenetic tumours and intramedullary metastases.

Table 3.3. Relative incidence of intramedullary canal tumours

Tumour type	Incidence	Comments
Astrocytoma	30%–40%(adults) 50%–80%/(children)	10%–25% grades III and IV
Ependymoma	55%–65%(adults) 30%(children)	
Oligodendroglioma	1%–3%	
Haemangioblastoma	1.5%–6%	Multiple in 10%–25% of patients with Hippel-Lindau disease
Miscellaneous	5%–10%	
Non-glial tumours (ganglioma, ganglioneuroma)	1%–3% 1%–6%	
Lymphomas Dysembryogenetic tumours (teratoma, lipoma, epidermoid, dermoid, cavernoma, angiolipoma, arterinvenous malformation)		
Metastatic tumours	1%-3%	

Intramedullary tumours most frequently occur in the cervical region (55%), followed by the thoracic cord (23%), the conus medullaris (12%) and the cervico-medullary junction (5%) as well as involving the whole cord in 5% of cases.

The majority of intradural extramedullary tumours are meningeomas and neurinomas, which both may transgress the compartment boundaries and have extradural components as well.

The purpose of spinal cord imaging of intradural lesions is to describe the morpholoical changes caused by the lesion, the location and compartment occupied by the lesion, the extent of the lesion, the internal structure of the lesion with regard to haemorrhage, necrosis, calcification, vascularity, cysts, syrinx formation etc., as well as secondary changes such as bone erosion or scalloping. Though it is rarely possible to arrive at a histological diagnosis by imaging alone, it is of great importance to rule out lesions that may mimic intramedullary or extramedullary neoplasms. Such conditions are: multiple sclerosis, AIDS-related myelitis, intramedullary abscess or tuberculoma, neurosarcoidosis, intramedullary lymphoma, arteriovenous malformations, ischaemic lesions (as in arteriovenous dural shunts or anterior spinal artery infarction), traumatic changes and congenital malformations (intramedullary lipoma or dermoids).

3.2
Imaging Modalities

3.2.1
Plain Radiography

Plain radiography plays a limited role as far as intramedullary tumours are concerned. In late phases of slowly developing tumours, scalloping of vertebrae may be seen. Plain films may be of help in differential diagnosis when concurrent vertebral anomalies are present.

3.2.2
Myelography

Myelography with water-soluble contrast medium has for many years been the best method of delineating the extent of intradural tumours, whether intra- or extramedullary. In extramedullary tumours, the nature of the cord compression is usually evident. The cord is compressed and often shifted to one side. Generally the extramedullary tumours are well delineated, leading to a typical dome shape of the tumour next to the spinal cord. In intramedullary tumours, swelling of the cord depicted in two orthogonal planes is myelographically convincing evidence of an intramedullary lesion. The obvious disadvantage of myelography, apart from its invasiveness, is the indirect depiction of the tumour: no internal structure can be defined, and the core of the lesion is not exactly indicated. Myelography is nevertheless an excellent method for depicting an increase in blood vessels in the arachnoid spaces, which may be helpful in finding the level of the feeders for spinal angiography. Myelography is also excellent for showing drop metastases to the caudal roots in leptomeningeal seeding.

3.2.3
CT Myelography

CT Myelography has improved myelography by providing the capacity for transverse sections and yielding at least some information about the internal structure of the lesion and the cord, e.g. cyst or syrinx formation. Often, unfortunately, only the swelling of the cord is seen. (Fig. 3.1)

3.2.4
Magnetic Resonance Imaging

When available, magnetic resonance imaging (MRI) is the modality of choice for the examination of patients with symptoms indicating spinal cord disease (BROTCHI et al. 1991). MRI provides excellent tissue contrast and good anatomical detail in every desired plane. It therefore meets the requirements of an ideal imaging modality able to answer the diagnostic questions summarized above. The choice of image parameters and examination planes is of great importance for adequate interpretation of pathological changes. Modern MR machines offer a wide variety of choices of pulse sequences, including features such as fat suppression, magnetisation transfer, MR angiography and diffusion imaging. For morphological description of pathology, T1-weighted spin echo (SE) images with high spatial definition are required. T2-weighted images can be obtained by using 2D or 3D SE techniques, turbo SE (TSE) techniques, gradient echo (GE) pulse sequences and combinations of TSE and GE (TSEGE) techniques. A dramatic improvement of MR imaging of intramedullary lesions was achieved when gadolinium DTPA became available as an intravenous contrast agent. Both sensivity and specificity of MR diagnosis improved considerably (SLASKY et al. 1987; VALK 1988; SZE 1988; PARIZEL et al. 1989). Each of these

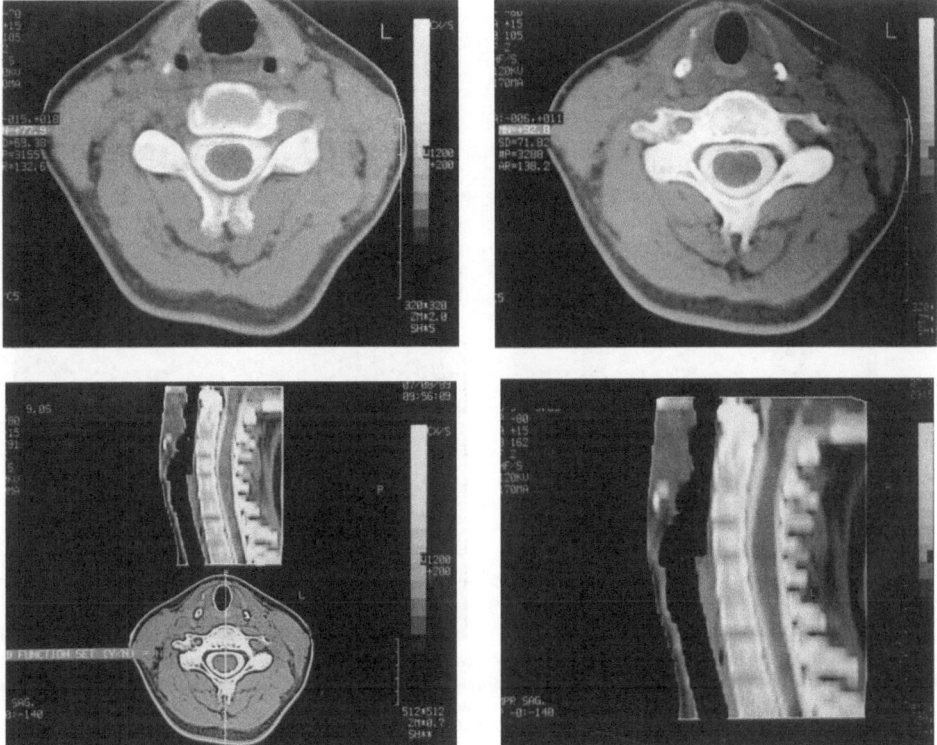

Fig. 3.1 a-d. Transverse and sagittally reconstructed images of CT myelography showing swelling of the cord. The inner structure of the abnormality cannot be assessed

techniques has its own advantages and disadvantages. As a rule, a shorter acquisition time is paid for by lower spatial resolution. The illustrations will show the effect of parameter settings on the images. The use of phased array coils has improved spinal imaging, allowing high-resolution images of the spine over a large trajectory (Fig. 3.2). This is achieved by four to six coupled "independent" coils, each with the high signal intensity of a single coil. By selecting combinations, larger segments of the spinal column can be imaged simultaneously with the high resolution of a single smaller coil (Fig. 3.3).

State-of-the-art MR techniques allow the following information about intramedullary lesions to be obtained:

1. Location of the lesion: level, segments involved
2. Compartment: extradural, intradural (extra- or intradurally)

3. Intrinsic structure of lesion: homogeneous, heterogeneous, necrotic areas, intratumoral cysts, pattern of enhancement
4. Additional features: calcifications, haemorrhage, syringohydromyelia, blocking of CSF pathways, exophytic components

Table 3.2. Normal behaviour of intramedullary components

	T_1	T_2/T_2^{*a}	IV contrast
Tumour	Intermediate/low	High	++/-
Haemorrhage	High	Low/High	-
Necrosis	Low	Low	+/-
Calcifications	Low/High	Low	-
Cyst	Low	High	-
Inflammation	Low	High	++/-

[a] Depending on age of haematoma

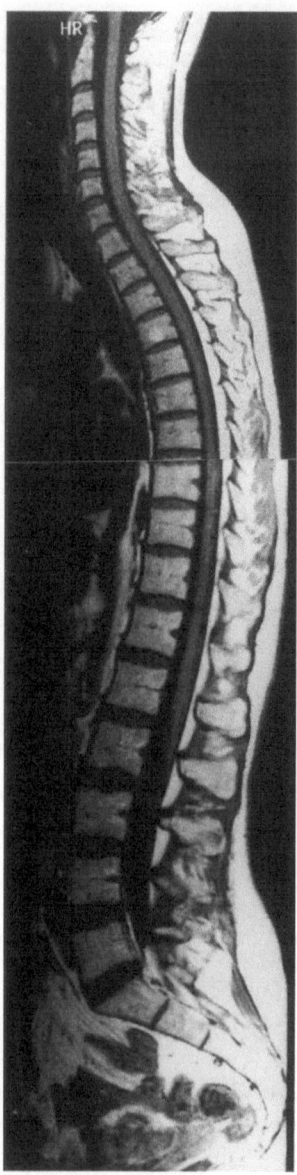

Fig. 3.2. Phased-array T1-weighted sagittal image covering the whole spine. Excellent detail has been obtained over a wide range

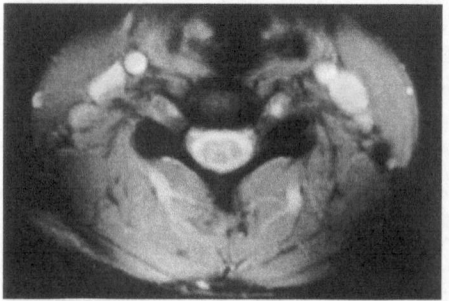

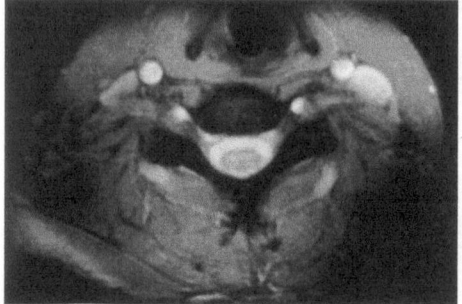

Fig.3.3a.b. Transverse T2-weighted gradient echo (FLASH) images through the cervical spinal cord at the level of intervertebral foramen C4-C5. The H-shaped grey-matter figure in the spinal cord can be seen very well

3.2.4.1
MRI and Spinal Compartments

As a rule, MRI allows adequate description of the location of a lesion in a spinal compartment (Fig. 3.4., 3.5.). There are, however, exceptions. Extradural masses may penetrate the dura and have intradural and possibly intramedullary extensions. Meningeomas and neurinomas may also extend beyond compartmental boundaries; neurinomas may extend from the intradural space, follow the neural roots through the intravertebral foramen and have a large mass outside the spinal canal hourglass or dumbbell shape). The illustrations show the separation and involvement of the spinal compartments.

3.2.4.2
MRI and Intramedullary Tumours

Morphological analysis of intramedullary tumours is, though sometimes complex, rather stereotyped (SCOTTI et al. 1987; CARSIN et al. 1987). Intramedul-

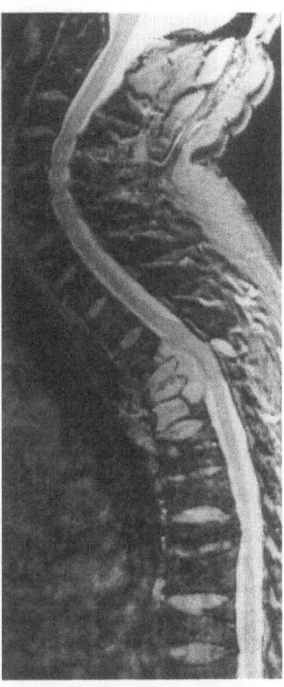

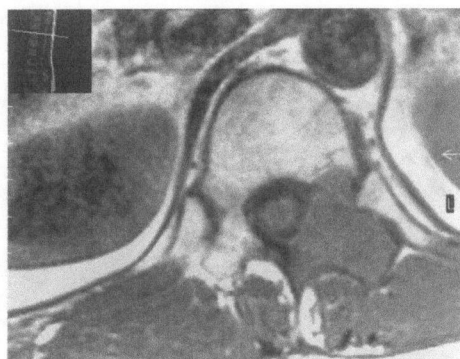

Fig.3.5. In T1-weighted transverse images the different compartments can be easily identified. Breast carcinoma meatstasis in a thoracic vertebra involving the left pedicle and transverse processus and invading the epidural space, displacing the dural sac without any involvement of the cord

Fig. 3.4. MRI allows easy diagnosis of the involved spinal compartments. T2-weighted sagittal image in a 19-year-old man with rhabdomyosarcoma metastasis in the thoracic vertebrae. The image shows the extradural component of the tumour, the displaced dural sac and the swollen and compressed spinal cord

lary tumours show thickening of the cord over a certain length. On MRI this should be demonstrated in at least two directions, usually sagittal and axial. Coronal images are sometimes helpful. Various pulse sequences show the internal structure of the tumour and the relationship with surrounding structures. Knowledge of the contrast obtained by the different pulse sequences is mandatory for a correct interpretation. Because intramedullary tumours are the main topic of this section, we will look in greater detail at the effects of various pulse sequences on the diagnostic work-up of intramedullary tumours (Table 3.2)

3.2.4.3
MRI specificity

The sensitivity of MRI in detecting spinal abnormalities is outstanding. The specificity is much lower; MRI does not distinguish reliably between benign and malignant lesions or predict the histological tumour type. Some clues, however, may be given.

3.2.5
T1-Weighted Images

The "anatomical" T1-weighted SE images may already show abnormal signal intensities (Fig. 3.6). Most intramedullary tumours are iso- or hypointense on T1-weighted images. Sometimes the lesion is homogeneous; in other cases the tumour consists of various tissue types. Tumour cysts are usually shown with a signal intensity identical to or slightly higher than that of CSF (VALK and KAISER 1986; WILLIAMS et al. 1987). Widening of the central canal at the apex of the tumour is the rule, with few exceptions. The resulting hydromelia may broaden the cord over a long trajectory. If haemorrhage or haemorrhagic necrosis is present, the areas involved show a high signal intensity (Fig. 3.7), unless the blood is very fresh (less than 3 days old). A high signal intensity may also be seen when lipomas or dermoids are present (Fig. 3.8). Rarely, this may also occur when calcifications are present. High signal intensities on T1-weighted images are usually seen in cavernous haemangiomas (FONTAINE et al. 1988).

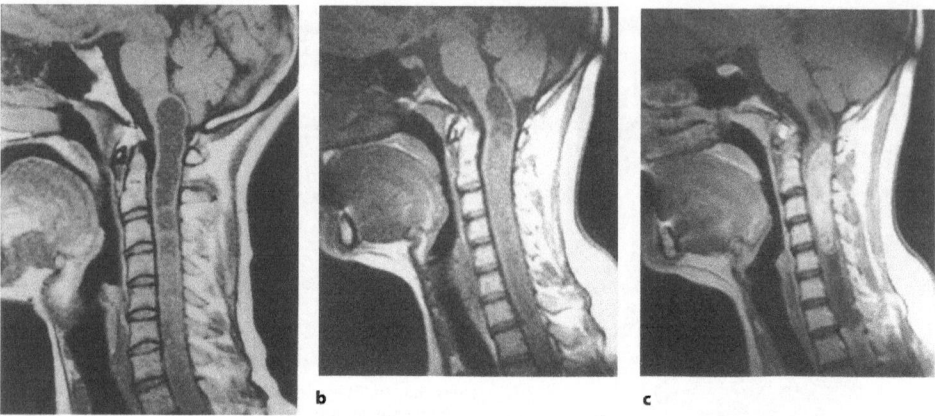

Fig. 3.6. a T1-weighted sagittal image of an intramedullary tumour. The image shows a number of characteristic features: swelling of the cord over the entire depicted range, inhomogeneous structure of the lesion with slightly hypointense massive tumour and cyst/syrinx formation at the upper border, extending upwards into the medulla oblongata. In most such cases the tumour will prove to be a low-grade astrocytoma. The T1-weighted transverse images b without and c with contrast enhancemnt show the extra information obtained by contrast injection. Here the core of the tumour is depicted. (MRI cannot, however, differentiate reliably between astrocytomas and ependymomas unless other features such as haemorrhage, calcification or pattern of enhancement make it possible to be more specific)

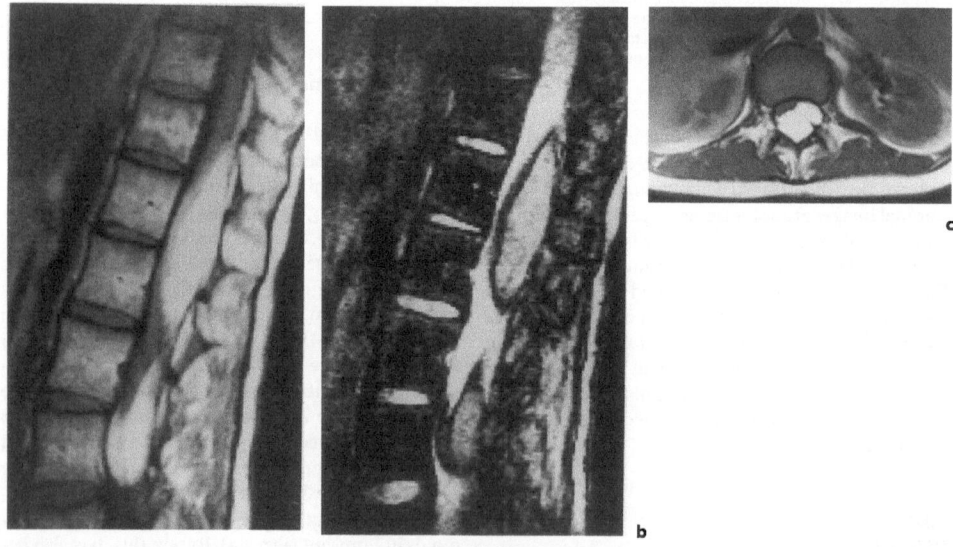

Fig. 3.7.a-c. Subdural haemorrhage in a patient on anticoagulative therapy after attempting epidural anaesthesia about 14 days earlier. a On the T1-weighted image blood of the same age shows a high signal intensity. b On the T2-weighted image the blood also has high signal intensity with a developing rim of low signal intensity caused by blood pigments. c The transverse T1-weighted image shows serious compression of the dural sac in the lumbar area

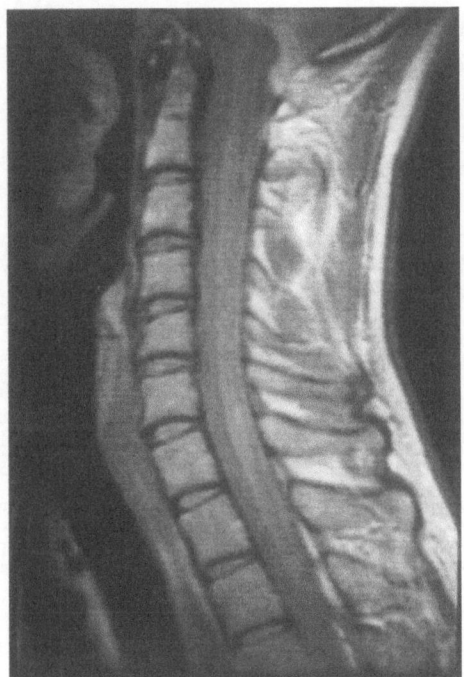

Fig. 3.9. Proton density image in the sagittal plane of the cervical spine. The CSF is isointense with the spinal cord, and the intramedullary lesion at the level of 6 is clearly seen. The disadvantage of PD images is also evident. The silhouette of the spinal cord is not seen, making exact localisation difficult

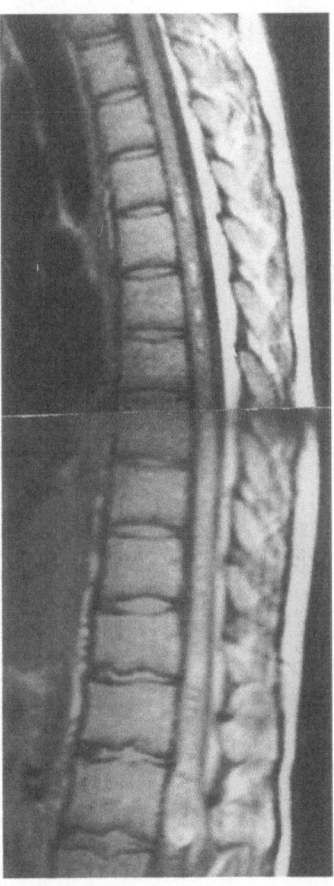

Fig. 3.8. On T1-weighted images fat has a high signal intensity. On this sagittal image multiple intramedullary lipomas with high signal intensity are seen. In the conus a dermoid was found at surgery. If necessary, diagnosis can be confirmed by a fat-suppression technique

3.2.6
Proton Density Images

By performing SE sequences with long TR and short TE, T1 and T2 weighting are reduced and the images mainly show the proton density (PD) of the tissue. A longer echo time will increase T2 weighting. The small differences in PD between healthy tissues make these components nearly isointense on PD images, whereas lesions will often stand out with high signal intensity (Fig. 3.9). The PD pulse sequence is very important in determining the nature of an intramedullary lesion.

3.2.7
T2-Weighted Images

On T2-weighted images, intramedullary tumours usually show high signal intensity (Fig. 3.10a), the CSF and fluid in cysts are also bright. Tumours, therefore, are easier to appreciate on PD images. The tumour signal on either sequence may be homogeneous or heterogeneous, depending on the internal structure of the tumour. Cysts will show high signal intensity on T2-weighted images. Haemorrhage will show either low signal intensity (<14 days) or high signal intensity (>14 days) depending on the age of the haemorrhage. Haemorrhagic necrosis will often appear dark on T2-weighted images. The fluid in hydromyelic cavities will usually be isointense with CSF or, when the pulsatile movement in the syrinx is less than in the CSF spaces, it will have a higher signal intensity (Goy et al. 1986; VALK and KAISER 1986).

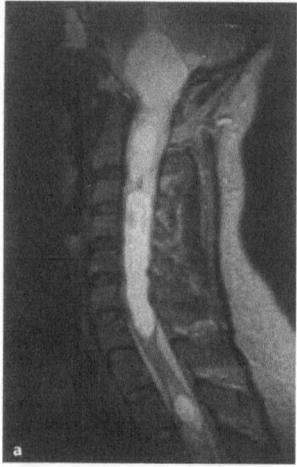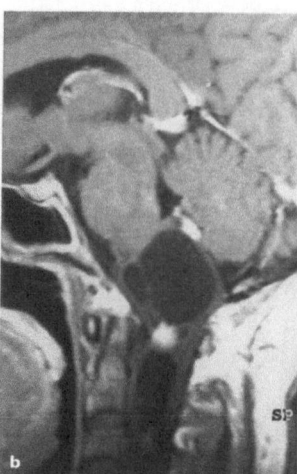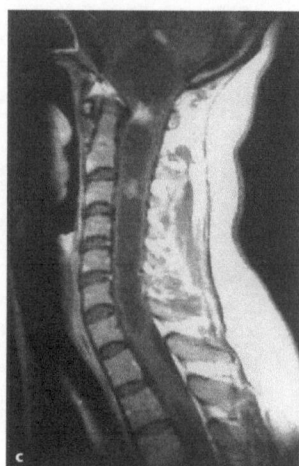

Fig. 3.10a-c. The usual MR appearance of an intramedullary tumour. **a** On the T2-weighted sagittal image swelling of the cord is seen with large cystic parts and extension of the cyst or syrinx into the medulla oblongata. The different compartments have different signal intensities depending on whether dephasing by pulsatile flow or concentration of proteinaceous fluid take place. **b,c** On the T1-weighted contrast-enhanced images nodular areas are seen with high signal intensity. At surgery this tumour proved to be a haemangioblastoma

3.2.8
Turbo or Fast Spin Echo Imaging

In conventional SE sequences all 180° refocussing pulses and steps in the phase-encoding direction are preceeded by a 90° excitation pulse, which is time-consuming. Much faster acquisition can be obtained by using fast or TSE sequences, where a single excitation pulse is followed by a number of 180° RF pulses and phase-encoding steps. In principle a single excitation pulse and as many phase-direction steps as necessary could be used. Signal intensity will decline with each echo and with degradation of the image. The solution is to combine a single excitation pulse with a limited number of phase steps, thereby saving quite a lot of time while preserving reasonable resolution (Fig. 3.11). The contrast in TSE imaging is different from SE contrast. Due to the pulse sequence, the fat signal is far less suppressed than in long TR, long TE SE imaging. The continuous refocussing pulses also cancel static magnetic susceptibility effects, so areas with previous haemorrhage, cavernous haemangiomas etc. may be less conspicuous. Conversely, the pulse sequence can be used for a myelography-like MR procedure with 3D acquisition which is useful in extramedullary and extradural lesions.

3.2.9
T2*-Weighted Images

By using gradient-recalled echoes rather than 180° refocussing pulses and adapting the flip angle over which the magnetisation vector is rotated (<15°), images can be made dependent on T2* relaxation (Fig. 3.11d). For practical purposes this means that images can be obtained faster (or with higher resolution) and that a greater deal of the magnetic suspectibility changes will be apparent on the images. The latter can detract from the quality of the image, yet is important for obtaining diagnostic information. Particularly in the presence of haemorrhage, the T2*-weighted images show dark areas where blood residue and therefore iron-containing blood pigments are present. This may be of diagnostic value in cavernous haemangiomas. The fast gradient echo technique can also be used in a 3D mode via a maximum intensity projection (MIP), thus being transformed into a 3D-myelography-like examination.

3.2.10
Fluid-Attenuated Inversion Recovery

The importance of FLAIR in MRI of the spinal cord is still unclear. Theoretically, FLAIR might be expected to be equally advantageous to imaging of the brain and spine. CSF, nulled in this sequence by the choice of a correct inversion time, will appear dark, while lesions will appear bright. With FLAIR and turbo FLAIR sequences, however, we have obtained rather poor results in imaging the spinal cord. The FLAIR sequence, though is implemented differently, and therefore may yield different results, on equipment from different manufacturers.

3.2.11
Contrast-Enhanced T1-Weighted Images

The use of intravenous paramagnetic contrast is mandatory in intramedullary tumours (VALK 1988;

BREGER et al. 1989; CHAMBERLAIN et al. 1991). It helps to show the core of the lesion, visualises exophytic tumour components and may differentiate the tumour from cysts, necrosis, oedema and hydromyelia (Fig. 3.10.b,c). The idea that contrast enhancement will show the true extent of the tumour is unfortunately overly simple, especially in astrocytomas. In low-grade glioma, often only part of the tumour enhances. Despite this restriction, contrast-enhanced studies will guide the neurosurgeon to locations with guaranteed tumour.

Other techniques currently standardly available on MR machines can be used to further improve contrast between tissues.

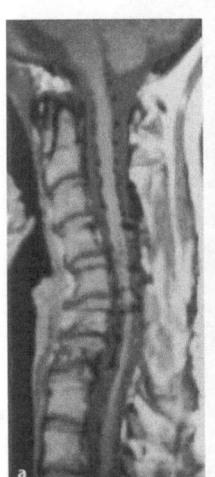 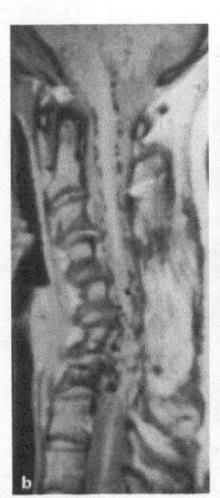 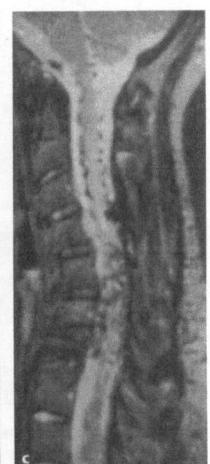

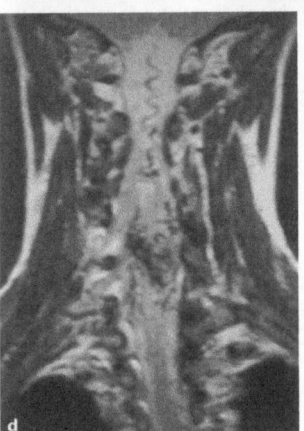 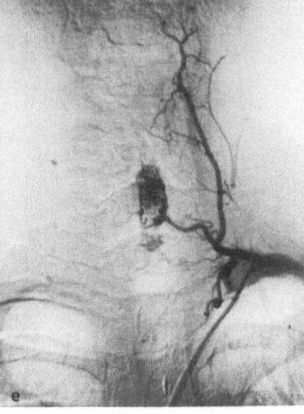

Fig. 3.11a-e. Demonstration of various MR techniques in a case of AVM of the cervical (thoracic spinal cord in a 13-year-old girl. **a** The T1-weighted sagittal image shows the kyphosis of the cervical spine, the loss of height of C6 and C7 due to a vertebral haemangioma and the flow voids in the many vessels surrounding the spinal cord. **b** The PD image better shows the vessels as well as focal cord destruction. **c** the T2-weighted image also shows the vessels at the local level of the nidus of the AVM. **d** In another (coronal) plane a gradient echo T2-weighted image clearly shows the AVM and the draining veins. **e** The AVM with multiple feeders was confirmed by angiography and treated incompletely by emolisation

3.2.12
Magnetisation Transfer

By an off-resonance pulse prior to the imaging sequence, protons bound in tight molecular structures can be saturated. Protons prepared in such a way can withdraw magnetisation from free protons, thus reducing signal intensity. This may help to suppress the background of the image and improve contrast between lesions and background.

3.2.13
Fat Suppression

Because there is a minute difference in resonance frequency between fat and water, it is possible to make separate fat (proton) and water (proton) images. This allows suppression of fat in the image and may sometimes be advantageous, for example in cases with tumour extension into the epidural fat, in the diagnosis of lipomas and dermoids, or following injection of contrast medium.

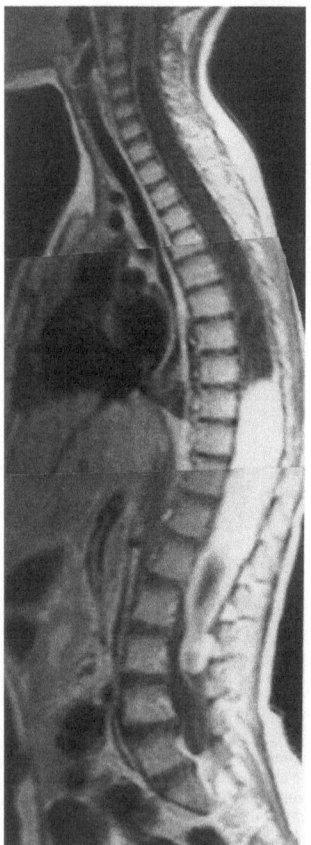

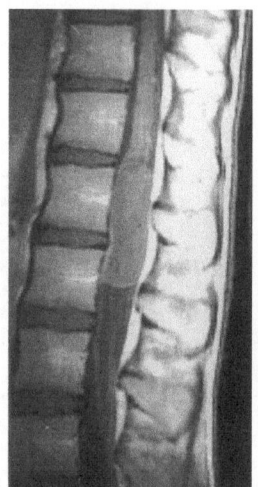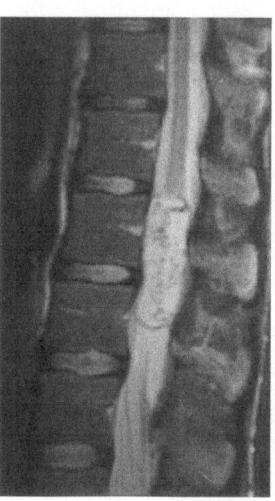

a

b

Fig. 3.13a,b. Sagittal a T1-weighted and b T2-weighted images of the conus region. A partially intramedullary tumour with an exophytic component is seen. The T2-weighted image suggests many vascular channels inside the tumour. The turnover seems to be well demarcated. Histologically, the tumour was a myxopapillary ependymoma

Fig. 3.12. Whole cord (or holocord) intramedullary tumour in a 7-year-old child. T1-weighted sagittal image after contrast enhancement shows the compact part of the lesion in the lower thoracic and lumbar region with homogeneous enhancement. Above this area hydromyelia has developed, reaching upwards into the brain stem. Histologically, the tumour was a low-grade astrocytoma

3.3
Intramedullary Tumours

Astrocytomas (Fig. 3.12) and ependymomas (Fig. 3.13) are the most frequently encountered intramedullary tumours, accounting for about 90% of all intramedullary tumours (Table 3.3). Most astrocytomas and ependymomas are benign and of low grade, first producing symptoms when they have already reached a considerable size. From a surgical point of view there is a major difference between these tumours: ependymomas are usually located centrally in the cord and have a cleavage plane with the surrounding healthy tissue, whereas astrocytomas diffusely infiltrate the surrounding parenchyma. In the latter case, there is no hope of total removal of the tumour. Differentiating astrocytomas from ependymomas by MR, important as it may be, is not always easy. Both tumours cause the cord to expand, may have cystic and necrotic parts, may cause hydromyelia and may have exophytic components. Ependymomas tend to haemorrhage and may show calcification, though generally much less than in the brain (FERRANTE 1992). Ependymomas have a preference for the conus and caudal regions. Both tumours enhance following injection of contrast medium. This is remarkable because in the brain low-grade astrocytomas usually do not enhance, with the exception of pilocytic astrocytomas. The enhancement of ependymomas is usually more intense and homogeneous than that of astrocytomas. When occuring in the cauda equina region, ependymomas can cause sacral bone destruction, especially the myxopapillary type (Fig. 3.14; McCormick et al. 1990). A somewhat unexpected secondary trait of caudally located ependymomas is the occurrence of communicating hydrocephalus along with this type of tumour. The hydrocephalus may be the presenting symptom. Subependymomas of the spinal cord have also been described. (PANI et al. 1992); on MR images they cannot be differentiated from ependymomas.

Haemangioblastoma is the third most frequent intramedullary tumour, though already rare. The usual appearance is that of a cyst-like tumour with an enhancing mural nodulus (Fig. 3.10), possibly presenting serpiginous structures with flow voids as the expression of vessels in the lesion (COLOMBO et al. 1986; FAHRENDORF et al. 1986; KAFFENBERGER et al. 1988; MOCK et al. 1990). MR angiography (MRA) may contribute to the diagnosis. In less typical cases it may be impossible to extract the correct diagnosis from the MR images, and MRA or conventional angiography has to be performed.

Next in frequency are intramedullary metastatic tumours. They most commonly occur in lung carcinoma, less often in breast carcinoma, melanoma and lymphoma. The metastatic lesion presents after contrast medium injection as well demarcated, strongly enhancing and surrounded by oedema (Fig. 3.15). All secondary features occurring in primary intramedullary tumours may also be seen in metastatic lesions (FOSTER et al. 1987).

Of even lower incidence are intramedullary lymphomas, but solitary intramedullary locations have been described (MITSUMOTO et al. 1980; HOLTAS et al. 1986; HOCHBERG and MILLER 1988; BLUEMKE and WANG 1990).

Intramedullary tumours of non-glial origin have been described as incidental findings. Their appearance on MR is aspecific.

Intramedullary lipomas are usually part of a complex congenital anomaly (JOHNSON and ROBERSON 1974).

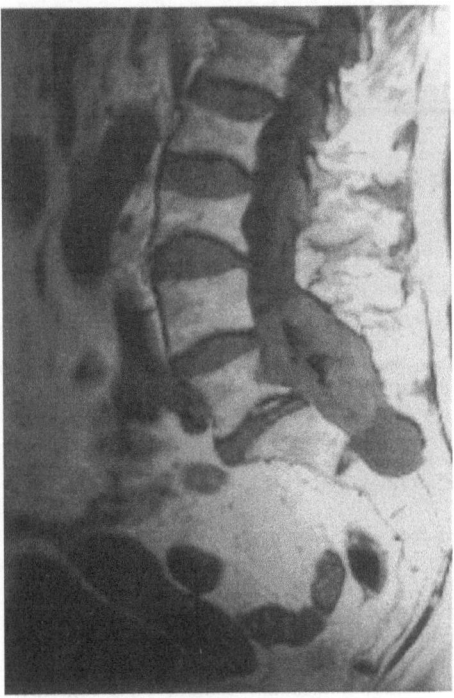

Fig. 3.14. Sagittal T1-weighted image of the lower caudal region showing another case of myxopapillary ependymoma, in this case with scalloping of L5 and partial destruction of the sacrum

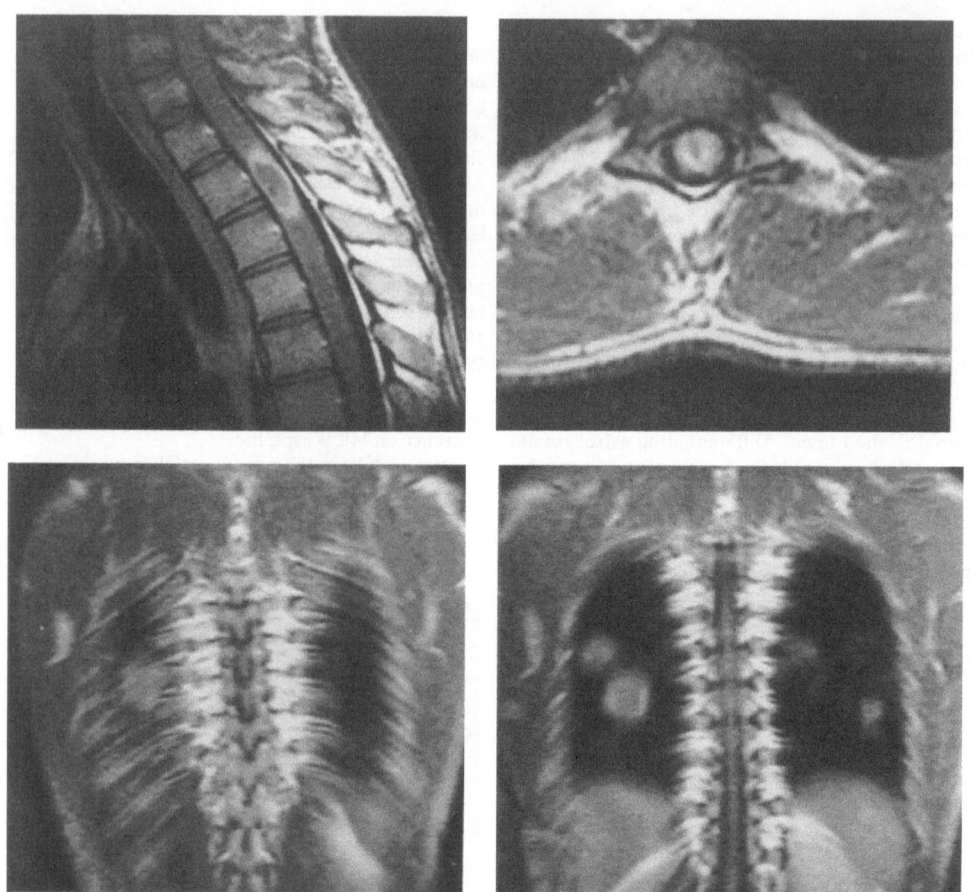

Fig. 3.15a-d. T1-weighted contrast-enhanced sagittal and transverse images of the upper thoracic spinal cord show an intramedullary lesion with ring-like enhancement and some degree of swelling. Chest MRI shows multiple rounded enhancing lesions. A combination of intramedullary and pulmonal metastases was considered. Histologically, the tumour was diagnosed as Wegener's granulomatosis

3.3.1
Differential Diagnosis

Intramedullary tumours have to be differentiated from intramedullary infections and inflammatory disease as well as from malformative disorders of the neural tube. In the infectious-inflammatory group, multiple sclerosis (FEASBY et al. 1981; MARAVILLA et al. 1985) and tropic spastic paresis (HIV-1 infection) may mimic intramedullary tumour (Fig. 3.16). AIDS-related myelitis also presents as an intramedullary lesion, often combined with a radiculitis (GRAFE and WILEY 1989; BARAKOS et al. 1990). The myelitis in AIDS can also be caused by cytomegalovirus (CMV) infection and by toxoplasmosis (HERSKOVITZ et al. 1989; HARRIS et al. 1990). In inflammatory and infectious diseases, there is usually no cyst formation. Enhancement is usually seen in active lesions. Intramedullary abscesses have also been reported (BLACKLOCK et al. 1982; KOPPEL et al. 1990), as well as intramedullary cysticercosis (CASTILLO et al. 1988), schistosoma mansoni infection, toxoplasmosis and herpes zoster. Neurosarcoidosis may present as an intramedullary mass (HITCHON et al. 1984; LEVIVIER et al. 1991).

Syringo-hydromelia formation may be part of a Chiari malformation or a myelo-dysplasia. It may also be present in degenerative disorders and post-traumatic cases. Ischaemic lesions of the cord may initially show swelling and enhancement. They are mostly due to obstruction of the anterior spinal artery. In follow-up studies, the affected site becomes atrophic. Arteriovenous malformations are usually easy to recognise because of the vessel structures in the lesion (DOPPMAN et al. 1987). Arteriovenous dural shunts lead to venous hypertension and central cord ischaemia, showing mild swelling of the cord with central excessively high signal intensity on T2-weighted images and central enhancement on delayed contrast-enhanced scans (Fig. 3.17). Cavernous angiomas or cavernomas of the spine can be familial or isolated, single or multifocal. They have specific MR features and can be identified readily (BICKNELL et al. 1978; SABIN et al. 1989; LOPATE et al. 1990; BOURGOUIN et al. 1992).

3.4
MRI of Extramedullary Expanding Lesions

Usually the topical diagnosis of extramedullary tumours on MRI is straightforward. Extramedullary

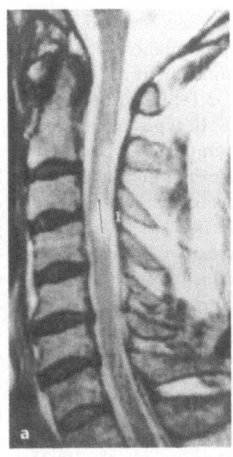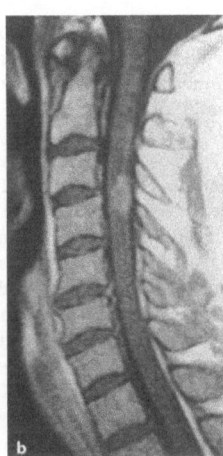

Fig. 3.16a,b. Sagittal a T2-weighted and b T1-weighted contrast-enhanced images of the cervical spine. The cervical spinal cord is slightly swollen; a lesion is seen with high signal intensity at the level of C3-C4 extending upwards. The C3-C4 component of the lesion enhances. Differential diagnosis: transverse myelitis, AIDS-related myelopathy, acute disseminated encephalomyelopathy, neurosarcoidosis or, most likely, multiple sclerosis. Clinical follow-up and response to treatment proved multiple sclerosis

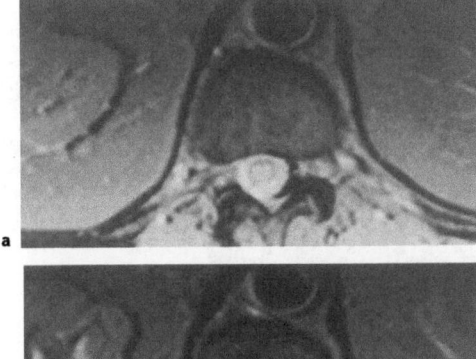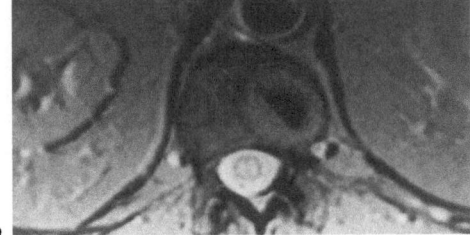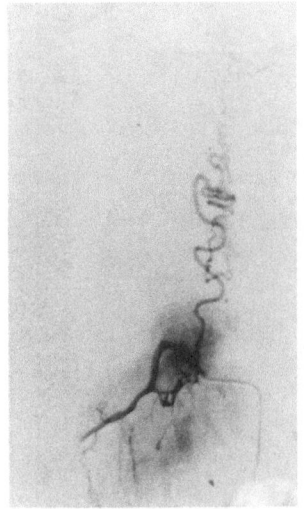

Fig. 3.17. a,b Transverse T2-weighted images at the level of the conus show swelling and a central area with high signal intensity. A lesion like this, especially when enhancemnt is late (20 minutes after injection), is highly likely to be an ischaemic lesion caused by an arteriovenous dural shunt with increased venous pressure. c Selective spinal angiography confirms this finding

tumours shift the spinal cord, which can be easily visualised by MRI in two or more planes. The most common tumours in this compartment are meningeomas and neurinomas (Fig. 3.18; DEMACHI et al. 1992; FRIEDMAN et al. 1992). Both types of tumours may be confined to the extramedullary compartment. Neurinomas, more often than meningeomas, may cross the boundaries of the intradural compartment and extend extradurally into the extraspinal compartments. The signal intensity of spinal neurinomas varies according to the histological substrate (HU and HUANG 1992). Both tumours are usually hypoisointense on T1-weighted images; meningeomas are usually dark on T2-weighted images, neurinomas bright (LEWIS and KINGSLEY 1987). Both tumours enhance after injection of contrast medium.

In the extramedullary compartment, ectopic tumours such as lipomas (TEKKÖK et al. 1992), dermoids and epidermoids are also found. Very rarely, these tumours are intramedullary. On MRI extramedullary epidermoids may be hard to demonstrate when the tumour has the same signal intensity as CSF on all pulse sequences. Epidermoids do not enhance unless they are infected. In imaging dermoids and epidermoids, care should be given to depict the possible cutaneous connection (dermal sinus), which may act as a porte d'entrée for infections.

Lipomas mostly occur along the filum terminale, in connection with the conus and as a gap-filling component in spina bifida cases. The characteristic signal of fat on MRI usually makes diagnosis simple. Fat suppression techniques may be helpful. Arachnoid and neurenteric cysts may behave as expanding lesions (Fig. 3.19; GEREMIA et al. 1988). Arachnoid cysts are usually secondary to other lesions or iatrogenic after surgery or myelography. Neurenteric cysts are developmental anomalies. They differ from arachnoid cysts in that they are lined by cuboid or columnar epithelium and may contain other structures such as serous glands and smooth muscle (STERN et al. 1991). The most frequent variety of neurenteric cysts occurs in the thoracic region, displacing the cord posteriorly (Fig. 3.19).

3.5
Leptomeningeal Spread of Tumour

Seeding of tumor along the CSF pathways occurs frequently in posterior fossa medulloblastomas or primitive neuroectodermal tumours (PNET) and incidentally in ependymomas (Fig 3.20; LIM et al. 1990). Meningeal spread has also been observed in lymphomas (BERNS et al. 1988). Diagnosis on MRI can only be achieved by injecting contrast material

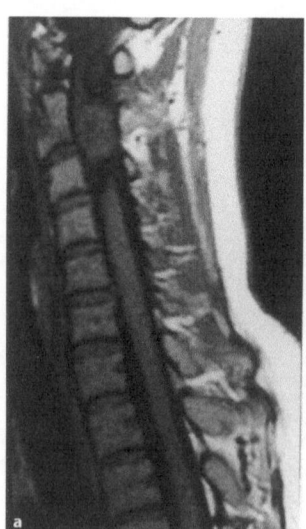
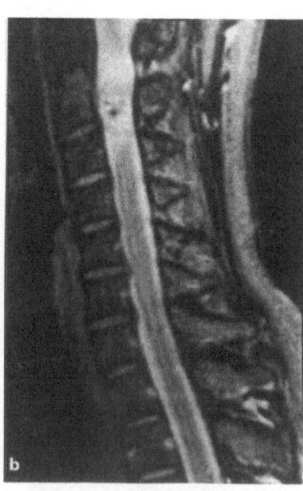
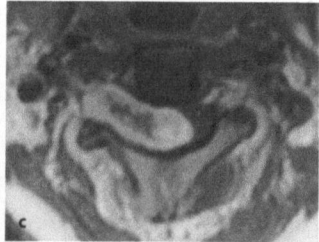

Fig. 3.18a-c. The sagittal a T1-weighted and b T2-weighted images show an intradural, extramedullary well-defined lesion at the level of C2-C3. c The transverse image shows that the neurofibroma extends through the widened foramen into the paravertebral region

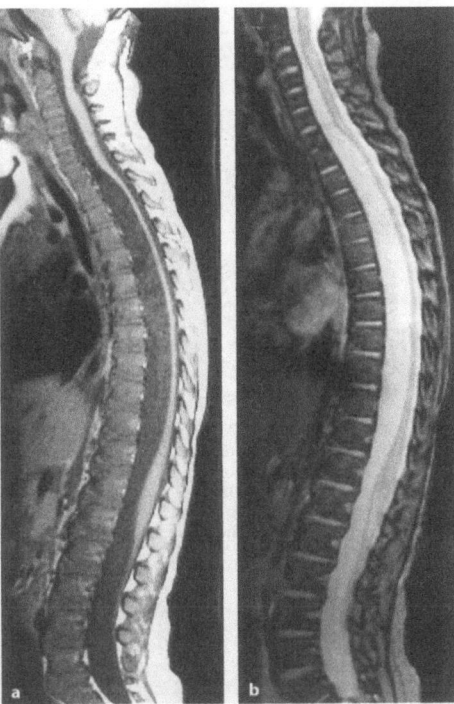

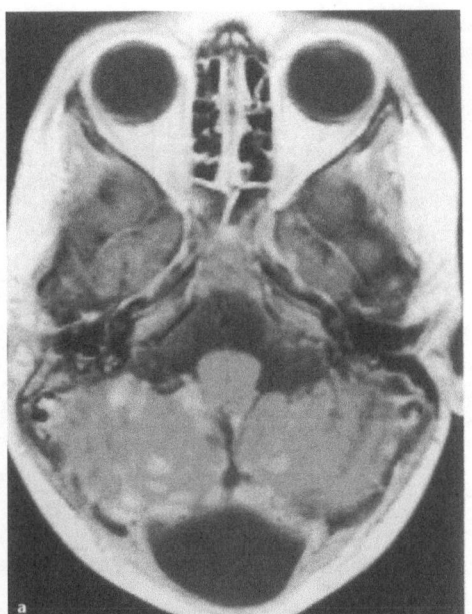

Fig. 3.19a,b. Characteristic sagittal a T1-weighted and T2-weighted images of a thoracic neurenteric cyst. The cyst compresses the thoracic cord against the dorsal border of the dural sac

in relatively high doses (0.2-0.3 mmol/kg body weight). MR images of meningeal spread are rather typical: the spinal cord shows a hyperintense layer on T1-weigted contrast-enhanced images, possibly presenting as a coating of irregular thickness. The caudal roots may show numerous rounded local thickenings often in association with coating of the entire surface of the roots. The end of the dural sac may be completely filled with tumour. Lesions may, however, also be discrete and confined to a single segment.

3.6
Postoperative Control

If no metallic implants or clips have been left in the patient, MRI is an excellent tool for postoperative control (Fig. 3.21). MRI allows differentiation of tumour invasion or resurrence from radiation myelitis (Fig. 3.22; MICHIKAWA et al. 1991). Because there is

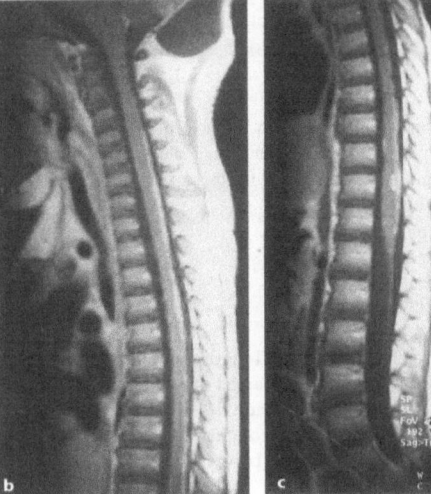

Fig. 3.20. a T1-weighted contrast-enhanced transverse image through the posterior fossa of a child treated for medulloblastoma. Multiple leptomeningeal metastases are present. **b,c** Sagittal T1-weighted images through the spine show a layer of enhancing tissue on the thoracic spinal cord and conus

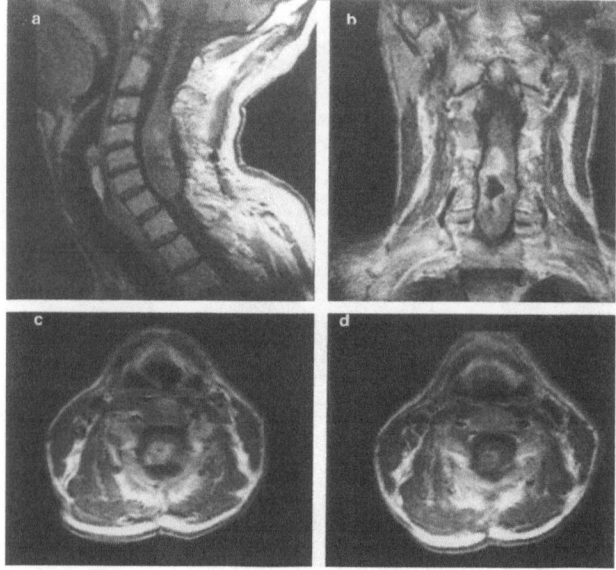

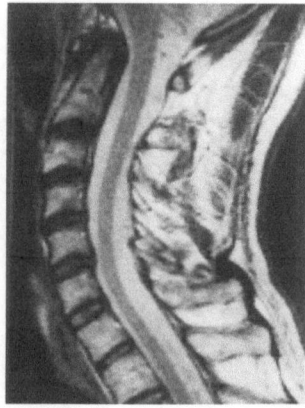

Fig. 3.22. MRI can help to differentiate between post-radiotherapy changes in the cord and compression or infiltration by tumour. In this case, 2 years after irradiation of the neck the spinal cord shows definite atrophy

Fig. 3.21a-d. Follow-up after surgery of a low-grade astrocytoma. Laminectomy of C3 to C7. Wide cervical canal. The spinal cord is thick and irregular (a,b) and shows partial enhancement, indicating residual tumour or recurrence

no hazardous radiation, the examination can be repeated as often as necessary. Furthermore, other imaging modalities in follow-up studies are rarely required.

3.7
Conclusion

In most cases, MRI will be the imaging modality of choice in patients suspected of having an intradural tumour. MRI will provide detailed diagnosis of the lesion and possible secondary features. In a limited number of cases, CT or plain radiography are still required.

References

Balériaux D (1986) Spinal cord tumors. In: Jeanmart L (ed) Radiology of the spine. Springer, Berlin Heidelberg New York, pp 39-45

Balériaux D, Parizel P, Segebarth C (1989) Pathologie intra-rachidienne et medullaire. In: Manelfe C (ed): Imagerie du rachis et de la moelle. Vigot, Paris, pp 499-545

Balériaux D, Parizel P, Bank WO (1992) Intraspinal and intra-medullary pathology. In: Manelfe C (ed) Imaging of the spine and spinal cord. Raven, New York, pp 513-564

Barakos JA, Mark A; Dillon WP, Norman D (1990) MR imaging of acute transverse myelitis and AIDS myelopathy. J Comput Assist Tomogr 14: 45-50

Berns DH, Blaser S, Ross JS, Masaryk TJ, Modic MT (1988) MR imaging with Gd-DTPA in leptomeningeal spread of lymphoma. J Comput Assist Tomogr 12: 499-500

Blacklock JB, Hood TW, Maxwell RE (1982) Intramedullary cervical spinal cord abscess. Case report. J Neurosurg 57; 270-273

Bluemke DA, Wang H (1990) Primary spinal cord lymphoma: MR appearance. J Comput Assist Tomogr 14: 812-814

Bourgouin PM, Tampieri D, Johnston W, Steward J, Melanson D, Ethier R (1992) Multiple occult vascular malformations of the brain and spinal cord: MRI diagnosis. Neuro-radiology 3: 110-111

Breger RK, Williams AL, Daniels DL et al (1989) Contrast enhancement in spinal MR imaging. AJR Am J Roentgenol 153: 387-391

Brotchi J, Dewitte O, Levivier M, et al (1991) A survey of 65 tumors within the spinal cord; surgical results and the importance of preoperative magnetic resonance imaging. Neurosurgery 29: 651-657

Carsin M, Gandon Y, Rolland Y, Simon J (1987) MRI of the spinal cord: intramedullary tumours. J Neuroradiol 14: 337-349

Castillo M, Quencer RM, Post MJD (1988) MR of intramedullary spinal cysticercosis. AJNR 9:393-395

Chamberlain MC, Sandy AD, Press GA (1991) Spinal tumours: gadolinium-DTPA-enhanced MR imaging. Neuroradiology 33: 469-474

Colombo N, Kucharczyk W, Brant-Zawadzki M, Norman D, Scotti G, Newton TH (1986) Magnetic resonance imaging of spinal cord hemangioblastoma. Acta Radiol Diagn 769: 734-737

Demachi H, Takashima T, Kadoya M (1992) MR imaging of spinal neurinomas with pathological correlation. J Comput Assist Tomogr 14: 250-254

Doppman JL, Di Chiro G, Dwyer AJ, et al (1987) Magnetic resonance imaging of spinal arteriovenous malformations. J Neurosurg 66:830-834

Edelson RN, Deck MDF; Posner JB (1972) Intramedullary spinal cord metastases. Neurology 22:1222-1231

Fahrendorf G, Sartor K, Gado, MH (1986) Magnetic resonance imaging of spinal cord hemangioblastomas and arteriovenous malformations. Acta Radiol Diagn 369:730-733

Feasby TE, Paty DW, Ebers GC, Fox AJ (1981) Spinal cord swelling in multiple sclerosis. Can J Neurol Sci 8: 151-153

Ferrante L (1992) Intramedullary spinal cord ependymomas: a study of 45 cases with long-term follow-up. Acta Neurochir (Wien) 119:74-79

Fontaine S, Melanson D, Cosgrove GR, et al (1988) Cavernous hemangiomas of the spinal cord: MR imaging. Radiology 166:839-841

Foster O, Crockard HA, Powell MP (1987) Syrinx associated with intramedullary metastasis. J Neurosurg Psychiatry 50:1067-1070

Friedman DP, Tartaglino LM, Flanders AE (1992) Intradural schwannomas of the spine: MR findings with emphasis on contrast-enhancement characteristics. AJR Am J Roentgenol 158:1347-1350

Geremia GK, Russell EJ, Clasen RA (1988) MR imaging characteristics of a neurenteric cyst. AJNR 9:978-980

Goy AMC, Pinto RS, Raghavendra BN (1986) Intramedullary spinal cord tumors:MR imaging, with emphasis on associated cysts. Radiology 161:381-386

Grafe MR, Wiley CA (1989) Spinal cord and peripheral nerve pathology in AIDS:the roles of cytomegalovirus and human immunodeficiency virus. Ann Neurol 25:561-566

Harris TM, Smith RR, Bognanno JR, Edwards MK (1990) Toxoplasmic myelitis in AIDS: gadolinium-enhanced MR. J Comput Assist Tomogr 14:809-811

Herskovitz S, Siegel SE, Schneider AT, et al (1989) Spinal cord toxoplasmosis in AIDS. Neurology 39:1552-1553

Hitchon PW, Ul Haque A, Olson JJ, et al (1984) Sarcoidosis presenting as an intramedullary spinal cord mass. Neurosurgery 15:86-90

Hochberg FH, Miller DC (1988) Primary central nervous system lymphoma. J Comput Assist Tomogr 10:111-115

Hu HP, Huang QL (1992) Signal intensity correlation of MRI with pathological findings in spinal neurinomas. Neuroradiology 34:98-102

Johnson RE, Roberson GH (1974) Subpial lipoma of the spinal cord. Radiology 111:121-125

Kaffenberger DA, Shah CP, Murtagh FR, Wilson C, Silbiger ML (1988) MR imaging of spinal cord hemangioblastoma associated with syringomyelia. J Comput Tomogr 12:495-498

Koppel BS, Daras M, Duffy K (1990) Intramedullary spinal cord abscess. Neurosurgery 66:145-146

Levivier M, Brotchi J, Baleriaux D, et al (1991) Sarcoidosis presenting as an isolated intramedullary tumor. Neurosurgery 25:271-276

Lewis TT, Kingsley DPE (1987) Magnetic resonance imaging of multiple spinal neurofibromata-neurofibromatosis. Neuroradiology 29:562-564

Lim V, Sobel DF, Zyroff J (1990) Spinal cord pial metastases:MR imaging with gadopentetate dimeglumine. AJNR 11:975-982

Lopate G, Black JT, Grubb RL (1990) Cavernous hemangioma of the spinal cord: report of two unusual cases. Neurology 40:1791-1793

Maravilla KR, Weinreb JC, Suss R, et al (1985) Magnetic resonance demonstration of multiple sclerosis plaques in the cervical cord. AJR Am J Roentgenol 144:381-385

McCormick PC, Torres R, Post KD, et al (1990) Intramedullary ependymoma of the spinal cord. J Neurosurg 72:523-532

Michikawa M, Wada Y, Sano MM, et al (1991) Radiaton myelopathy: significance of gadolinium-DTPA enhancement in the diagnosis. Neuroradiology 33:286-289

Mitsumoto H, Breuer AC, Lederman RJ (1980) Malignant lymphoma of the central nervous system: a case of primary spinal intramedullary involvement. Cancer 46:1258-1262

Mock A, Levi A , Darke JM (1990) Spinal hemangioblastoma, syrinx, and hydrocephalus in a two-year-old child. Neurosurgery 27:799-802

Pagni CA, Canavero S, Giordana MT (1992) Spinal intramedullary subependymomas: case report and review of the literature. Neurosurgery 30:115-117

Parizel PM, Balériaux D, Rodesch G, et al (1989) Gd-DTPA enhanced MR imaging of spinal tumors. AJR Am J Roentgenol 152:1087-1096

Rigamonti D, Hadley MN, Drayer BP, et al (1988) Cerebral cavernous malformations: incidence and familial occurrence. N Engl J Med 319:343-347

Sabin HI, Duniel S, Wild AM, et al (1989) Cavernous angioma of the thoracic spinal cord with intra and extramedullary components. Br J Neurosurg 3:123-126

Scotti G, Scialfa G, Colombo N, Landoni L (1987) Magnetic resonance diagnosis of intramedullary tumors of the spinal cord. Neuroradiology 29:130-135

Slasky BS, Bydder GM, Niendorf HP. et al (1987) MR imaging with gadolinium-DTPA in the differentiation of tumor, syrinx, and cyst of the spinal cord. J Comput Assist Tomogr 11:845-850

Stern Y, Spiegelamn S, Sadeh M (1991) Spinal intradural arachnoid cysts. Neurochirurgie 34: 127-130

Sze G (1988) Gadolinium-DTPA in spinal disease. Radiol Clin North Am 26:1009-1024

Sze G, Krol G, Zimmerman RD, et al (1988) Intramedullary disease of the spine: diagnosis using gadolinium-DTPA-enhanced MR imaging. AJR Am J Roentgenol 151:1193-1204

Tekkök IH, Palaoglu S, Erbengi A, et al (1992) Intramedullary epidermoid cyst of the cervical spinal cord associated with an extraspinal neurenteric cyst: case report. Neurosurgery 31:121-125

Valk J (1988) Gd-DTPA in MR of spinal lesions. AJR Am J Roentgenol 150:1163-1168

Valk J, Kaiser M (1986) Magnetic resonance imaging in the differentiation of spinal cord tumours and hydromyelia. Acta Radiol Diagn 369:242-244

Williams AL, Haughton VM, Pojunas KW, et al (1987) Differentiation of intramedullary neoplasms and cysts by MR. AJR Am J Roentgenol 149:159-164

4 Diagnostic Imaging of Vertebral Metastases

P.R. ALGRA

CONTENTS

4.1
Metastatic Bone Disease

Cancer is the second leading cause of death and the incidence of cancer is still rising (BORING et al. 1992). Currently available therapy can now cure approximately 50% of cancer patients. The majority of patients die of the effects of metastatic disease. Following lung and liver, the skeletal system is the third most common site of metastasis. Up to 80% of all cancer patients will have skeletal disease at autopsy. Metastatic neoplasms vastly outnumber primary tumors of the skeleton. Excluding multiple myeloma, primary bone tumors account for only 0.3% of all malignancies.

P.R.ALGRA, MD, PhD, Department of Radiology, Medical Center Alkmaar, POB 501, 1800 Alkmaar, The Netherlands

The spine is the most common site of bone metastases, irrespective of the primary tumor that is involved. Spinal metastases have considerable clinical significance. They are a major cause of suffering in patients with cancer by producing severe pain, vertebral instability, and disruption of neural function with loss of urinary or sphincter control or complete paralysis.

These facts, coupled with increasing financial pressures to optimize the use of diagnostic resources, have led radiologists and oncologists to scrutinize the use of radiologic procedures and to look systematically at the benefits of a variety of staging procedures.

4.2
Distribution of Bone Metastases

Metastatic disease predominantly occurs in the axial or central skeleton. This is most probably related to the fact that the axial skeleton contains the majority of the red marrow. The distribution of metastases over the vertebral column is, in order of frequency, lumbar, lower thoracic, upper thoracic, sacral and cervical spine (Fig. 4.1).

The primary "soil" of metastatic bone disease is the bone marrow, and radiographic evidence of bone metastases is the result of invasion and destruction of the bone matrix by osteoclasts mediated by tumor cells from the marrow cavity. CT and MR studies confirm that metastatic deposits in the vertebral column are usually located in the vertebral body. Here marrow is more abundant than in the posterior parts of the vertebrae, such as the pedicles, and provides a fertile field for the earliest metastatic deposits. CT findings of metastatic spread to vertebral bodies rather than pedicles correlate well with pathologic findings. The plexus of vertebral veins provides ample blood supply for hematogenous metastases to lodge in vertebral body marrow. While relative lack of marrow in the pedicles may predispose to radiographic visualization of metastases, CT shows earlier changes in the vertebral body (ALGRA et al. 1992a).

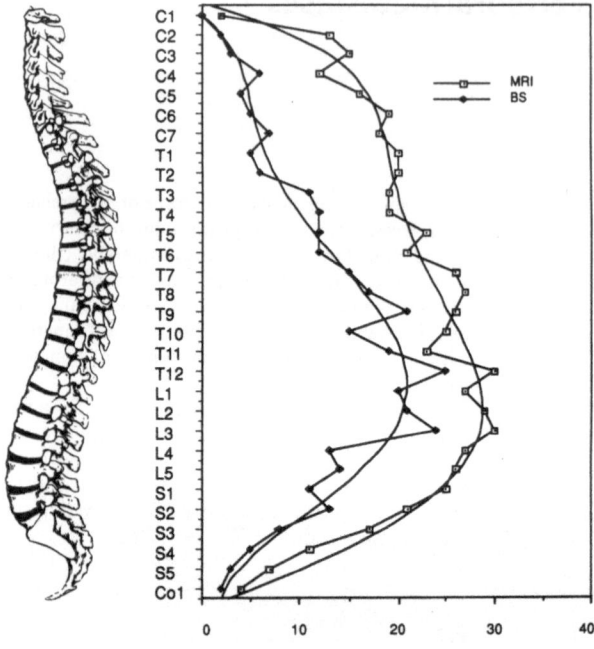

C1
C2
C3
C4
C5
C6
C7
T1
T2
T3
T4
T5
T6
T7
T8
T9
T10
T11
T12
L1
L2
L3
L4
L5
S1
S2
S3
S4
S5
Co1

——□—— MRI
——•—— BS

0   10   20   30   40

Fig. 4.1. The distribution of vertebral metastases in respect to the spinal level. In a group of 71 patients, the entire spine was examined both by bone scintigraphy (*left curve*) and by MR imaging (*right curve*). At each spinal level, MR imaging showed more abnormal vertebrae than did bone scintigraphy. Distribution of metastases over the spinal column as identified by MR imaging almost parallels that determined with bone scintigraphy. Most lesions are found in the lower thoracic and the lumbar spine. (From ALGRA 1992, with permission)

4.3
Pathogenesis of Bone Metastases

The fact that the lungs and liver are frequently involved in the metastatic process is readily understandable, since the lung receives the venous drainage from the caval system, and the liver the portal drainage. The reason for the frequent involvement of the bone is not as evident as the involvement of liver and lung.

Historically, two theories on the pathogenesis of bone metastatic disease are noteworthy; the seed and soil theory of PAGET (1889): "some tumor cells find certain organs provide a more fertile soil for metastatic growth;" and the first-station theory of EWING (1928): "mechanics of circulation."

4.3.1
Seed and Soil

PAGET believed that certain organs had a diminished resistance or prediposition to metastasis. In 1889 he stated: "When a plant goes to seed, its seeds are carried in all directions; but they can only live and grow if they fall on congenial soil."

It is evident that some predisposing factors must prevail to promote the generation of bone metastatic disease, considering the fact that the skeleton receives only 10% of the cardiac output; muscle and spleen, for example, receive a far greater amount of the cardiac output yet are rarely affected by metastatic disease. This finding supports the seed and soil theory of PAGET, i.e. metastases from certain primary tumors have a particular tendency to develop in the bone marrow.

4.3.2
Mechanics of Circulation

RECKLINGHAUSEN (1885) was the first to attribute the frequency of secondary carcinoma of the bone marrow to the favorable conditions afforded by the sluggish current in the sinusoidal capillaries of the marrow for the effective lodgment of blood-borne tumor cells. The theory explaining the relative frequency of metastatic bone disease as a result of mechanics (EWING), is supported not only by the presence of slow blood flow in the sinusoids, but also by the fenestrated membrane of the endothelium lining the vessels, together with other factors promoting the development of metastastic disease.

Anatomic studies, originally carried out by BATSON (1940), suggest a preferential drainage to the vertebral column of certain organ sites, e.g. breast, prostate, colon and rectum, by means of a vertebral venous plexus system. Batson suggested that tumor cell emboli from the prostate might enter the vertebral venous system and be carried directly to the bones of the spine, pelvis and skull, by-passing the lungs entirely.

Both theories (EWING and PAGET) have been well validated and are no longer considered mutually exclusive. The mechanical and seed-and-soil theories can be integrated if the enhanced suspectibility of red marrow is due to special hemodynamic and microanatomical aspects of its vasculature. "Mechanical-circulatory" factors of the bone marrow can account for the suitability of the "soil" of the bone marrow for the development of metastases.

Unlike the gradual transitions that are present in other organs, the medullary small arteries abruptly give off smaller vessels with thin double-layered walls, which then gradually branch into the single-layered medullary sinusoids and cortical capillaries.

Furthermore, the marrow sinusoids are composed of endothelical cells supported by fine reticular fibers, and they lack both a basement membrane and the cement substance that lines the edges of typical endothelial cells.

4.4
Prognosis of Metastatic Bone Disease and Metastatic Epidural Cord Compression

The expected survival for patients with bone metastasis must be taken into account when treatment is planned. Assessment of the prognosis of patients suffering from metastatic bone disease is important when considering palliative procedures or excisional procedures for the purpose of improving their period of survival. Extensive treatment in the terminally ill must be avoided, whereas many patients may live for years and greatly benefit from active treatment. (Table 4.1)

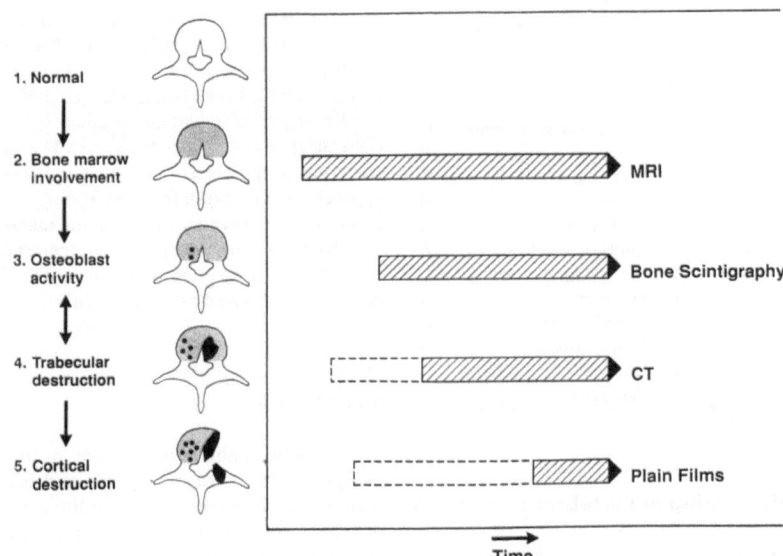

Fig. 4.2. The time course of imaging findings (*horizontal axis*) correlated with the presumed cascade of events (*vertical axis*) in skeletal metastatic disease. Blood borne metastases invade the bone marrow (visible with MR imaging) and cause an increase in bone turnover (visible in bone scintigraphy). Initial bone destruction (trabecular or cortical bone) can be seen with CT. Usually, osteoblast activity precedes bone destruction. However, as is the case in rapid metastatic destruction lysis of bone can be noted without new bone formation (*dashed lines*, CT). Large cortical lesions or gross trabecular destruction will be seen on plain films. In case of pure lytic metastases, plain films can reveal destruction of bone while bone scintigraphy is still negative (*dashed lines*, plain films). (From ALGRA 1992 with permission)

Table 1. Factors that influence survival rates in patients suffering from spinal metastases. Survival rates should be taken into account in deciding on treatment and thus on diagnostic procedures

Nature of primary tumor
General condition of patient
Number of extraspinal bone metastases
Number of vertebral metastases
Ñumber of extraskeletal metastases
Severity of spinal cord palsy

It is generally agreed that two factors are the major determinants for the outcome of treatment of spinal metastases. The first is the nature of the primary tumor (Table 4.2) with particular reference to the radiosensitivity, which is positively correlated to the treatment response. The other factor is the clinical and neurologic status before treatment (KIM et al. 1990; TOKUHASHI et al. 1990).

Table 2. Five-year survival rates for selected primaries. Percentages are adjusted for normal life expectancy. Numbers are based on cases diagnosed in 1981–1987. Rates adapted from Surveillance, Epidemiology and End Results (SEER) National Cancer Institute (BORING et al. 1992)

Primary tumor	%	Primary tumor	%
All sites	53		
Thyroid	94	Oral carvity/pharynx	54
Testis	93	Kidney/renal/pelvis	53
Corpus uteri	84	Non-Hodgkins' lymphoma	51
Melanoma skin	82	Ovary	39
Urinary bladder	79	Leukemia	36
Breast (female)	78	Multiple myeloma	26
Hodgkin's lymphoma	77	Brain/spinal cord	24
Prostate	76	Stomach	16
Cervix uteri	68	Lung/bronchi	13
Larynx	68	Esophagus	9
Colon	58	Liver	5
Rectum	55	Pancreas	3

4.5
Diagnostic Imaging of Vertebral Metastases

The following paragraphs provide an overview of the current state of the art of diagnostic imaging of spinal metastases. Fig. 4.2 shows the cascade of events in the metastatic process as it is visible by diagnostic imaging. Irrespective of items such as sensitivity and specificity, the diagnostic steps to be taken should be tailored according to the actual clinical problem.

4.5.1
Plain Films

Plain films are an easy, fast and non-invasive means to rule out a variety of spinal lesions and are also needed in case of pre-operative and pre-radiation evaluation. As plain films can establish remineralization, conventional radiographs are useful in monitoring therapy.

No specific pattern of vertebral collapse permits confident conclusions as to the cause (SARTORIS et al. 1986). Angling of endplates was found to be highly predictive of underlying malignancy, whereas concavity was more suggestive of benign disease. The contours of collapsed vertebral bodies can suggest the nature of the underlying disease, but conventional radiography alone is unreliable in the differentiation between benign and malignant causes of vertebral body collapse.

The major limitation of conventional radiography is poor visualization of soft tissues because of the markedly limited contrast resolution of this technique. Furthermore, conventional radiographs have a very low yield in depicting bone metastases when these are still located in the bone marrow. Experimental studies have shown that only metastases that cause destruction of more than 50%-70% of trabecular bone within the vertebral body can be seen on plain radiographs (EDELSTYN et al. 1967).

The origin of metastatic deposits is within the bone marrow of the vertebral body. The fact that destruction of the vertebral pedicle is far more easily appreciated on standard plain radiographs than is loss of density because of lytic bone metastases may have led to the misconception that metastatic disease is located more frequently in the pedicle than in the vertebral body (ALGRA et al. 1992a).

4.5.2
Myelography

Myelography enables visualization of the arachnoidal space, spinal cord, nerve roots, and, in an indirect manner, the immediate surroundings. Screening of the entire spinal canal can be accomplished by myelography, unless obstruction(s) in the archnoidal space prohibits sufficient flow of contrast material to pass the impediment. Myelography should not be restricted to the symptomatic spinal segment, but rather be extended to evaluate the entire spine as it may reveal additional epidural lesions. Epidural metastases can be clinically asymptomatic. Asymptomatic epidural metastases not associated with vertebral metastases will be present in 7%-11% of the patients with epidural disease.

A major drawback of myelography is that in cases of a complete block, a second puncture might be needed to establish the total longitudinal extent of the compressive lesion. CT myelography can replace a supplementary cervical myelography in the majority of patients with epidural metastases causing a complete block.

Myelography is not without risks (HILZ et al. 1990); lumbar and cervical puncture carry the risk of arterial bleeding. Punctures can be particular harmful in patients with coagulopathies. Inadvertent needle placement within the cord is an additional risk in the case of cervical puncture.

On rare occasions, an increase in neurological deficit may occur acutely after myelography which is thought to be the result of downward herniation of the spinal cord induced by a reduction of CSF pressure below the lesion. This has been described to occur in 14%-26% of the cases when the puncture was performed below a complete subarchnoid block.

Other complications are trauma due to hyperextension of the neck in cervical myelography and inadvertent puncture of the cord.

Except for the mechanical complications, myelography performed with modern non-ionic contrast agents has very few side effects. Arachnoiditis is not a common complication anymore. However, myelography carries the risk of inadvertent administration of ionic hyperosmolar contrast medium. Reported neurological complications range from mild and temporary to severe and even fatal.

4.5.3
CT and CT Myelography

The major advantage of CT over alternative imaging modalities lies in its ability to define subtle cortical and trabecular destruction. Bone marrow infiltration, which precedes bone destruction, can be established by CT or quantitative CT. A difference of more than 20 HU in CT density between the marrow of two different sites is likely to represent a pathologic process at the site with the higher density.

CT can be of value in the follow-up of therapy of lytic metastases as it can establish the earliest signs of remineralization. The changes in mineralization after therapy can be measured by double-energy CT.

Closed needle biopsy of spinal lesions under CT guidance is a safe and convenient technique for all levels of the spine. The use of CT to guide the biopsy procedure can eliminate the risks that have frequently accompanied the technique of closed needle biopsy using conventional roentgenographic guidance. Using CT guidance, the angulation and depth of the needle path are predetermined. This is especially important for vertebral body lesions with the aorta lying just anteriorly. In cases where the standard postero-lateral approach is difficult, an alternative route is the transpedicular approach.

The principal limitation of CT is the potential failure to disclose a second site of cord compression, which can be present at first presentation in as many as 8%-9% of patients. The second site of compression can be separated from the first site by a mean of 12 vertebral segments.

4.5.4
Bone Scintigraphy

Radionuclide bone scintigrams are very sensitive in detecting the altered local metabolism in areas of bone remodelling associated with metastatic deposits. The radionuclide study requires as little as a 5%-10% change in the lesion-to-normal bone ratio for an abnormal focus to be appreciated on the scintigram.

However, Tc-MDP bone scintigraphy can yield false-negative findings in the case of rapidly growing metastases, entirely osteolytic metastases, when the lesion is less than 2 mm, and in patients with multiple myeloma.

Bone reacts to most stimuli, e.g. tumor invasion, infection and injury, by the production of reactive new bone. Therefore, any such lesion will produce an increased uptake of bone-seeking isotopes. This explains why bone scintigraphy is a nonspecific investigation and why bone scintigrams should not be read without considering clinical and radiological parameters. Since only a bone scan with multiple (three or more) new abnormalities is strongly suggestive of metastatic disease, correlative radiographs are especially important when bone scans show one or two new lesions. It was found that only 14% of patients with cancer in whom bone scans showed one or two new lesions actually had metastases. When correlative radiographs of bone scans with one or two abnormalities show foci suggestive of metastases, the presence should be confirmed by MR imaging, CT, bone biopsy or, if clinically appropriate, follow-up (JACOBSON et al. 1990 a,b).

4.5.5
MR Imaging of Normal Bone Marrow

The *age-related changes* in the composition of the bone marrow are described as a successive decrease in red marrow and a corresponding increase in fat content. (Dooms et al. 1985; Moore and Dawson 1990; Ricci et al. 1990; Dawson et al. 1992; Zawin and Jaramillo 1993; Richardson and Patten, 1994).

The change in composition is greatest during the first decade of life and after the age of 65 years. As patient ages, the MR signal intensity of bone marrow changes. Bone marrow becomes increasingly hypocellular with age, and decreasing T1 and T2 relaxation times of vertebral marrow with age have been reported.

The process of red to yellow conversion is normally completed by the age of 25 years, when the adult marrow distribution pattern is reached. At that time, red marrow predominates only in the axial skeleton. Variation in this pattern exist. After the adult marrow pattern is attained, the balance of red and yellow marrow may change with age.

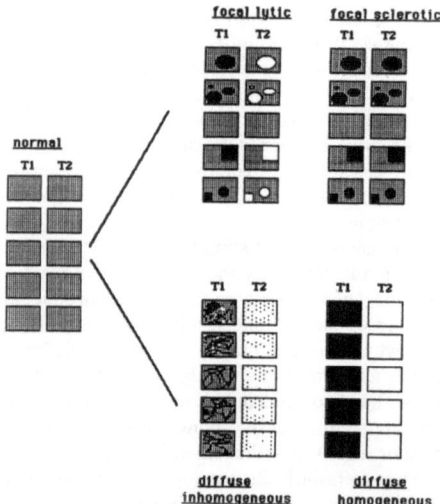

Fig. 4.3. The four patterns of MR appearance of metastases. Focally lytic lesions show focal areas of low signal intensity on T1-weighted images and a increased signal intensity on T2-weighted images. Focal sclerotic lesions will show focal areas of low signal intensity on both T1- and T2-weighted images. In the diffuse patterns the abnormal signal intensity may be homogeneous or inhomogeneous. Both the focal and diffuse patterns of metastases can also be seen in non-malignant disease. (From Algra et al. 1990, with permission)

Reconversion from inactive yellow marrow to active red marrow can take place when there is a need for additional hematopoiesis (e.g. in chronic anemia, smoking, and chronic heart failure). Red marrow consists of 40% water, 40% fat, and 20% protein. Yellow marrow contains 80 % fat. (Dooms et al. 1985; Moore and Dawson 1990; Ricci et al. 1990; Dawson et. al 1992; Zawin and Jaramillo 1993; Richardson and Patten 1994).

Physiologic changes may alter signal intensities of the bone marrow.

T1 and T2 signal intensities are slightly *lower for females* than for males. This could be due to the loss of bone and mineral content, which is more rapid and significant in women. Increase of bone marrow fat can also attribute to this difference in relaxation times.

The T2 relaxation time of lumbar vertebral body decreases after prolonged *bedrest*. The observed decrease in relaxation time is explained by the replacement of hematopietic marrow by fatty marrow. A decrease in red blood cell production is a known consequence of bedrest, and the amount of marrow fat is inversely related to red blood cell production. Altered *weight bearing* causes also the appearance of marrow edema on MR images. *Window setting* can influence the appearance of bone marrow signal intensity. Ideally, MR images should be reviewed at multiple window settings. Furthermore, relaxation times vary with *field strength*. At high field strengths T1-relaxation times increase, whereas T2 relaxation times are not affected by the main magnetic field strengths. However, qualitative age-related changes are probably constant at a given field strength. (Le Blanc et al. 1988; Poulton et al. 1993; Schweitzer and White 1996).

4.5.6
MR Characterization of Vertebral Metastases

Bone marrow contains a large portion of mobile protons in fat and water in cellular hematopoietic and stromal tissue. It is therefore ideally suited for MR imaging. Especially in the case of lytic bone marrow metastases, the high contrast between fat-containing bone marrow and the high concentration of water in the cytoplasm of metastatic cells renders ideal circumstances for MR imaging.

When analyzing the MR appearances of metastatic disease of the vertebral column, one can distinguish at least four metastatic patterns (Fig. 3) (Algra et al. 1990; Ruzal-Shapiro et al. 1991; Petren-

Fig. 4.4. Parasagittal T1-weighted spin echo images. Two contiguous slices of the lumbar spine reveal focal areas of low signal intensity in vertebral bodies and T12, L1 and L3 pedicles. Loss of cortical definition of these pedicles indicates destruction of the bone. Both involvement of the pedicles and destruction of the cortical bone are highly suggestive of metastasic disease. Note also retroperitoneal lymphadenopathy

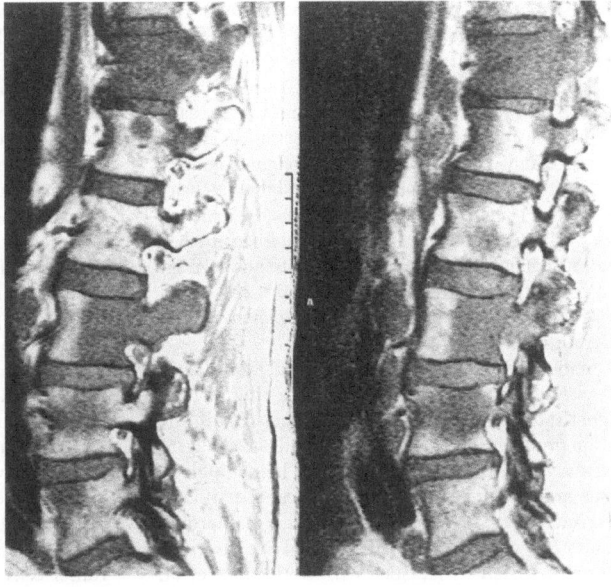

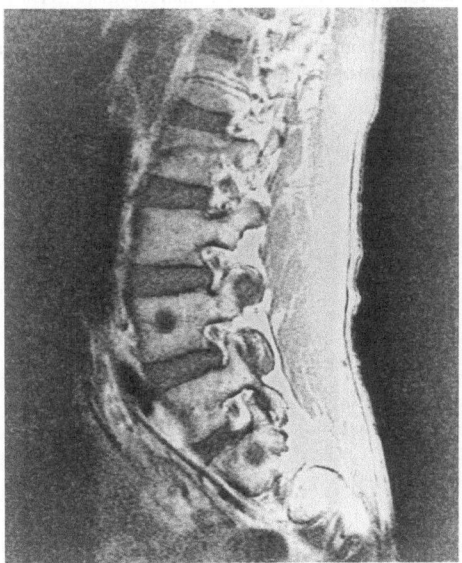
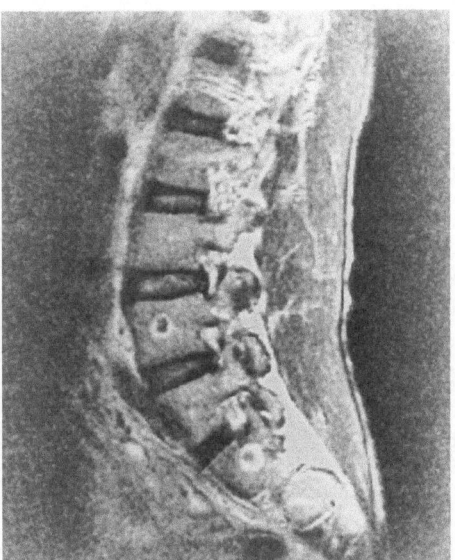

a   b

Fig. 4.5. Parasagittal images of the lumbar spine show focal areas in L4 and S1 of low signal intensity on a T1-weighted image (a) surrounded by a rim of high signal intensity on a T2-weighted image (b). These lesions (halos) are highly suggestive for metastases

MALLMIN et al. 1992; BLOEM and ALGRA 1993); two focal (focal lytic and focal sclerotic, or a combination thereof and two diffuse patterns (diffuse homogeneous and diffuse inhomogeneous).

Focal lytic metastases show a focal area of decreased signal intensity on T1-weighted images (Fig. 4) and an increased signal intensity on T2/T2*-weighted images. Focal sclerotic lesions will exhibit low signal intensity on both T1-and T2/T2*-weighted images. In some cases these focal abnormalities in signal intensity may indicate benign disease; bone islands will show low signal intensity on both T1-weigthed and T2-weighted images; and it may be difficult to distinguish these from sclerotic metastases by MR imaging.

In the case of focal areas of low signal intensity on T1-weighted images, surrounded by a ring of high signal intensity on T2-weighted images (halo), the lesion probably represents metastatic disease (Fig. 5) (SCHWEITZER et al. 1993). Islands of hematopoietic bone marrow often demonstrate a focal area of fatty marrow. The MR imaging equivalent is termed "bull's eye" and may be used as a negative discriminator of osseous metastases (SCHWEITZER et al. 1993).

In the diffuse patterns of bone marrow metastases (Fig. 6), the bone marrow of the spine will show a diffuse low signal intensity on T1- and a high signal intensity on T2/T2*-weighted images. These diffuse patterns can be inhomogeneous, irregular or homogeneous and smooth. In diffuse bone marrow lesions, the intervertebral disk may show a relative high signal intensity on T1-weighted SE images. This sign of

diffuse bone marrow pathology was first described in three patients in whom the vertebrae were of low signal intensity on T1-weighted images, thereby making the disks appear brighter ("bright intervertebral disk sign") (CASTILLO et al. 1990). The bright intervertebral disk sign should be interpreted with care, as calcified disks may also show up bright on T1-weighted images (MAJOR et al. 1993; BANGERT et al. 1995; QUINT 1995).

Again, as is the case with focal lesions, diffuse patterns of abnormal signal intensity of the bone marrow can be seen in a number of non-malignant diseases for example, increased iron storage, which can occur in anemia of chronic disease, can result in diffuse low signal intensity of the bone marrow (GEREMIA et al. 1990).

The location of abnormal signal intensity within the vertebra can give valuable clues to the nature of the disease. Involvement of the pedicles and posterior parts of the vertebra (spinous process and transverse process; Fig. 4) indicates metastases and is not seen in degenerative lesions (ALGRA et al. 1992a).

Tumor cells lodge and grow in the hematopoietic bone marrow of the vertebrae. Cancer cells are more likely to invade the vertebral canal through the foramina of the basivertebral veins than to destroy cortical bone. Loss of visibility on MR imaging of the basivertebral vein ("basivertebral vein sign"), can be an early sign of diffuse bone marrow disease. Disappearance of the basivertebral vein may be more conspicuous than abnormal signal intensity in early bone marrow involvement (Fig. 7) (ALGRA et al. 1991b).

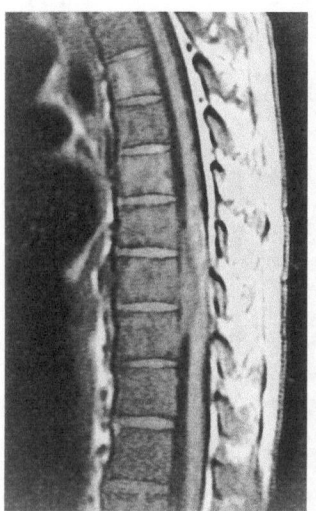 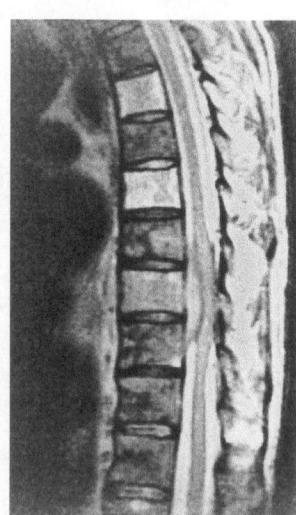

Fig. 4.6. Sagittal T1-weighted (a) and T2-weighted (b) images of the thoracic spine in a patient with metastases from lung carcinoma. Low signal intensity of the bone marrow on T1-weighted images gives rise to the "bright intervertebral disc sign". Note also that there is a extension of tumor into the spinal canal causing compressive myelopathy

a   b

Fig. 4.7. Sagittal T1-weighted (**a**) and T2-weighted (**b**) images show abnormal signal intensity of the bone marrow of L4, L5 and the sacrum. On the T2-weighted image, L4 shows a loss of definition of the basivertebral vein ("Basivertebral vein sign") as well as a slight convexity of the posterior body ("convex posterior body sign"). These findings probably represent an early stage of tumor tissue growing towards the spinal canal via the nutrient foramen of the basivertebral vein.

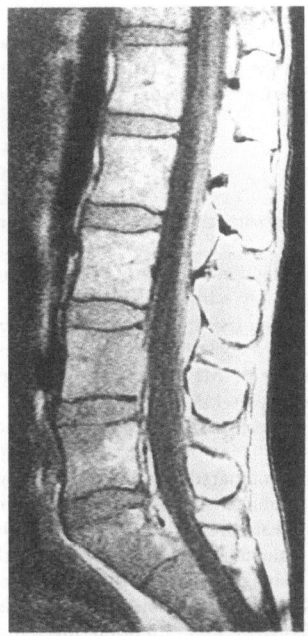 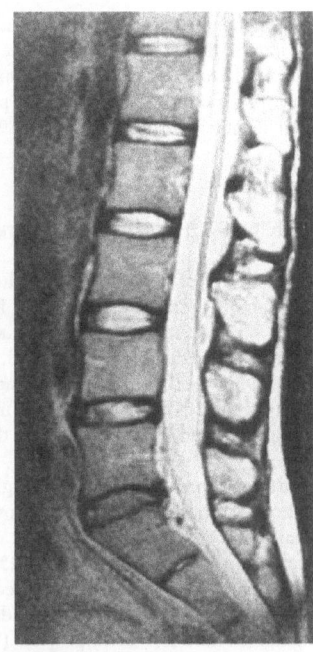

a

b

Fig. 4.8. Transverse T1-weighted image of T11. Apart from the abnormal low signal intensity of the bone marrow, there is a loss of definition of the cortical bone. Furthermore, tumor tissue extends into the spinal canal in a bilateral fashion ("curtain sign")

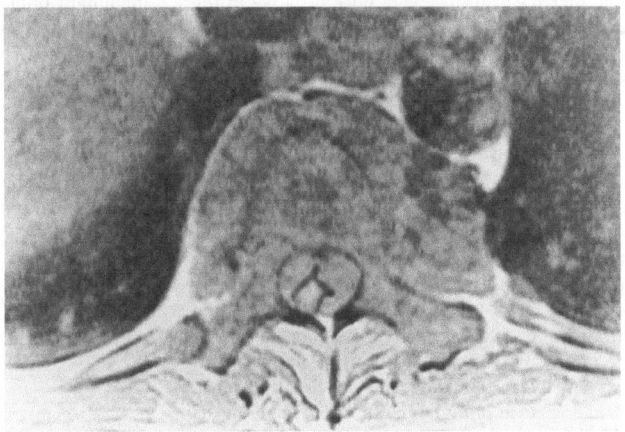

The early stage of tumor extension towards the spinal canal can be seen as tumor tissue growing from the posterior part of the vertebral body ("rounded posterior body sign" or "convex posterior body sign") (Fig. 7). Although the convex posterior body sign indicates the presence of disease, it is not specific for metastases. Spondylitis may also give rise to a convex posterior body.

Intraspinal epidural carcinomatous infiltrations tend to respect the sagittal midline, even if the infiltration is bilateral. The radiological representation of epidural infiltration is similar to theater curtains to draw open. Other non-metastatic anterior epidural space occupying lesions can also produce a "curtain sign" (Fig. 8). On the contrary, intradural pathology will not present a midline sparing. The curtain sign may be related with the existence of a posterior longitudinal ligament-midline septum complex (ligament of Trolard) which would connect the posterior face of the vertebral body with the posterior longitudinal ligament (SCHELLINGER et al. 1990).

4.5.7
Sensitivity of MR Imaging in Vertebral Metastases

The sensitivity of MR imaging in the detection of bone marrow metastases compares favorably with Tc-MDP bone scintigraphy (AVRAHAMI et al. 1989). In a prospective study (ALGRA et al. 1991 a) comparing 99mTc-MDP bone scintigraphy with MR imaging in the detection of vertebral metastases, MR imaging showed 60% more lesions than scintigraphy.

The high sensitivity of MR imaging compared with bone scintigraphy in the detection of bone marrow metastases can have important clinical consequences. In a prospective study of 25 patients with small cell lung carcinoma, four proved to have bone marrow metastases which were only detected by MR imaging. Both bone scintigraphy (Tc-MDP) and bone marrow aspirates were false negative in these patients. MR imaging changed the diagnosis in these patients from limited disease to extensive disease (JELINEK et al. 1990).

The high sensitivity of MR imaging in the detection of bone metastases may be explained by the fact that the lesion itself (malignant bone marrow infiltration) is directly visualized. The high contrast between fat and metastatic deposits, which have a high water content, allows MR imaging to detect lesions at a relatively early stage. There is a significant correlation between the T1 value and bone marrow cellularity. As is known from pathological studies, intratrabecular metastases can be present in which the metastatic deposits are limited to the marrow spaces between the trabeculae, leaving the trabeculae and cortical bone intact. In order for bone scintigraphy to be positive, metastases must have given rise to an osteoblastic response in the surrounding bone (Fig. 2).

4.5.8
Specificity of MR Imaging in Vertebral Metastases

MR imaging is the most reliable imaging modality in the distinction between benign versus malignant disease. By means of MR imaging it is usually possible to make a reliable distinction between degenerative bone disease and malignant infiltration (MODIC et al. 1988; PETREN-MALLMIN et al. 1992). Morphologic characteristics and alterations in signal intensity must be taken into account. Loss of height of the intervertebral disc can be seen in degenerative disease and in discits, whereas the shape and height of the disc is usually preserved in metastatic diseases. The shape and homogeneity of the T1 and T2 signal abnormalities of bone marrow (particularly in relation to the relation to the vertebral endplates) may allow distinction between benign and metastatic compression fractures (MODIC et al. 1988).

Secondary signs such as increased signal intensity on T1-weighted images, fractures at multiple levels with preservation of normal bone marrow, vertebral body fragmentation, and disc rupture indicate benign disease. Multiple vertebrae with bone marrow with abnormal signal intensity, and vertebrae with abnormal signal intensity in posterior elements, are indicative for malignant disease. Paraspinal masses can be seen in both traumatic and malignant cases.

MR imaging cannot distinguish between metastatic disease and bone marrow alterations caused by multiple myeloma, lymphoma, and other forms of malignant bone marrow infiltration such as leukemia. Furthermore, hematologic disorders such as aplastic anemia and polycythemia vera can show diffuse abnormal signal intensity of bone marrow which cannot be differentiated from multiple bone marrow metastases by MR imaging. Increased iron accumulation resulting in diffuse low signal intensity of the bone marrow can be seen in anemia of chronic disease and hemosiderosis (Tables 3, 4).

Table 3. A number of non-neoplastic diseases which can cause altered signal intensity of the bone marrow. Depending upon the clinical setting, these diseases should be considered when the spinal bone marrow shows abnormal signal intensity on MR imaging

Osteonecrosis	Anemia in chronic disease:
Osteomyelitis	– Heart failure
Fractures, bruises	– Smoking
Transient osteoporosis	– Aids
Marrow edema	Radiation therapy
Bone marrow hyperplasia (regeneration)	Osteopetrosis
Myelofibrosis	Polycythemia vera
Gaucher's disease	Bone infarction (sickle cell disease)
Mastocytosis	Disc degeneration
Iron deposition	Focal fatty degeneration
Bone marrow transplantation	Spondylitis, spondylodiscitis

Table 4. Summary of MR imaging characteristics of abnormal signal intensity (SI) of the vertebral bone marrow. Lesions are characterized by SI, location of abnormal SI within vertebral body (VB) and within the spinal column, destruction or perseverance of anatomical structures, and condition of the other vertebrae (entire spine). MR imaging signs should be interpreted in the correct clinical setting (age of patient; known to have primary tumor; known to have metastases elsewhere, etc.). Furthermore, discriminative signs are heuristic rather than absolute

	Benign	Malignant
Abnormal SI of Bone marrow	– confined to endplates – confined to anterior part of VB, with sparing of posterior part VB and pedicles (posterior band)	– focal within body – Involvement of entire VB extending into pedicles and posterior part
High SI on T1-W in centre of lesions (bull's eye)	+	–
High SI on T2-W around lesion (halo)	–	+
Bright SI discs on T1wSE	–	+ (in diffuse metastases)
Vertebral collapse		
– acute	Abnormal SI adjacent to fractured bone	Abnormal SI of entire VB, pedicle and posterior part
– chronic	Normal SI	Abnormal SI entire VB
Cortical destruction	–	+
Destruction of discs	Only in (spondylo-) discitis	Seldom
Convex posterior body		+
Soft tissue extension	Absent in osteoporotic fractures, can be present in spondylodiscitis	+
Condition of other vertebrae	No abnormalities	Signs of metastases
Gadolinum		
– enhancement pattern	Linear	Globular
– dynamic	Slope < 30 %	Slope > 30 %
Basivertebral vein	Usually identifiable	May be absent
No of lesions	Usually solitary	Usually multiple
Distribution of lesions	Predominantly below T7	Below and above T7
Additional findings		
– Lymphadenopathy	–	+
– Primary tumor	–	+
– Liver, lung, brain metastases	–	+
– Leptomeningeal metastases	–	+

4.5.9
MR Imaging Contrast Agents

Gd-GTPA-enhanced images are obligatory if leptomeningeal spread is expected. However, with conventional spin echo (SE) techniques Gd-DTPA may obscure metastatic lesions within the bone marrow as some metastases will become iso-intense to normal bone marrow (Fig.9; 11). This phenomenon can be circumvented using fat suppression techniques or simply by obtaining pre-contrast enhanced T1-weighted images (STIMAC et al. 1988; SZE et al. 1988, 1989, 1990; MIROWITZ et al. 1994; MEHTA et al. 1995).

Enhancement of normal anatomic structures in the spine depends on the vasculature and on whether or not the capillary endothelium is fenestrated. Fenestrated endothelium allows Gd-DTPA to pass through the capillary walls into the interstitial space. After intravenous administration of Gd-DTPA certain structures within the spinal column will show contrast enhancement. Among these normal structures are the epidural plexus and the dorsal root ganglion. On sagittal views, the penetrating basivertebral venous plexus appears as a linear enhancing structure that pierces the vertebral body at its posterior cortex (JINKINS et al. 1995).

Enhancement of normal bone marrow is seen in children aged less than 7 years, and marked enhancement is noted in children younger than 2 years. Normal adult bone marrow will not enhance after injection of GD-DTPA. In contrast, reactive hematopoietic regions will show marked enhancement after intravenous Gd-DTPA (BREGER et al. 1990; AMANO et al. 1994).

Intramedullary spinal cord metastases are an unusual complication of malignancies arising outside the central nervous system, and is estimated at 1% of the patients with cancer. Intramedullary metastases

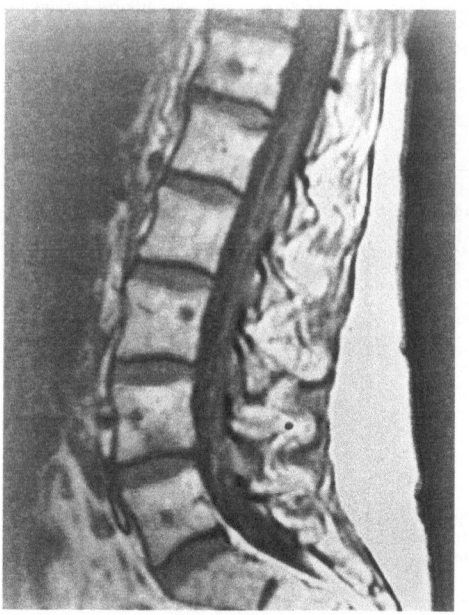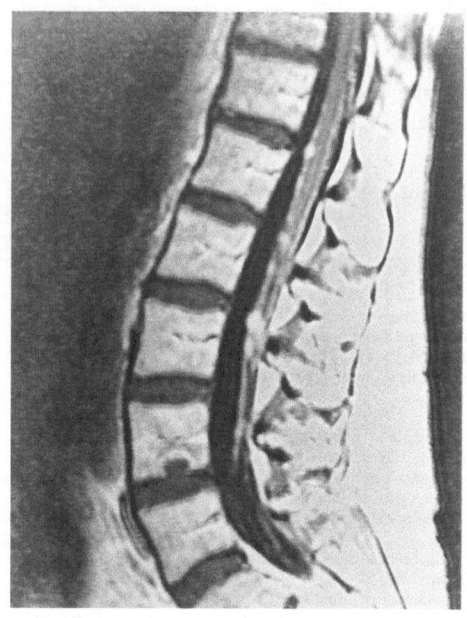

a   b

Fig. 4.9. Sagittal T1-weighted image before (a) and after (b) contrast enhancement. Administration of intravenous Gd-DTPA shows leptomeningeal metastases to better advantage, but tends to make bone marrow metastases (T12, L3, L4 and L5) isointense to normal bone marrow

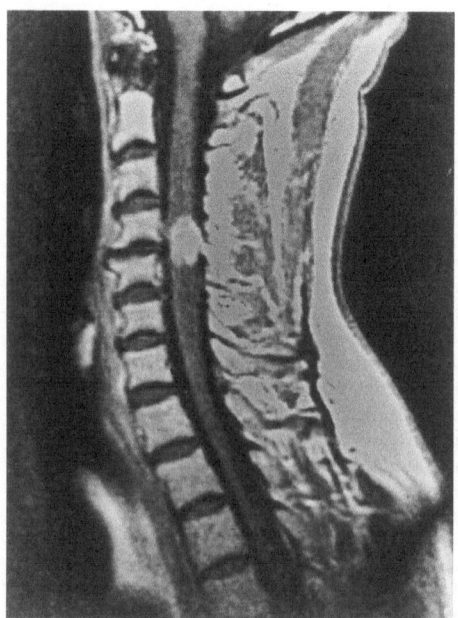

are seen with MR imaging as lesions causing enlargement of the cord on T1-weighted images, and with a high signal intensity on T2-weighted images. After intravenous administration of Gd-DTPA a marked enhancement of the tumor nidus will be seen. (STIMAC et al. 1988; SZE et al. 1988, 1989, 1990; ERLEMANN et al. 1989; LIM et al. 1990) (Fig. 10).

The mechanism of contrast enhancement in extramedullary tumors is different from intramedullary lesions, since extramedullary pathology does not have a blood-brain-barrier. Therefore, the degree of T1 shortening after intravenous injection of Gd-DTPA is a function of tumor vascularization (Fig. 11). Gd-DTPA can be helpful as an adjunct when epidural tumors are considered. Gd-DTPA can delineate epidural tumor spread, establish extension of abscesses, differentiate disc herniation from tu-

Fig. 4.10. Sagittal T1-weighted image after administration of intravenous Gd-DTPA shows a high-signal-intensity lesion in the cervical cord at the C3–4 level. Administration of intravenous Gd-DTPA is useful to depict intramedullary lesions. Intramedullary lesion can also be revealed using T2-weighted sequences

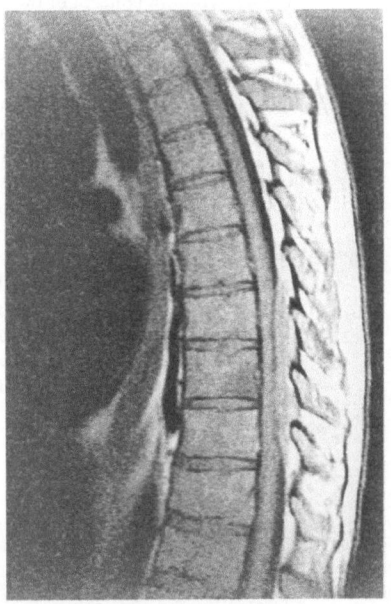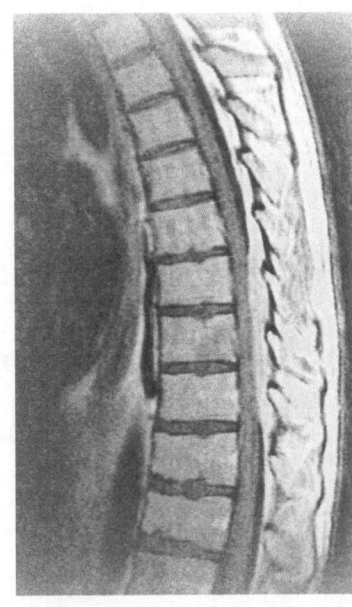

a   b

Fig. 4.11. Sagittal T1-weighted images of the thoracic spine before (a) and after (b) Gd-DTPA administration. T1-weighted images before contrast show abnormally low signal intensity of the bone marrow. Note also epidural tumor extension dorsal to the thoracic cord. Marked enhancement is seen of both bone marrow and soft tissue extension

mor, guide biopsy as it indicates viable tumor, out-linig areas of cord compression, and demonstrate tumor response to therapy.

Enhancement may also prove useful in the follow-up of patients treated for epidural tumor. Decrease in uptake of contrast agent after radiation therapy may be due to decreased vascularity. Serial images must be compared with a baseline, since untreated epidural neoplasms can vary in degree of enhance-ment.

Gd-DTPA administration in combination with fast imaging sequences enables dynamic study of bone marrow perfusion. Malignant tumors tend to show slopes higher than 30% per minute, whereas benign tumors are characterized by slopes lower than 30% per minute. Dynamic techniques enables assessment of the malignant potential of a tumor (accuracy 79.4%). Necrotic areas and peritumoral edema show lower signal intensity and more gradual increase in signal intensity than adjacent neoplastic tissue. Other studies using fast spin echo techniques in combination with Gd-DTPA report no significant distinction between benign and malignant musculoskeletal masses (ERLEMAN et al. 1989, 1990).

4.5.10
Loss of Height of Vertebral Body

The use of MR imaging in the differential diagnosis between malignant and benign cause of vertebral body collapse, has been the subject of many studies (YUH et al. 1989, BAKER et al. 1990, HOROWITZ et al. 1991, LAREDO et al. 1995, CUENOD et al. 1996).

An important feature helpful to distinguish old osteoporotic, traumatic and malignant causes of vertebral body collapse is signal intensity of residual bone marrow (Fig. 12). Complete replacement of bone marrow indicates malignancy, whereas benign fractures without history of trauma usually show preservation of normal bone marrow. The homogeneous, diffuse abnormal signal intensity in pathologic fractures reflects complete bone marrow replacement. This is probably a condition necessary for fractures to occur. Fractures with a history of trauma can show incomplete replacement with an irregular signal intensity pattern. The accuracy of MR imaging in the differentiation between benign and malignant fractures was reported in one study as 94% (CUENOD et al. 1996).

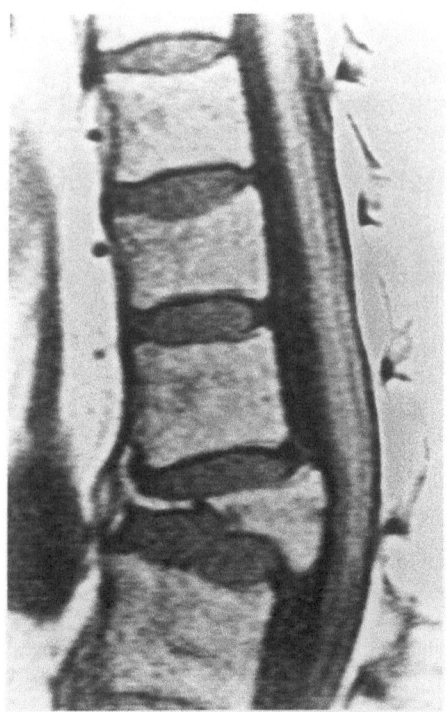

Fig. 4.12. Sagittal T1-weighted image of lower thoracic spine shows wedge-shaped collapsed vertebral body. Posterior part of the body protrudes into the spinal canal. Normal signal intensity of the bone marrow within fractured body indicates non-malignant disease, e. g hronic osteoporotic vertebral collapse

Care must be taken in interpreting MR examinations in recently collapsed vertebral bodies, as they can show signal intensities indistinguishable from metastatic disease. Marrow signal intensity in patients with benign fractures varies according to fracture age. Chronic benign compressions fractures are characterized by homogeneous signal intensity isointense to normal bone marrow. Acute benign fractures demonstrate inhomogeneous low signal intensity on T1-weighted images and inhomogeneous high signal intensity on T2-weighted images (FRAGER et al. 1988). Signal intensity abnormalities in MR images of acute compression fractures can revert to normal marrow signal intensity. This has been noted over periods of 1-3 months (Fig. 13).

Other signs for differentiation of benign from malignant causes of vertebral collapse are based on

the three-column concept of the spine. Benign compression fracture is a failure of the anterior column (anterior two-thirds of vertebral body, anterior longitudinal ligament and anterior annulus fibrosus) under compression. The middle column (posterior one-third of vertebral body, posterior annulus fibrosus, posterior longitudinal ligament and anterior pedicles) is intact in benign compression fractures and acts as a hinge. Metastatic disease may invade the vertebral column through the nutrient artery supply to the midportion of the vertebral body or basivertebral vein. A sharply delineated isointense vertical band of preserved normal bone marrow along the dorsal aspect of the compressed ("posterior band sign") body indicates benign compression fracture (HOROWITZ et al. 1991) (Table 5).

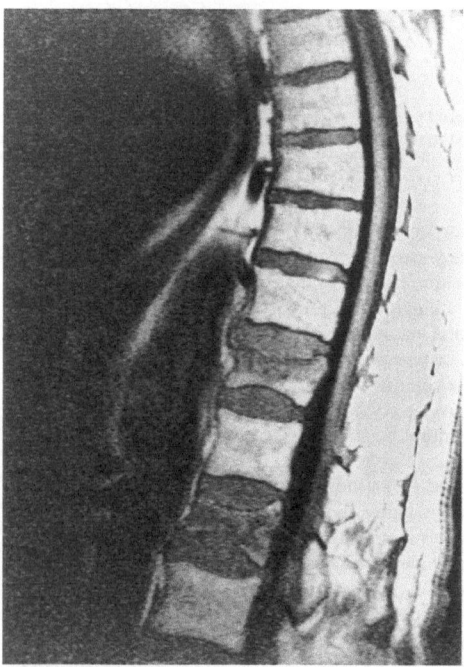

Fig. 4.13. Sagittal T1-weighted image of the thoracolumbar spine shows collapsed T12 and L2 bodies. Signal intensity of the bone marrow in affected bodies is abnormally low. The entire bone marrow of L2 is replaced by low signal intensity tumor tissue, whereas the abnormal bone marrow in T12 is confined to the fractured endplate. The latter appearance is suggestive for recent benign fracture

Table 5. Summary of MR imaging characteristics of acute vertebral body collapse: benign versus malignant causes. Discriminative signs are heuristic rather than absolute

	Benign	Malignant
Morphology		
Shape	Smooth angles	Obtuse angles
Epidural soft tissue mass	–	+
Convex posterior body	±	+
Retropulsion bone fragments	++	–
Signal intensity		
T1	– Isointense with normal bone marrow	No residual normal SI, low SI
	– Abnormal SI adjacent to fractured site	extending into pedicles and posterior parts
	preservation of normal SI, opposite to fracture site, usually bandlike	
	or restricted to the posterior part of the body (posterior band sign)	
T2	– Isointense with normal bone marrow	– Iso to slightly hyperintense with bone marrow
Gd-DTPA	– Isointense with normal bone marrow	– Inhomogeneous enhancement to hyperintense with bone marrow
Abnormal SI in noncollapsed bodies	–	+
Involvement of pedicles, neural arch	–	+

_, absent; +, present; SI signal intensity

4.5.11
Compressive Myelopathy

MR imaging is the modality of choice to rule out compressive myelopathy as it allows imaging of the tissues surrounding the cord (CARMODY et al. 1989). MR imaging will accurately depict the level of compression of the cord (Fig. 14). Especially in the case of cord compression at multiple levels, MR imaging will obviate the need for punctures at each level to perform myelography. Compressive myelopathy can be seen on T2- and T2*- weighted sagittal images of the spine, which will show a high-signal-intensity intramedullary lesion.

The entire spine (cervical, thoracic and lumbar) should be examined in case of spinal metastases, as clinically silent metastases are usually present in patients with vertebral metastatic disease. In addition , one may consider having the pelvis and proximal femora examined in a routine protocol in patients with metastatic disease. This may yield important metastatic lesions causing pathologic fractures. (JELINEK et al. 1990).

Having the entire vertebral column examined by MR imaging will also avoid the problem of the verification of the vertebral level scanned. This can also be achieved by obtaining a scout view of the entire spine. In cases where only a segment of the spine is examined by MR, recognition of the surrounding anatomy (e.g. vascular anatomy, renal arteries) may be helpful in the establishment of the "true" vertebral level (HAHN et al. 1992; RALSTON et al. 1992; SPIRNAK et al. 1995).

MR imaging is superior to myelography, CT and plain films in detecting bone and epidural involvement by tumor and is valuable in clinical decision making (DU BOULAY et al. 1990).

4.6
Follow-up After Systemic Therapy

Response to chemotherapy can be evaluated with plain films and CT. Lytic metastases respond in a definite sequence: sclerotic rim, filling in, uniformly blastic, uniform fading. Increase in size or number of

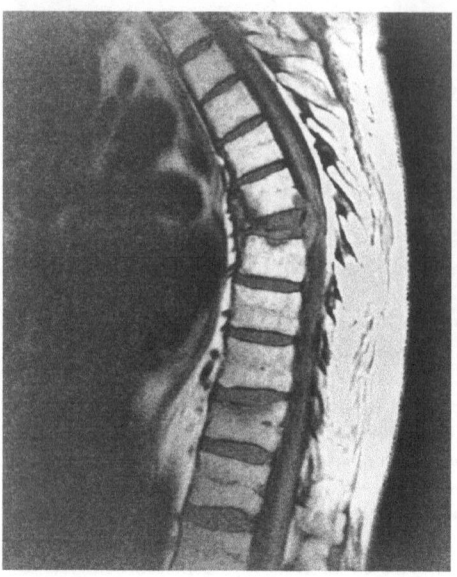

Fig. 4.14. Sagittal T1-weighted image of the thoracolumbar spine reveals a wedge-shaped compression fracture of a midthoracic vertebral body. Together with soft tissue extension of tumor, the vertebral fracture gives rise to compressive myelopathy

lytic lesions, as well as destruction in previously responding areas, signals worsening of the metastatic disease.

Response to therapy correlates well with radiographic improvement (91%), but less well with changes with bone scans (57 %).The value of bone scans is limited by the frequent false results. Response may be associated with a flare of increased intensity of "hot spots" mimicking progression, and some progressive lesions may appear "cold" on scans due to extensive destruction of bone tissue mimicking regression.

Evaluation based on the total area of hot spots seems to increase the reliability of bone scans as a follow-up tool. There is also a concordance between clinical and radiographic findings in the cases of progressive metastatic disease.

Although changes in MR signal intensity will be seen during treatment, controversy exists regarding the value of MR imaging in monitoring systemic therapy (JENSEN et al. 1990; ALGRA et al. 1992b; VAN DE BERG et al. 1995).

4.7
Differential Diagnosis of Bone Marrow Disease

Bone marrow lesions visualized with MR imaging can result from a wide variety of benign and malignant disease. MR images, as all other diagnostic images, should not be read in isolation without appropriate clinical information. In the context of the actual clinical setting, it will usually be possible to determine the true status of the lesion(s) visualized by MR imaging. However, a great number of benign disorders can cause changes in the signal intensity of bone marrow. In the group of patients in whom vertebral metastases are suspected, degenerative disease and osteoporotic compression fractures must be differentiated from metastases as both of these conditions are likely to occur simultaneously with metastases.

4.7.1
Degenerative Disease

Signal intensity changes of bone marrow in conjunction with degenerative changes of the adjacent intervertebral disc represent benign bone marrow lesions and can usually be distinguished from metastases. Alterations in bone marrow signal intensity adjacent to   the intervertebral discs can be seen in 50 % 6 the patients with degenerated discs (MODIC et al. 1988).

Bone marrow adjacent to degenerated discs may show low signal intensity on T1-weighted images and high signal intensity on T2-weighted images. This is attributed to granulation tissue or vascularized fibrous tissue. This pattern of bone marrow abnormality is known as type 1 lesion. Type 1 bone marrow alteration has been shown to exhibit enhancement after injection of Gd-DTPA. These areas of abnormal signal intensity can be differentiated from infection by the absence of an increased signal intensity of the intervertebral disc.

Increased signal intensity on T1- and isointense or slightly hyperintense signal on T2-weighted images is caused by local increase in marrow fat. Fat deposition is usually bandlike and located along the endplates. This type 2 of degeneration will not show contrast enhancement.

Isolated focal fatty degeneration can also be seen elsewhere within the vertebral body, unrelated to degenerated discs. These areas are seen as rounded, well-delineated zones ranging from 0.5 to 1.5 cm in diameter, usually located in either the peripheral portions of the vertebral bodies adjacent to the discs or in the posterior osseous elements. The frequency of focal fatty infiltration increases with advancing age.

Type 3 changes are represented by decreased signal intensity on both T1-and T2-weighted images, which correlates with sclerosis on plain radiographs. The lack of signal intensity in type 3 reflects the absence of marrow in areas of advanced sclerosis (MODIC et al. 1988).

4.7.2
Radiation Therapy

Ionizing radiation exerts a depressive effect on the hematopoietic cells in the irradiated volume. Irradiated bone marrow becomes edematous and hypocellular with destruction of vasculature, followed by fatty marrow replacement, resulting in an increase of signal intensity on T1-weighted images. Eventually, as a late result of radiation therapy, MR imaging shows areas of increased signal intensity of T1-weighted images of bone marrow corresponding to radiation ports (STEVEN et al. 1990) (Fig. 15).

The earliest detectable changes following radiation of the bone marrow are areas of high signal intensity on short tan inversion recovery (STIR) images, 1-2 weeks after radiation therapy. These changes probably represent edema, hemorrhage and necrosis. SE images will not show any signal intensity at this stage. After 3-6 weeks, irradiated bone marrow shows increasing heterogeneity in signal intensity on T1-weighted SE images and an increase in the central marrow fat. These changes are attributed to fibrosis and fatty degeneration. Six weeks after the initiation of radiation therapy, increase of signal intensity on T1-weighted images and evidence of early fatty infiltration can be seen in most cases. Eventually two distinct patterns are described: progressive homogeneous increase in signal intensity, and a band pattern with a peripheral region of intermediate signal intensity surrounding a central zone of bright signal intensity on T1-weighted images. The latter pattern may represent peripheral hematopoietic marrow with central marrow fat. This pattern is seen in younger patients and may suggest that the ability of marrow to regenerate after radiation therapy is age dependent.

The radiation-induced modifications of the MR images in the bone marrow are tightly linked to the administered radiation dose and length of the time since the treatment (STEVENS et al. 1990; LIEN et al. 1995).

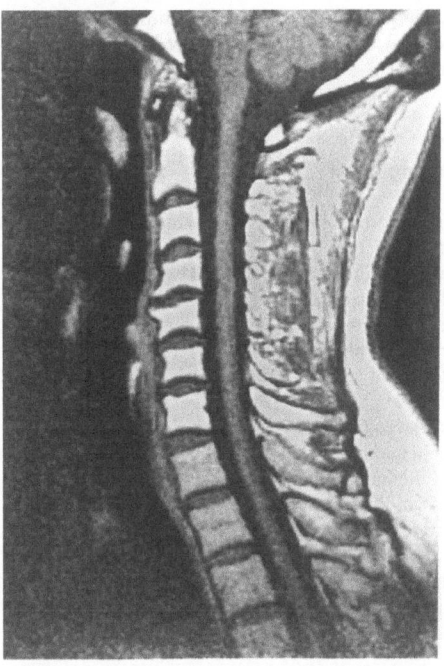

Fig. 4.15. Sagittal T1-weihted image after administration of Gd-DTPA to the cervical spine in a patient who was treated with radiation therypy for intramedullary metastases (same patient as in Fig. 10). Vertebrae C1–7 show abnormally high signal intensity of the bone marrow. This high signal intensity results from fatty degeneration caused by the radiation therapy. Note also that the intramedullary tumor is no longer visible. Loss of the normal intumescence indicates atrophy of the cervical cord

4.7.3
Spondylitis, Spondylodiscitis

Spondylodiscitis has characteristic findings on MR imaging: narrowed disc space, low signal intensity in the marrow of at least two adjacent vertebrae, subligamentous or epidural soft tissue masses and erosion of cortical bone (AHMADI et al. 1993). Evidence on MR imaging of involvement of two consecutive vertebrae and the intervening disc is virtually diagnostic of infective spondylitis. Rim enhancement around abscess loculations within the vertebral bodies and/or paraspinal soft tissues is strongly suggestive of tuberculous spondylitis.

Spondylodiscitis can cause abnormal signal intensity of the bone marrow adjacent to the abnormal disc. Infection of the vertebra will be visible as low signal intensity of the bone marrow on T1-weighted images and increased signal intensity on T2-weighted images and on T1-weighted enhanced images.

4.7.4
Hemangiomas

Hemangiomas are slowly growing, benign hamartomas, which, in bones, are most commonly found in the calvarium and the vertebral bodies. Histopathologically they consist of thin-walled blood-filled vessels and sinuses. Vertebral hemangiomas can show variable signal intensities on MR imaging. Low signal intensity corresponds to fatty stroma, while normal to slightly increased signal intensity indicates vascularization or hypervascularization. Fatty vertebral hemangiomas represent inactive forms of vertebral hemangiomas, while vascularized hemangiomas indicate more active lesions with potential to compress the spinal cord.

The more cellular components of the tumor probably give rise to the increased signal intensity on T2-weighted images (LAREDO et al. 1990, 1995).

4.7.5
Multiple Myeloma

Multiple myeloma is a malignancy composed of plasma cells showing variable degrees of differentiation. It primarily involves bone marrow and is usually multicentric. In contrast to metastatic disease, multiple myeloma deposits usually do not cause osteoblastic bone response; therefore, bone scintigraphy yields a high proportion of false negative results. The lack of osteoblastic response in the case of multiple myeloma is probably related to the inhibiting factors produced by the multiple myeloma cells. These factors diminish the proliferation of osteoblastic cells and decrease their metabolic activity. Initial evaluation of the spine by plain radiography has been recommended because of the high proportion of false negative findings of bone scintigraphy in the detection of myelomatous lesions.

Multiple myeloma exhibits low signal intensity on T1-weighted images and high signal intensity on T2-weighted images and cannot be differentiated from lytic metastases. No reliable differentiation is possible between leukemias (myeloproliferative and lymphoproliferative disease) and a variety of benign hematological disorders by MR imaging: Signal intensity reflects marrow cellularity, as has been shown in patients with diffuse infiltrative diseases (LIBSHITZ et al. 1992; MOULOPOULOS et al. 1994; STÄBLER et al. 1996).

4.7.6
Diffuse Disorders

Diffuse bone marrow disorders can alter, according to the stage of the disease, the MR signal intensity of the bone marrow. Abnormal signal intensity of the bone marrow has been described in patients with acute lymphatic leukemia, aplastic anemia, osteopetrosis, Gaucher's disease, polycythemia vera; myelofibrosis, bone infarction in sickle cell disease and myelolymphoproliferative diseases such as lymphoma and plasmacytoma (VAN DE BERG et al. 1995; JENSEN et al. 1990; KAPLAN et al. 1990; LIBSHITZ et al. 1992).

Increased retention of iron within the bone marrow due to anemia of chronic disease and transfusional state are known to cause low signal intensity on both T1- and T2-weighted images (GEREMIA et al. 1990). Diffuse low signal intensity on T1-weighed SE images can be seen in patients with sickle cell anemia and may be a reflection of hematopoietic marrow hyperplasia or secondary hemosiderosis. Focal areas of low signal intensity on T1-weighted images and high signal intensity on T2-weighted images are attributed to marrow infarction, whereas focal areas of low signal intensity on both T1- and T2-weighted images are seen in old infarcts and fibrosis.

Lymphoma and avascular necrosis of the vertebral body may give either diffuse abnormal signal intensity or foci of abnormal signal intensity on MR imaging.

References

Ahmadi J, Bajaj A, Destian S, Segall HD, Zee CS (1993) Spinal tuberculosis: atypical observations at MR imaging. Radiology 189:489-493
Algra PR (1992) MR imaging and CT of vertebral metastases. Thesis, Amsterdam. ISBN 90-9005678-5
Algra PR, Bloem JL, Verboom L, Arndt JW, Vogel HJP, Tissing H (1990) Detection of vertebral metastases: MRI versus bone scintigraphy. Preliminary results. In: Higer HP, Bielke G (eds). Tissue characterization in MR imaging. Springer, Berlin Heidelberg New York, pp 193-197
Algra PR, Bloem JL, Verboom LJ, Tissing H, Falke THM, Arndt JW, Verboom LJ (1991a) MRI vs scintigraphy in the detection of vertebral metastases. Radiographics 11:219-232

Algra PR, Bloem JH, Valk J (1991b) Loss of visibility of the basivertebral vein: a new MR sign of diffuse bone marrow disease. AJR 157:1129-1130

Algra PR, Heimans JJ, Valk J, Nauta JJ, Lachniet M, Van Kooten B (1992a) Do metastases begin in the body or pedicle? AJR 158:1275-1279

Algra PR, Postma T, Van Groeningen CJ, Van der Valk P, Bloem JL, Valk J (1992b) MR imaging of skeletal metastases from medulloblastoma. Skeletal Radiol 21:425-430

Algra PR, Bloem JL (1992c) MR imaging of metastatic disease and multiple myeloma. In: Bloem JL, Sartoris JD (eds) MRI and CT of the musculoskeletal system. Williams and Wilkins, Baltimore, pp 218-236

Amano, Y, Hayashi H, Kumazaki T (1994) Gd-DTPA enhanced MRI of reactive hematopoietic regions in marrow. J Comput Assist Tomogr 18: 214-217

Avrahami E, Tachmor R, Dally O, Hadar H (1989) Early MR demonstrations of spinal metastases in patients with normal radiographs, CT and radionuclide bone scans. J Comput Assist Tomogr 13:598-602

Baker LL, Goodman SB, Perkash I, Lane B, Enzman DR (1990) Benign versus pathologic compression fractures of vertebral bodies: assessment with conventional spin echo, chemical shift and STIR MR imaging. radiology 174:495-502

Bangert BA, Modic MT, Ross JS (1995) Hyperintense disks on T1-weighted MR: correlation with calcification. Radiology 195:437-443

Batson OV (1940) The function of the vertebral veins and their role in the spread of metastases. Ann Surg 112:138-149

Berg BC van de, Schmitz PJ, Scheiff JM, Filleul BJ, Michaux JL, Ferrant A, Jamart J, Malghem J, Maldague BE (1995) Acute myeloid leukemia: lack of predictive value of sequential quantitative MR imaging during treatment. Radiology 197:301-305

Bloem JL, Algra PR (1993) Imaging of osseous metastases. Acta Clin Belg 48:43-46

Boring CC, Squires TS, Tong T (1992) Cancer statistics. CA 42:19-38

Boulay GH du, Hawkes S, Lee CC, Teather BA, Teather D (1990) Comparing the cost of spinal MR with conventional myelography and radiculography. Neuroradiology 32:124-136

Breger RK, Williams AL, Daniels DL, Czervionke LF, Mark LP, Haughton VM, Papke RA, Coffer M (1990) Contrast enhancement in spinal MR imaging. AJNR 10:633-637

Carmody RF, Yang PJ, Seeley GW, Seeger JF, Unger EC, Johnson JE (1989) Spinal cord compression due to metastatic disease: diagnosis with MR imaging versus myelography. Radiology 173:225-229

Castillo M, Malko JA, Hoffman JC (1990) The bright intervertebral disk, an indirect sign of abnormal spinal bone marrow on T1-weighted MR images. AJNR 11:23-26

Cuénod CA, Laredo JD, Chevret S, Hamze B, Naouri JF, Chapaux X, Bondeville JM, Tubiana JM (1996) Acute vertebral collapse due to osteoporosis or malignancy: appearance on unenhanced and gadolinium-enhanced MR images. Radiology 199:541-549

Dawson, KL Moore SG, Rowland JM (1992) Age-related marrow changes in the pelvis: MR and anatomic findings. radiology 183:47-51

Dooms GC, Fisher MR, Hricak H, Richardson M, Crooks LE, Genant HK (1985) Bone marrow imaging: MR studies related to age and sex. radiology 155:429-432

Edelstyn GA, Gillespie PJ, Grebell FS (1967) The radiological demonstration of osseous metastases:experimental observations. Clin Radiol 18: 158-162

Erlemann R, Reiser M, Peters PE, Vasallo P, Nommensen B, Kusnierz-Glaz CR, Ritter J, Roessner A (1989) Musculoskeletal nesplasms: static and dynamic Gd-DTPA-enhanced MR imaging. Radiology 171:767-773

Erlemann R, Vassallo P, Bongartz G, Müller-Miny H, Rummeny E, Stöber U, Peters PE (1990) Musculoskeletal neoplasms: fast low-angle shot MR imaging with and without Gd-DTPA. Radiology 176:489-495

Ewing J (1928) Metastasis. In: Ewing J (ed) Neoplastic diseases: a textbook on tumors, 3rd edn. Saunders, Philadelphia, PP 77-89

Frager D. Elkin C, Swerdlow M, Bloch S (1988) Subacute osteoporotic compression fracture: misleading magnetic resonance appearance. Skeletal Radiol 17:123-126

Geremia GK, Mc Kluney KW, Adler SS, Charletta DA, Hoile RD, Huckmann MS, Ramsey RG (1990) MR hypointensity of the spine in AIDS. J Comput Assist Tomogr 14:785-789

Hahn PY, Strobel JJ, Hahn FJ (1992) Verification of lumbosacral segments on MR images: identification of transitional vertebrae. Radiology 182:580-581 and 185:616

Hilz MJ, Huk W, Schellmann B, Sörgel F, Druschky KF (1990) Fatal complications after myelography with meglumine diatrizoate. Neuroradiology 32:70-73

Horowitz S, Fine M, Azar-Kia B (1991) Differentiation of benign versus metastatic vertebral body compression fractures. Neuroradiology 33[Suppl]:114-116

Jacobson AF, Stomper PC, Cronin EB, Kaplan WD (1990a) Bone Scans with one or two new abnormalities in cancer patients in no known metastases: reliability of interpretation of initial correlative radiographs. Radiology 175:503-507

Jacobson AF, Cronin EB, Stomper PC, Kaplan WD (1990b) Bone Scnas with one or two new abnormalities in cancer patients with no known metastases: frequency and serial scintigrapic behaviour benign malignant lesions. Radiology 175:229-232

Jelinek JS, Redmond J III, Perry JJ, Burell LM, Benedikt RA, Geyer CA, Peller PJ, Wacks LL, Wise BJ, Ghaed VN (1990) Small cell lung cancer: staging with MR imaging. Radiology 177:837-842

Jensen KE, Thomsen C, Henriksen O, Hertz H, Johansen HK, Yssing M (1990) Changes in T1 relaxation processes in the bone marrow following treatment in children with acute lymphoblastic leukemia. A magnetic resonance imaging study. Pediatr Radiol 20:464-468.

Jinkins JR, Rauch RA, Gee GT, Bazan C, Xiong L, Kashanian FK, Hanna EP (1995) Lumbosacral spine: early and dealyed MR immaging after administation of an expanded dose of gadopentetate dimeglumine in healthy, asymptomatic subjects. Radiology 197:247-251

Kaplan KR, Mitchell DG, Steiner RM, Murphy S, Vinitski S, Rao VM, Burk DL, Rifkin MD (1992) Polycythemia vera and myelofibrosis: correlation of MR imaging, clinical, and laboratory findings. Radiology 183:329-334

Kim RY, Spencer SA, Meredith RF, Weppelman B, Lee JY, Smith JW, Salter MM (1990) Extradural spinal cord compression. Analysis of factors determining functional prognosis: prospective study. Radiology 176:279-282

Laredo J-D, Assouline E, Gelbert F, Wybler M, Merland JJ, Tubiana JM (1990) Vertebral hemangiomas: fat content as a sign of agressiveness. Radiology 177:467-472

Laredo J-D, Lakhdari K Bellauiche L, Hamze B, Jaklewicz P Tubiana J-B (1995) Acute vertebral collapse: CT findings in bening and malignant nontraumatic cases. Radiology 194:41

Le Blanc AD, Schonfeld E, Schneider VS, Evans HJ, Taber KH (1988) The spine: Change in T2 relaxation times from disuse. Radiology 169:105-107

Libshitz HI, Malthouse SR, Cunningham D, Mac Vicar AD, Husband JE (1992) Multiple myeloma: appearance at MR imaging. Radiology 182:833-837

Lien HH, Taksdal I, Scheistron M, Knutse H (1995) Focal regeneration of irratiated bone marrow: a pitfal in MR imaging. AJR 165:742-743

Lim V, Sobel DF, Zyroff J (1990) Spinal cord pial metastases: MR imaging with gadopentetate dimeglumine. AJNR 11:975-982

Major NM, Helms CA, Genant HK (1993) Calcification demonstrated as high signal intensity on T1-weighted MR images of the disks of the lumbar spine. Radiology 189:494-496

Metha RC, Marks MB Hinks RS (1995) MR evaluation of vertabral metastases: T1-weighted short-inversion-time inversion recovery, fast spin-echo, and inversion recovery fast spin-echo sequences. AJNR 16:281

Mirowitz SA, Apicella P, Reinus WR, Hammerman AM (1994) MR imaging of bone marrow lesions: relative conspicuousness on T1-weighted, fat suppressed T2-weighted, and STIR images. AJR 162:215-221

Modic MT, Masaryk TJ, Ross JS, Carter JR (1988) Imaging of degenerative disk disease. State of the art. Radiology 168:177-186

Moore SG, Dawson KL (1990) Red and yellow marrow in the femur: age related changes in appearance at MR imaging. Radiology 175:219-223

Moulopoulus LA, Dimopoulos MA, Alexanian R, Leeds NE, Libshitz HI (1994) Multiple myeloma: MR patterns of response to treatment. Radiology 193:441-446

Paget S (1889) The distribution of the secondary growth in cancer of the breast. Lancet 1:571-573

Petrén-Mallmin M, Nordström B, Andréasson I, Nyman R, Jónsson H, Rauschning W, Hemmingsson A (1992) MR imaging with histopathological correlation in vertebral metastases of breast cancer. Acta Radiol 33:213-220

Poulton TB, Murphy WD, Duerk JL, Chapek CC, Feiglin DH (1993) Bone marrow reconversion in adults who are smokers: MR imaging findings AJR 161:1217-1221

Quint DJ (1995) Hyperintense disks on T1-weighted MR: are they important? Radiology 195:325-326

Ralston MD, Dykes TA, Applebaum BI (1992) Verification of lumbar vertebral bodies (letter). Radiology 185:615-616

Recklinghausen F von (1885) Über die venöse Embolie und den retrograden Transport in den Venen und in den Lymphgefässen. Virchows Arch 100:503-539

Ricci R, Cova M, Kang YS, Yang A, Rahmouni A, Scott WW, Zerhouni EA (1990) Normal age-related patterns of cellular and fatty bone marrow distribution in the axial skeleton: MR imaging study . Radiology 177:83-88

Richardson ML, Patten RM (1994) Age-related changes in marrow distribution in the shoulder: MR imaging findings. Radiology 192:209-215

Ruzal-Shapiro C, Berdon WE, Cohen M, Abramson SJ (1991) MR imaging of diffuse bone marrow replacement in pediatric patients with cancer. Radiology 181:587-589

Sartoris DJ, Clopton P, Nemcek A, Dowd C, Resnick D (1986) Vertebral body collapse in focal and diffuse disease: patterns of pathologic processes. Radiology 160:479-483

Schellinger D, Mauz HJ, Vidic B, Patronas NJ, Deveikis JP, Muraki AS, Abdullah DC (1990) Disk fragment migration. Radiology 175:831-836

Schweitzer ME, Levine C, Mitchell DG, Gannon FH, Gomella LG (1993) Bull's-eyes and halos: useful MR discriminators of osseous metastases. Radiology 188:249-252

Schweitzer ME, White LM (1996) Does altered biomechanics cause marrow edema? Radiology 198:851-853

Spirnak JP, Nieves N, Betz TA (1995) Identification of vascular anatomy on the sagittal scout MR images. Radiology 194:285-288

Stäbler A, Bauer A, Bartl R, Munker R, Lametz R, Reiser MF (1996) Contrast enhancement and qualitative signal analysis in MR imaging of multiple myeloma. AJR 167:1029-1037

Stevens SK, Moore SG, Kaplan ID (1990) Early and late bone marrow changes after irradiation: MR evaluation. AJR 154:745-750

Stimac GK, Porter BA, Olson DO, Gerlach R, Genton M (1988) Gadolinium-DTPA enhanced MR imaging of spinal neoplasms. Preliminary investigations and comparsion with unenhanced spin-echo and STIR sequence AJR 151:1185-1192

Sze G, Krol G, Zimmermann RD, Deck MDK (1988) Malignant extradural spinal tumors: MR imaging with Gd-DTPA. Radiology 167:217-223

Sze G, Bravo S, Krol G (1989) Spinal lesions: quantitative and qualitative temporal evolution of gadopentetate dimeglumine enhancement in MR imaging. Radiology 170:849-856

Sze G, Stimac GK, Bartlett C, Dillon WP, Haughton VM, Orrison W, Kashaniam F, Goldstein H (1990) Multicenter study of gadopentetate dimeglumine as an contrast agent: evaluation in patients with spinal tumors. AJNR 1:967-974

Tokuhashi Y, Matsuzaki H, Toriyama S, Kawano H, Ohsaka S (1990) Scoring system for the preoperative evaluation of metastatic spine tumors prognosis. Spine 15:1110-1113

Yuh WTC, Zachar CK, Barloon TJ, Sato Y, Sickles WJ, Hawes DR (1989) Vertebral compression fractures: distinction between beningn and malignant causes with MR imaging. Radiology 172:215-218

Zawin JK, Jaramillo D (1993) Conversion of bone marrow in the humerus, sternum and clavicle: changes with age on MR images. Radiology 188:159-164

5 Imaging of Extradural Tumors: Primary Tumors

M.A. VAN BUCHEM, V.P.M. VAN DER HULST, and J.L. BLOEM

CONTENTS

5.1
General Considerations

Spinal tumors frequently occur outside the dura. In a review of 4885 cases of spinal tumors in the literature, NITTNER (1976) reported that 30% of all spinal neoplasms were extradural . This frequency is likely to be even higher, since hemangiomas and metastases, the most frequent extradural tumors, were not taken into account in NITTNER's series (RASMUSSEN et al. 1940). Due to the high incidence of spinal hemangiomas, i.e., an estimated 11% in the general population (SCHMORL 1971), primary extradural tumors are the most frequent tumors of the spine including the spinal contents.

M.A. VAN BUCHEM, MD, Department of Radiology, Leiden University Medical Center, Albinusdreef 2, 2333 AA Leiden, The Netherlands
V.P.M. VAN DER HULST, MD, Department of Radiology, Onze Lieve Vrouwe Gasthuis, 1e Oosterparkstraat 179, 1090 HM Amsterdam, The Netherlands
J.L. BLOEM, MD, Department of Radiology, Leiden University Medical Center, Albinusdreef 2, 2333 AA Leiden, The Netherlands

5.1.1
Tissues of Origin of Extradural Tumors

By definition, extradural tumors occur in the spinal tissues that are located outside the dura mater. Since the extradural spine contains diverse cell and tissue types, and since most of these can give rise to the development of tumors, the diversity of primary extradural tumors is considerable. In order to get a better understanding of the type of tumors that can be expected, the extradural cells and tissues of the spine will be briefly reviewed.

The extradural spine can be divided into two compartments: the epidural space, containing soft tissues, and the osseous vertebral column. Owing to their different histologic compositions these compartments are home to different populations of primary tumors.

In the spine, the epidural space is a real space, due to the fact that, contrary to the situation in the skull, the inner and outer laminae of the dura mater are separated. The outer lamina covers the inner surface of the spinal osseous structures, whereas the inner lamina is adjacent to the arachnoidea. The epidural space is a closed compartment, since the inner and outer lamina fuse in the neural foramina (ST. AMOUR et al. 1994). The epidural compartment is filled with loose connective tissue containing fat cells, an abundance of arterial and venous vascular networks, and nerves. All these epidural constituents can give rise to primary spinal tumors (Table 5.1). In addition, embryonal ectodermal and hematopoietic "rests" in the epidural space may be the origin of tumorous lesions. Finally, tumors originating from spinal dural tissue may occur in the epidural space. Their epidural presence is the result of either extradural expansion of a durally based meningioma, or of the development of a meningioma in the epidural space not associated with the dura.

Like osseous structures elsewhere in the body, the vertebral column contains bone, bone marrow, cartilage, ligaments, blood vessels, and nerves. Bone is present in two forms: a shell of cortical bone, and,

Table 5.1. Histologic classification of extraosseous primary epidural tumors of the spine

Tissue	Neoplasm		Non-neoplastic lesion
	Benign	Malignant	
Dura	(Ectopic) meningioma	Malignant meningioma	
Nerves			
Nerve sheath	Neurofibroma Schwannoma	Malignant Schwannoma	
Adipose tissue			
Lipocytes	Lipoma Lipomatosis Angiolipoma Angiomyolipoma	Liposarcoma	
Blood vessels			

Endothelial cells
    Perithelial cells
    Smooth muscle cells
	Hemangioma	Hemangioblastoma
		Hemangiopericytoma
		Leiomyosarcoma	

Epidural embryonal rests	Teratoma	Malignant teratoma	(Epi)dermoid
Hematopoietic tissue	Extramedullary hematopoiesis	Lymphoma Chloroma	
Others	Fibromatosis	Rhabdomyosarcoma	

Table 5.2. Histologic classification of osseous primary tumors of the spine

Tissue	Neoplasm		Non-neoplastic lesion
	Benign	Malignant	
Cortical and woven bone			
Osteoblasts	Enostosis Osteoblastoma Osteoid osteoma	Osteosarcoma	Fibrous dysplasia

Osteoclasts	Giant cell tumor
	  (grades I and II)
	Paget's disease
		Giant cell tumor
		  (grades III and IV)
		Paget's sarcoma	

Cartilage			
Chondroblasts	(En)chondroma Osteochondroma Chondroblastoma Chondromyxoid fibroma	Chondrosarcoma	
Bone marrow			

Histiocytes
    Fibroblasts/fibrohistiocytes
    Lipocytes
    Hematopoietic cells
	Eosinophilic granuloma
	
	Lipoma
	Mast cell disease
		True histiocytic lymphoma
		MFH/fibrosarcoma
		Liposarcoma
		Lymphoma
		Leukemia/chloroma
		Myeloma
		Ewing's sarcoma	

Intraosseous vascular system			
Endothelial cells	Hemangioma Hemangiomatosis	Hemangioendothelioma Hemangiosarcoma	Aneurysmal bone cyst

Perithelial cells
    Perivascular smooth
      muscle cells
	Leiomyoma	Hemangiopericytoma
		
		Leiomyosarcoma	

Notochord			
Notochordal cells		Chordoma	
Uncertain origin			Solitary bone cyst

within this shell, a network of trabecular bone. Bony tissue consists of cellular components and an extracellular matrix. The cellular components are osteoprogenitor cells, osteoblasts, osteocytes, and osteoclasts. Osteoprogenitor cells and osteoblasts play a role in bone production, while osteoclasts resorb the bony matrix. Neoplasms may arise from each of these cell types (Table 5.2).

The space between the trabeculae is the marrow cavity, which contains the bone marrow. Bone marrow consists of a system of thin-walled anastomosing blood vessels and sinuses containing blood-forming cells and surrounded by stroma of reticular cells, reticular fibers, macrophages, and adipose cells (BLOOM and FAWCETT 1994). Each of the constituents of the bone marrow may give rise to primary tumors: the vascular system to vascular tumors, the hematopoietic cells to hematologic neoplasms, and the stroma to several types of tumor (Table 5.2).

The amount of hematopoietic tissue present in the bone marrow is a function of age and demand (KRICUN 1993). Depending on the amount of hematopoietic tissue present in bone marrow, a distinction is made between red marrow, containing mainly highly vascularized hematopoietic tissue, and yellow marrow, containing mainly fatty tissue. Under normal circumstances in adults, the vertebral body predominantly contains red marrow, whereas the posterior elements predominantly contain yellow marrow (KRICUN 1993). Therefore, vascular and hematologic neoplasms have a tendency to occur preferentially in the vertebral body.

Under normal circumstances, cartilage is present in the spine of adults as hyaline cartilage plates lining the superior and inferior aspects of the vertebral body and as hyaline cartilage in the synovial intervertebral joints (SCHMORL 1971). These structures rarely, if ever, give rise to cartilaginous tumors. Cartilaginous tumors tend to originate in the epiphyseal plate cartilage during growth or in misplaced islands of cartilage shed into the osseous medulla by the growing epiphyseal plate (MIRRA et al. 1989).

The intervertebral discs consist of two compartments: the fibrocartilaginous annulus fibrosus and the nucleus pulposus. The nucleus pulposus is a derivative of the embryonal notochord and consists of a soft matrix rich in hyaluronic acid. During childhood, notochordal cells may be found in this matrix. However, their number diminishes with time, and, in general, after the age of 20 years none are found (BLOOM and FAWCETT 1994). Since intervertebral discs give rise to disc herniations and protrusion, they are a frequent source of mass lesions within the spinal canal, but true neoplasms seldom, if ever, arise from the intervertebral discs (ROSENBERG and SCHILLER 1990). For reasons unknown, spinal tumors originating from rests of the notochord arise from the vertebral bodies, but never from intervertebral discs (MIRRA et al. 1989).

Ligaments are abundant in the spine. The ligaments that are present within the spinal canal over its entire length are the posterior longitudinal ligament and the flaval ligaments. These structures may become hypertrophic and may even ossify, which may cause compression of the thecal sac and spinal cord. However, they rarely, if ever, give rise to neoplastic disease.

In the extradural spine, peripheral nerves are present in the bone as well as in the epidural space. Nerves in the epidural space and those located in the periosteum lining the bone have a myelinated sheath consisting of Schwann cells. However, nerves invading the bony cortex lose their myelinated sheath beneath the level of the periosteum, and thus the bone itself contains only naked nerve fibers (MIRRA et al. 1989). Since tumors originating from peripheral nerves arise in the nerve sheath, they never arise in the bone of the spine. In general, they arise in the epidural space or in the periosteum. When intraosseous localization of a nerve sheath tumor occurs, it is usually the result of direct extension from a soft-tissue or periosteal primary lesion, or it has reached the bone by metastatic spread (MIRRA et al. 1989).

5.1.2
Histologic Classification of Extradural Tumors

The extradural site of the spine is home to two different categories of primary neoplasms. Most of the tumors arising in the loose connective tissues of the epidural space belong to the category of soft tissue tumors. The vertebral column with its osseous, cartilaginous, and ligamentous components is essentially part of the musculoskeletal system, and the tumors originating from this system are members of the family of bone tumors. The bone and soft tissue tumors in the spine differ not only histologically, but also in growth pattern, clinical consequences, and radiologic appearance. Due to the high incidence of hemangiomas and myeloma localizations in the osseous spine, bone tumors are more frequent in the spine than soft tissue tumors (SCHÄFER 1976).

The classification of spinal bone tumors provided in Table 5.2 is based on a generally accepted histologic classification of primary bone tumors. In this system, tumors are classified according to their supposed tissue and cell of origin. The nature of the cells of origin is derived from the cellular morphology, their antigenic characteristics, and the extracellular substance they seem to produce. Bone tumors are usually divided into true neoplasms, being benign or malignant, and non-neoplastic tumorous lesions (Table 5.2). The latter category contains lesions that might be mistaken for a neoplastic condition on the basis of radiologic and/or pathologic evidence (MIRRA et al. 1989), and sometimes even on the basis of behavior (MULDER et al. 1993).

Thanks to the description of several large series of bone tumors in the literature, the statistics on the incidence of bone tumors are rather reliable. From these statistics the incidence of many spinal bone tumors may be derived. Still, one should be aware of two drawbacks. First, the incidence of spinal hemangiomas in these series is far too low. This is the consequence of the fact that the published bone tumor series cover or include the era before the introduction of MRI, when spinal hemangiomas were much less frequently detected. Second, spinal localizations of hematologic diseases such as myeloma, leukemia, and lymphoma are the rule rather than the exception and are, if not giving rise to myelum compression, in general not radiologically documented. In addition, when they are radiologically investigated, they are usually not a diagnostic problem, since diagnosis has already been performed on clinical grounds. Therefore, these patients are mostly treated without consultation of a specialist in bone tumors, so these tumors are underrepresented in series of bone tumors reported by specialists as well.

Due to the very high incidence of vertebral hemangiomas, benign bone tumors are more frequent in the spine than malignant bone tumors. Apart from metastases, myeloma is the most frequent malignant bone tumor of the spine. Compared to hemangioma and myeloma, the other bone tumors of the spine are quite rare. In a series of 6873 bone tumors from the Netherlands Committee on Bone Tumors, 319 tumors of the spine other than hemangioma and hematologic diseases are described (Table 5.3; MULDER et al. 1993). In this series more than 80% of the spinal bone tumors are represented by 8 types of tumors. In decreasing order of frequency these are: giant cell tumor, chordoma, osteoblastoma, chondrosarcoma, aneurysmal bone cyst, osteoid osteoma, Ewing's sarcoma, and osteosarcoma. It is also apparent from this series that certain bone tumors are preferentially located in the spine (Table 5.3). More than one third of all bone

localizations of the following tumors concerns the spine: schwannoma, chordoma, hemangiopericytoma, and osteoblastoma.

The tumors arising in the epidural space are listed in Table 5.1. Most of these tumors belong to the category of soft tissue tumors because they arise from extraskeletal tissue of mesodermal origin (ENZINGER and WEISS 1988). By convention this category also includes the peripheral nervous system. The classification of soft tissue tumors in the epidural space provided in Table 5.1 is based on the WHO histologic classification of soft tissue tumors. Just as in bone tumor classification, these tumors are classified on a histogenetic basis according to the adult tissue they resemble. By definition, some tumors in the epidural space do not belong to the category of soft tissue tumors, not being of mesodermal origin (hematopoietic tissue, teratoma, dermoids and epidermoids) or being considered part of the central nervous system (dural-based

Table 5.3. Incidence of bone tumors and tumor-like lesions of the spine in a series of 6873 primary bone tumors of the Netherlands Committee on Bone Tumors

	Incidence among spinal tumors[a] (no. of vertebral / sacral lesions)		Rate of occurrence in the spine[a]
Benign tumors			
Giant cell tumor	15.1	(32/16)	10.3
Osteoblastoma	11.0	(34/1)	33.3
Osteoid osteoma	7.5	(23/1)	12.6
(En)chondroma	4.4	(13/1)	1.8
Schwannoma	1.6	(4/1)	83.3
Chondroblastoma	0.3	(1/-)	0.6
Malignant tumors			
Chordoma	13.8	(18/26)	78.6
Chondrosarcoma	11.0	(22/13)	4.9
Ewing's sarcoma	6.6	(13/8)	5.6
Osteosarcoma	6.0	(11/8)	1.6
Hemangioendothelioma /-sarcoma	1.9	(4/2)	12.5
MFH	1.6	(2/3)	3.2
Fibrosarcoma	0.9	(2/1)	1.7
Hemangiopericytoma	0.6	(2/-)	40
Paget's sarcoma	0.6	(2/-)	6.3
Radiation sarcoma	0.3	(1/-)	3.1
Synovial sarcoma	0.3	(1/-)	1.4
Non-neoplastic lesions			
Aneurysmal bone cyst	10.7	(20/14)	13.1
Eosinophilic granuloma	3.8	(12/-)	6.9
Fibrous dysplasia	1.3	(4/-)	1.0
Myositis ossificans	0.6	(2/-)	3.1
Hematoma	0.3	(1/-)	4.8

[a] In percentage

meningiomas). In addition, dural based meningiomas are by definition not extradural. However, since the behavior and consequences of these non-mesenchymal epidural tumors differ by no means from mesenchymal soft tissue tumors, we have included them in this category. In Table 5.1, soft tissue tumors are classified as malignant, benign, and, analogous to the classification of spinal bone tumors, as non-neoplastic tumorous lesions. Reliable statistics on the incidence of soft tissue tumors in general, and those of the epidural space in particular, are lacking (ENZINGER and WEISS 1988).

Blood vessels and fat cells occur both in the osseous spine and in the epidural space, and in both compartments these tissues can give rise to primary spinal tumors. Therefore these tumors are mentioned in the context of bone tumors as well as epidural tumors. Although occurring in both spaces, some of these tumors have a tendency to occur preferentially in one or the other. Hemangiomas predominantly occur in the vertebrae, while lipomas originate more frequently in the epidural space.

Some benign tumors have a potential for becoming malignant. In the extradural spine these are: neurofibromas associated with neurofibromatosis type 1 (Recklinghausen), Paget's disease of bone, hereditary multiple osteochondromatosis, and enchondromas – notably in Ollier's disease or in Maffucci's syndrome. The initially benign nerve sheath tumors in Recklinghausen's neurofibromatosis can develop into very aggressive malignant nerve sheath tumors. Malignant degeneration of vertebral Paget lesions can result in osteosarcoma, and less frequently in chondrosarcoma. In hereditary multiple osteochondromatosis, the chance of developing chondrosarcoma in the cartilage cap of an exostosis is considerably higher than with isolated osteocartilaginous exostoses. Finally, enchondromas can dedifferentiate into chondrosarcoma, the chance of which is increased in Ollier's disease and Maffucci's syndrome. Patients affected with these diseases require life-long follow-up, even when initially the benign nature of the tumors has been demonstrated (SCHMIDEK and SCHILLER 1990).

since the spine contains anatomic structures that are relatively efficient barriers to tumor spread. The barriers to expansion in the axial plane are the osseous cortex, the spinal ligaments, and especially the inner lamina of the dura. In the longitudinal plane, the intervertebral discs are an efficient barrier to tumor spread. Due to the presence and location of these barriers, growth patterns of tumors originating in the epidural space tend to differ from those of tumors arising in the osseous spine. Upon expansion, tumors in the epidural space experience no barriers in the longitudinal plane, and may easily spread upwards and downwards in the loose connective tissue of the epidural space. In the axial plane these tumors experience resistance from the spinal ligaments and the inner dural lamina, and therefore in this plane tumors tend to encirculate the thecal sac within the confines of the spinal canal. Epidural tumors may also expand outside the spinal canal by growing through the intervertebral foramina. The lack of tumor-resistant borders in the foramina also permits tumor growth in the opposite direction and makes the epidural space prone to expansion of paravertebral tumors. In contrast to epidural tumors, those originating in the osseous spine experience resistance in both the axial and longitudinal plane. As a result, bone tumors tend to grow in a more segmented fashion, and in addition they are initially more likely to remain localized. It is evident that when tumors expand beyond the borders of the compartment they arose from, the growth pattern of this extracompartmental extension is influenced by its new environment.

The extradural part of the spine shelters the vital and vulnerable parts of the nervous system. The principal danger of extradural tumor growth is its tendency to affect these fragile structures. Bone tumors may endanger the nervous system in two ways. First, they may disturb the stability of the spinal column and predispose for myelum compression due to vertebral collapse or spondylolisthesis. Second, neural structures may be damaged as a result of local expansion. Epidural tumors tend to affect neural structures by local expansion without endangering of the spine's stability.

5.1.3
Growth Patterns of Extradural Tumors

The growth pattern of an extradural tumor depends on its specific biologic character on the one hand, and its anatomic location on the other. The anatomic location influences the pattern of tumor extension,

5.1.4
Clinical Manifestations of Extradural Tumors

Apart from hemangiomas, extradural tumors are seldom an incidental finding (MACDONALD 1990). In general, patients with these tumors present with a combination of pain and neurologic dysfunction (MACDONALD 1990).

Pain is usually the first symptom and dominates the clinical picture of patients with extradural tumors. It may herald the presence of the tumor days, weeks, months, or even years before diagnosis. The origin and resulting character of the pain these patients experience is diverse. First, it may result from infiltration and destruction of the osseous structures of the spine by the tumor, and notably from distension of the periost. These phenomena give rise to pain that is localized to the area of vertebral involvement (MACDONALD 1990). The pain can develop gradually or, when resulting from vertebral collapse, have an acute onset following minor trauma. Second, pain may result from stretching, compression, or infiltration of nerve roots and plexuses. This type of pain tends to be radicular along the course of the involved nerve root, or confined to the distribution of a plexus. Third, pain may result from compression of the sensory tracts in the spinal cord. It is then confined to the distribution of the long sensory tracts of the myelum. Finally, pain may be due to reflex spasms of paraspinal muscles adjacent to a spinal tumor.

In general, signs and symptoms of neurologic dysfunction occur late in the course of disease of an extradural tumor. The signs consist of a loss of motor, sensory, and autonomic functions in various combinations, which may be accompanied by spasticity in the case of myelopathy. Neurologic dysfunction may result from compression and infiltration of the spinal cord, nerve roots, and plexuses. The way these structures respond to compression, and the resulting prognosis, depend on the severity, duration, and speed of onset of compression. Mild compression and compression of short duration or gradual onset may give rise to edema and local demyelination of the nervous system. Especially the spinal cord may resist severe compression and deformity without axonal loss, provided that the onset of compression is gradual. The signs and symptoms resulting from these changes may be reversible following decompression. However, when compression is severe, of long duration, and, particularly, of acute onset, axonal damage may result. Axonal damage in nerve roots and plexuses may be functionally reversible following decompression due to axonal sprouting and regeneration. However, the regenerative capacity of the spinal cord is minimal, and axonal damage of the cord is, functionally, largely irreversible. Thus the presence of signs and symptoms of neurologic dysfunction in a patient with an epidural tumor is an emergency, particularly when indicative of cord compression of acute onset. Decompression, either by surgery or radiation therapy, should be performed without delay in order to limit axonal loss. Since both therapeutic options require radiologic examination to determine the nature and location of compression, this situation also constitutes a radiologic emergency.

5.1.5
Imaging of Extradural Tumors

In the work-up of patients clinically suspected of having an extradural tumor, imaging plays a pivotal role. Radiologic techniques are used to detect the lesion responsible for the signs and symptoms, to perform differential diagnosis, and, if the lesion is a tumor, to grade and stage the tumor.

5.1.5.1
Detection

Use of the different diagnostic modalities in spinal tumors has been treated in a previous chapter. In the context of this chapter it should be emphasized that both MRI and CT have a role in detecting and characterizing extradural tumors, due to the intimate relation between soft tissues and osseous structures in the extradural compartment. The role of plain radiographs is limited. The superior soft tissue discrimination of MRI compared to CT makes MRI more suitable for the detection of tumors or extension of tumors in the epidural space and paravertebral tissues. In addition, MRI is superior in the detection of lesions in the bone marrow. Finally, the possibility of performing an examination in the sagittal plane with MRI is an advantage when the location of a spinal lesion is hard to predict from the clinical signs and symptoms. On the other hand, CT provides more detailed information about the bony reaction on the interface of the tumor with normal bone, periosteal reactions, and mineralization in the tumor matrix. Thus, the information provided by MRI and CT is complementary.

5.1.5.2
Diagnosis

Once the presence of a spinal lesion has been established, radiologic properties and nonradiologic data guide the radiologist towards a differential diagnosis, and sometimes a firm diagnosis. The data that should be taken into account are: location of the tumor, aspects of the interface between tumor and normal tissue, type of periosteal reaction, tumor matrix, tumor extension, multiplicity of lesions, the presence of predisposing factors, and the patient's age.

5.1.5.2.1
LOCATION

Since every compartment of the spine has its own pathology, determining the location of the lesion narrows the spectrum of possible diagnoses. First, it should be established whether a spinal tumor is intra- or extradural. Often the extradural origin of the lesion is apparent by the position of its epicenter. When an extradural tumor abuts the dura mater, visualization of the displaced dura on MRI as a low-intensity band between the spinal cord and tumor (TAKEMOTO et al. 1988), and replacement of epidural fat by tumor, giving rise to a fatcap on the opposite site in the spinal canal (HORNER and PINTO 1989), may point to the extradural origin. In attempting to discriminate intra- and extradural tumors using roentgen techniques, myelography may be of help. On both conventional and CT myelography, an extradural lesion displaces the contrast-filled subarachnoid space away from the osseous contour of the spinal column.

Since within the extradural compartment the nature of disease in the epidural space and the vertebral column differs, the second localizing step consists of determining in which of these spaces the lesion originated. Tumors occurring at the interface of these spaces may complicate determination of the site of origin. Again, determination of the location of the epicenter often indicates the site of origin. On MRI the relation of the posterior longitudinal ligament or the ligamentum flavum with the tumor may also be an indicator. And when bone destruction occurs, the site of cortical destruction may be of help. Primary skeletal tumors initially cause endosteal cortical destruction, whereas epidural tumors initially erode the outer cortical surface (MADEWELL and MOSER 1988).

When the origin of a tumor has been determined to be the osseous spine, the location within this compartment may suggest certain diagnoses, since bone tumors may preferentially occur at certain locations. These locations may be characterized both by spinal level and by the specific site within individual vertebrae. The most relevant feature regarding the spinal level is whether the tumor is located in the spine or in the sacrum. As can be derived from Table 5.3, most bone tumors in the sacrum are malignant (ratio malignant:benign = 2:1), whereas most bone tumors in the spine are benign (ratio = 1:2). Chordoma occurs preferentially in the sacrum. However, osteoblastoma, osteoid osteoma, chondroma, and eosinophilic granuloma seldom originate in the sacrum and have a definite preference for the spine (Table 5.3). With regard to the individual vertebrae, the locations relevant for differential diagnosis are the vertebral body, the posterior elements, and the junction between the pedicles and the body. Due to the different histologic properties of these skeletal compartments, they are sites of predilection for different types of tumor.

In the epidural compartment, the dural or nerve sheath origin of a tumor may be suggested by an intimate relation between a tumor and dura or spinal nerve root, respectively.

5.1.5.2.2
MARGIN

The interface between tumor and normal tissue reflects the biologic behavior of the tumor. With regard to bone tumors, LODWICK and colleagues (1980) demonstrated that the radiographic properties of this interface reflect the tumor's manner and rate of growth . These authors found that benign tumors tended to have well circumscribed margins, reflecting a tendency to expand within the osseous tissues without infiltration. This pattern was described as geographic. In contrast, the margins of malignant tumors were often found to be ill defined due to infiltration of the surrounding tissues, and the degree of indistinctness of these margins tended to correlate with the degree of malignancy. The margins typically found in infiltrative tumor growth are referred to as "moth-eaten" or permeative. A moth-eaten pattern consists of multiple, often clustered, small lytic areas that vary in size, tend to coalesce, and have indistinct margins. In a permeative marginal pattern the lesions consist of innumerable, minuscule oval or linear lucencies that fade, without a distinct margin, into the surrounding bone. In addition to reflecting the tumor's tendency to infiltrate, the marginal pattern may also reflect the growth rate. In slow-growing tumors, the margin may be very distinct due to the formation of a sclerotic rim, whereas at higher growth rates time may be insufficient to create such a rim. Apart from being of help for diagnostic purposes, the findings of LODWICK and coworkers (1980) served as a basis for a staging system of bone tumors. This system has become an accepted standard. While using this system, it should be borne in mind that Lodwick based his findings on radiographic images.

Although an elaborate classification based on tumor margins has not been developed for soft tissue tumors, the radiographic aspects of the interface of these tumors with their environment may also provide a clue to the diagnosis. Again, these margins may be well circumscribed or ill defined. The former are more consistent with a benign and the latter with a malignant lesion. These margins may exist between the tumor and the surrounding epidural space contents, and may only be perceived with MRI. However, the tumor may also abut the surrounding osseous structures, resulting in a margin that may be visualized by radiographic techniques. The adjacent bone may show scalloping, with a well-circumscribed margin favoring a benign tumor. When the tumor is slow-growing, this margin may be sclerotic. However, an ill-defined erosion, cortical destruction, and even marrow extension are suggestive of a malignant tumor (MADEWELL and MOSER 1988).

5.1.5.2.3
PERIOSTEAL REACTION

Both tumors arising in the osseous structures of the spine and those originating in the epidural soft tissues may give rise to periosteal new bone formation. Tumors originating in the bone may penetrate the cortex and irritate the periosteum from within. Based on radiographic appearance, the resulting periosteal reaction may have a lamellar or spicular pattern or give rise to Codman's triangles (MULDER et al. 1993). A smooth and uninterrupted lamellar periosteal reaction suggests a slow-growing benign lesion, while interrupted, fuzzy lamellar reactions are likely to indicate malignancy. Spicular reactions and Codman's triangles are an indication of aggressive tumor growth. Combinations of more than one type of periosteal reaction are more often encountered in malignant tumors.

Epidural tumors adjacent to bone may also give rise to periosteal reactions. Especially hypervascular tumors of both benign and malignant nature are notorious for this tendency. In general, periosteal new bone formation found in benign tumors tends to show up as solid cortical thickening, whereas single

or multilamellar and interrupted reactions are more frequently encountered in malignant lesions. As mentioned above, the posterior lining of the vertebral bodies has a relative lack of periosteum, and thus lesions occurring at that site may lack a periosteal reaction.

5.1.5.2.4
MATRIX

Apart from its margins, tumor tissue itself may have a radiologic appearance indicative of its nature. Traditionally, bone tumors are scrutinized for the presence of calcifications by means of radiographic techniques. These calcifications may have characteristic appearances. Mineralization may occur as a result of maturation of the matrix, the extracellular substance of the tumor. Tumor matrices that are prone to mineralization are osteoid, produced by osteoblasts, and chondroid, produced by chondroblasts. Mineralization of the osteoid matrix gives rise to ossification, of which the radiographic appearance, depending on the amount of mineralization, varies from a diffuse increase in radiodensity to a well-defined trabecular pattern. This pattern may be distinguished from the amorphous calcifications, often arranged in rings and arcs, that result from mineral deposition in the chondroid matrix. The presence of these calcifications proves the presence of chondroblasts and osteoblasts in the lesion. However, the absence of mineralization does not exclude the presence of these cells, since they may be too undifferentiated to produce matrix.

Apart from being part of matrix maturation, mineralization may also occur in the absence of a matrix. In the spine, this may occur in hemangiomas and angiolipomas in the form of phleboliths.

5.1.5.2.5
OTHER RADIOLOGIC DATA

In primary bone tumors, extensive infiltration in the surrounding soft tissues, either paravertebrally or epidurally, is a sign of rapid growth and suggestive of a malignant nature of the tumor. Extensive soft tissue involvement is often found in lymphoma and Ewing's sarcoma. Multiplicity of lesions may occur in the absence of metastatic disease. This may particularly be the case with certain benign lesions, such as neurofibromas, giant cell tumors, and hemangiomas.

5.1.5.2.6
CLINICAL DATA

Finally, nonradiologic data influence the composition of differential diagnosis. Although almost every tumor may occur at any age, notably bone tumors have a strong tendency to occur at certain periods of life. Therefore, a patient's age influences the order of differential diagnosis. Finally, the patient may have a condition that increases the risk of certain tumors. Examples of such conditions are bilateral retinoblastoma predisposing for the development of osteosarcoma; Paget's disease and the increased incidence of osteosarcoma and fibrosarcoma; the higher risk of developing chondrosarcomas in multiple osteocartilaginous exostoses and in Ollier's disease; and the development of sarcomas in patients who have been subjected to radiation therapy.

5.1.5.3
Staging

In addition to its role in the detection and interpretation of extradural tumors, radiology plays an important role in their staging. Staging of a tumor provides indispensable information regarding the state and extent of disease with which treatment may be planned. An accepted staging system for musculoskeletal tumors is the one designed by ENNEKING (1990) Since this system also covers soft tissue tumors, it is highly suitable for staging spinal extradural tumors. Enneking's system is based on the interrelationship of three factors: grade (G), site (T), and metastases (M). Each of these factors is stratified by components that influence both prognosis and response to treatment .

5.1.5.3.1
GRADE

Grading provides an estimate of the degree of malignancy of the tumor. In the Enneking system, this estimate is based not only on histologic findings, but also on radiologic and clinical data, because notably in bone tumors histologic features are often poor indicators of biological behavior (ENNEKING et al. 1980, ENNEKING 1985, 1990). Especially the grading of benign tumors and the distinction between benign masses and low-grade malignancies may be difficult or impossible on histologic grounds. In these cases radiologic and clinical data may determine the estimated tumor grade. Radiologic grading is based

on the description of tumor margins as described by LODWICK et al. 1980.

5.1.5.3.2
SITE

In the Enneking system three anatomic settings are described according to the presence and integrity of a (pseudo)capsule and the integrity of the boundaries of the compartments the tumor arises from. These settings are referred to as T0, T1, and T2, and in the spine they are based mainly on radiologic examinations.

T0 lesions are intracapsular and intracompartmental. A tumor is intracapsular when it is surrounded by an intact capsule or pseudocapsule. In the extradural part of the spine, T0 tumors arise in the epidural space or in the osseous spine and respect the boundaries of these compartments. The boundaries considered to be relevant in this context are the cortex and spinal ligaments for the osseous compartment, and the spinal ligaments and dura for the epidural space. The intervertebral disc is an irrelevant boundary, and therefore bone tumors expanding through the disc are intracompartmental as long as they respect the integrity of the annular and longitudinal ligaments. Although in T0 lesions the boundaries of the compartments remain intact, they may be distorted.

T1 lesions are extracapsular and intracompartmental. Extracapsular refers to expansion of the tumor beyond its (pseudo)capsule. This growth occurs per continuum or as isolated satellites. Lesions are intracompartmental when both the tumor, the satellites, and the reactive zone are contained within the compartment of origin. In the spine T1 lesions are always bone tumors. Epidural and paravertebral soft tissue tumors with extracapsular growth are considered as extracompartmental (T2) lesions since these spaces have no longitudinal barriers to tumor extension.

T2 lesions are extracompartmental. This group includes bone tumors that expand into the surrounding soft tissues and epidural and paravertebral soft tissue tumors that expand beyond their capsule and/or their compartmental boundaries.

5.1.5.3.3
METASTASES

According to the presence of metastases, tumors are classed as M0 or M1. M0 indicates no evidence of metastases, whereas M1 refers to the presence of metastases. Since in sarcomas prognosis is similar concerning metastatic involvement of regional lymph nodes and distal organs, no specification is provided for these situations. Obviously, radiologic examinations play a crucial role in the search for metastases.

5.2
Specific Pathology

5.2.1
Tumors of Cortical and Woven Bone

5.2.1.1
Enostosis

Enostosis, or bone island, probably develops in the immature skeleton, but is found in all age groups as an incidental finding. There is no gender predilection. Enostosis consists of normal compact bone. It probably develops secondary to deficient bone resorption in the process of enchondral ossification. It causes no symptoms and is therefore almost always an incidental finding. The estimated prevalence is 1%, but prevalence in the spine may be as high as 14% (RESNICK and NIWAYAMA 1988). In the spine enostiosis can be encountered in the vertebral body as well as in the posterior complex.

On radiographs, enostosis appears as a solid osteoblastic lesion with characteristic spicules merging with surrounding trabecular bone (Fig. 5.1). Since osteoblastic activity may be present, the lesion may show increased tracer uptake on technetium bone scintigrams. For the same reason it may also increase or decrease in size over time.

Active bone islands, especially in the spine, may be mistaken for metastases. Bone islands, however, frequently do not show increased tracer uptake on bone scintigrams, and the peripheral spicules seen on radiographs or CT are fairly characteristic of enostosis. Although some work groups differentiate osteopoikilosis from multiple enostoses, for all practical purposes multiple enostoses can be considered similar in appearance and behavior to osteopoikilosis. Other lesions that may look like enostosis are osteoma, fibrous dysplasia, and osteoid osteoma. Of these, only osteoid osteoma may cause some confusion in differential diagnosis in the spine, when the nidus of osteoid osteoma is not visualized.

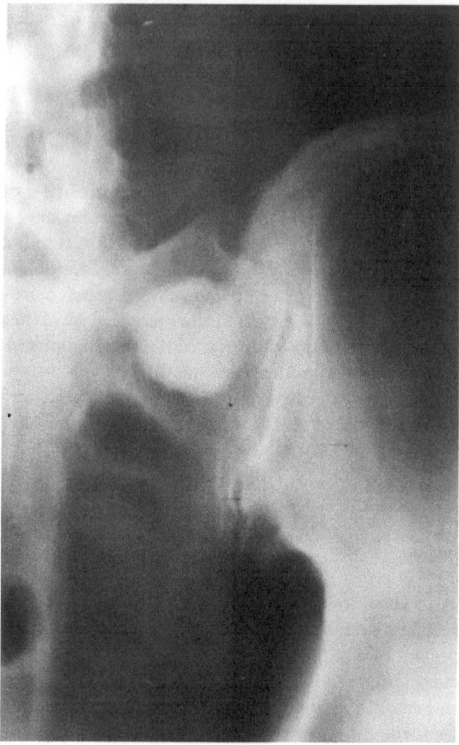

Fig. 5.1. Enostosis in a 35-year-old asymptomatic man Conventional tomography of the left pelvis shows a solid osteoblastic lesion. This incidental finding did not change during several years of follow-up

5.2.1.2
Osteoid Osteoma

Most (90%) of the patients with osteoid osteoma are between 7 and 33 years of age with a peak incidence at 15 years (MULDER et al. 1993). There is a 2:1 male predominance. The incidence is approximately 4% of all primary bone tumors, excluding myeloma, and 10% of all benign primary bone tumors (MULDER et al. 1993). Approximately 8% of all primary spinal bone tumors other than hemangioma and hematologic diseases are osteoid osteomas, and 13% of osteoid osteomas are found in the spine (Table 5.3).

The so-called nidus is the actual lesion and is composed of well-vascularized connective tissue containing trabeculae, osteoid, and calcified bone surrounded by osteoblasts. The presence of sensory nerve endings is thought to be responsible for the characteristic spontaneous pain and the pain experienced at biopsy.

Pain is characteristically worse at night and responds well to salicylates. A scoliosis concave to the affected side is often present. When located in the spine, the median duration of symptoms is 10 months, which is longer than that of osteoid osteoma located in the appendicular skeleton. Traditionally, treatment has consisted of surgical removal of the nidus. Currently, osteoid osteomas are successfully treated in many centers with CT-guided percutaneous cauterization. This procedure needs to be performed under general anesthesia because of unbearable pain when the needle tip enters the nidus.

Osteoid osteoma is more frequently found in the lumbar spine than in the cervical or thoracic spine. These tumors invariably arise in the posterior column and not in the vertebral body. Osteoid osteoma varies in size from a few millimeters to 1.5 cm and is therefore easily missed on plain radiographs. Usually the reactive sclerosis, and not the nidus itself, is first detected (Fig. 5.2a) The well-defined nidus may be purely lytic or may contain central calcification(s) and is best seen on CT with thin collimation. Reac-

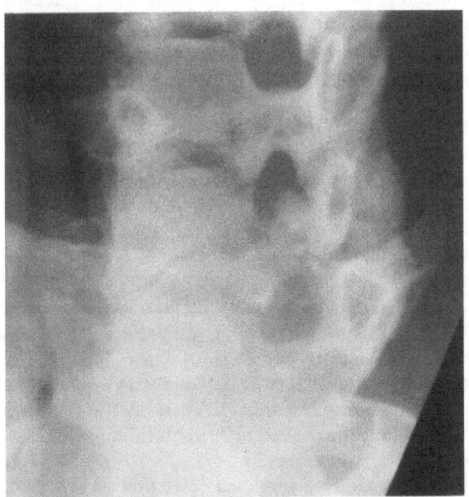

a

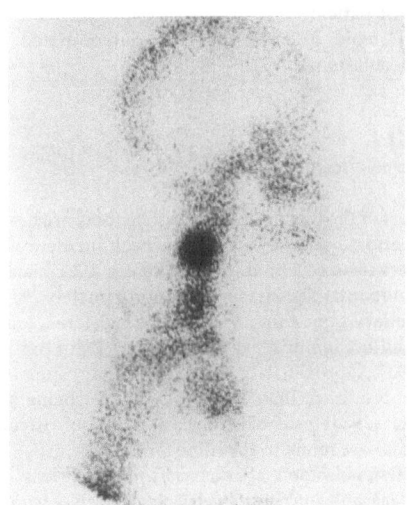

b

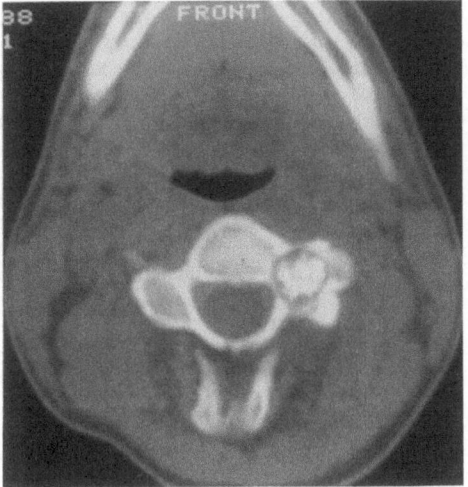

c

Fig. 5.2 a–c. A 22-year-old man presenting with backpain. a Oblique radiograph of upper cervical spine exhibits sclerosis of the left arch of C3. b Tc-99m-HDP scintigraphy shows high tracer uptake in the upper cervical spine. c CTimage of C3. Reactive sclerosis; broadened left arch contains a sclerotic lesion with osteolytic margin caused by nidus

tive osteosclerosis may be extensive or minimal, is often seen as a sclerotic pedicle, and may even extend beyond the bone bearing the nidus.

Technetium bone scintigraphy will show an intense focal increased tracer uptake and is the method of choice for localizing a suspected osteoid osteoma when radiographs are equivocal or negative (Fig. 5.2b). After localization with technetium bone scintigraphy or plain radiographs, thin collimation (preferably 1 mm) CT is indicated to visualize the nidus (Fig. 5.2c). On MRI the nidus is usually difficult to visualize, but extensive bone marrow and soft tissue edema are easily appreciated in all symptomatic patients.

Osteoid osteoma must be differentiated from osteoblastoma.

5.2.1.3
Osteoblastoma

Most of the patients with osteoblastoma are between 10 and 20 years of age with a peak incidence at 15 years (MULDER et al. 1993). There is a 2:1 male predominance. The incidence is approximately 2% of all primary bone tumors, excluding myeloma, and 6% of all benign primary bone tumors (MULDER et al. 1993). Approximately 11% of all primary spinal bone tumors other than hemangioma and hematologic diseases are osteoblastomas, and 33% of osteoblastomas are found in the spine (Table 5.3).

Osteoblastoma characteristically is at least 2 cm in size, and consists of well vascularized osteoid and connective tissue. Giant cells and osteoblasts are seen throughout the tumor, and mitotic figures without atypia are also present. Histologic differentiation between osteoblastoma and osteoid osteoma may be difficult and is not always possible. Another more clinically relevant problem is histologic differentiation between (aggressive) osteoblastoma and well differentiated osteosarcoma.

Pain without the typical features of that experienced secondary to osteoid osteoma is characteristically the presenting symptom. As in osteoid osteoma, a scoliosis concave to the affected side is not infrequently seen. Local excision or curettage, if necessary in combination with cryosurgery, is the treatment of choice. Recurrences tend to occur, especially in aggressive osteoblastoma.

The spine (lumbar, thoracic, and cervical) is the most common localization of osteoblastoma. Since osteoblastoma invariably originates from the posterior elements, involvement of only the vertebral

body is rare. Up to 25% of osteoblastomas are reported to involve both the posterior elements and the vertebral body.

On radiographs, a geographic pattern of bone destruction is characteristically appreciated. In 10% of cases the lesion may show aggressive features such as moth-eaten destruction and rapid growth. Almost 80% of spinal osteoblastomas are expansile and are enclosed by an intact calcified shell. Extension into the vertebral canal may easily cause neurologic symptoms. Usually calcifications, sclerosis, and ridges are seen in the osteolytic lesion.

CT is the method of choice for showing local extension prior to surgery (Fig. 5.3a). MRI is usually not indicated, but when performed, will show the lesion as well as muscle wasting and bone marrow and soft tissue edema (Fig. 5.3b,c).

The radiologic differential diagnosis includes osteoid osteoma, aneurysmal bone cyst, and giant cell tumor.

5.2.1.4
Giant Cell Tumor

Most (75%) of the patients with giant cell tumor are between 15 and 45 years of age, with a peak incidence in the third decade (MULDER et al. 1993). In one series almost 30% of patients with spinal giant cell tumor were less than 20 years of age (KRICUN 1993). There is a slight female predominance. The incidence is approximately 10% of all primary bone tumors, excluding myeloma (MULDER et al. 1993). Approximately 15% of all primary spinal bone tumors other than hemangioma and hematologic diseases are osteoblastomas, and 10% of osteoblastomas are found in the spine (Table 5.3).

Giant cell tumors are well-vascularized tumors containing closely packed epitheloid mesenchymal cells and many multinucleated giant cells. The presence of giant cells alone is not specific, since these are frequently found in other conditions as well. We use a four-point histologic grading system (MULDER et al. 1993). Grades I and II are benign, grade III is borderline, and grade IV is malignant. More than half of giant cell tumors are grade II, grade IV is rare (3%) (MULDER et al. 1993).

Patients present with atypical pain or local tenderness. Treatment is aimed at preventing recurrence while avoiding iatrogenic morbidity. When possible, curettage with local adjuvants (cement with phenol) is performed. Radiation therapy can be used, especially in high-grade giant cell tumor, when surgical therapy is not feasible. Depending on the grade and the therapy used, the recurrence rate varies between 27% and 50% (MULDER et al. 1993). The mortality rate likewise varies from 0.9% to 29% (MULDER et al. 1993).

Within the spinal column, the thoracic and sacral regions are preferential sites (MULDER et al. 1993). Other investigators have reported that sacral localizations are four times as common as spinal localizations (KRICUN 1993). Giant cell tumor is, after chordoma, the most common primary tumor of the sacrum. In more than 50% of cases the tumor is located in the vertebral body, in approximately 40% of cases the tumor is located in the vertebral body and posterior column. Localization only in the posterior column does occur, but is rare. As elsewhere in the body, giant cell tumor may be multifocal and may therefore be seen in more than one vertebra.

The destruction of bone is of the geographic type in 100% of grade I lesions, but in only 50% of grade IV lesions (Fig. 5.4a). In 50% of grade IV lesions, at least a moth-eaten destruction pattern is seen in part of the lesion. The tumor tends to be more osteolytic in the higher grades, whereas ridges are more frequently seen in low-grade tumors. Ballooning of new cortical bone is often seen. Cortical bone may be intact in low-grade lesions, but irregular destruction of cortical bone may be encountered in high-grade tumors.

MRI is used for local staging of the lesion (Fig. 5.4b,c). Extensive bone marrow and soft tissue edema are often seen and must be differentiated from true tumor extension.

The differential diagnosis may include osteoblastoma, aneurysmal bone cyst, and chordoma.

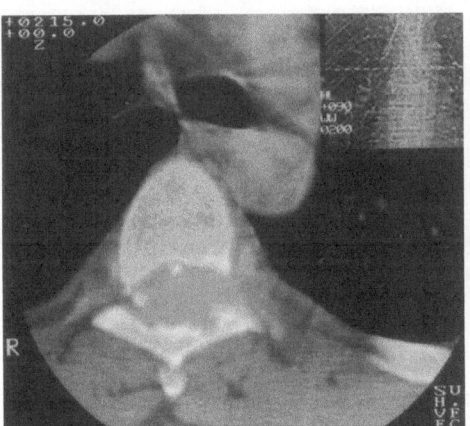

a

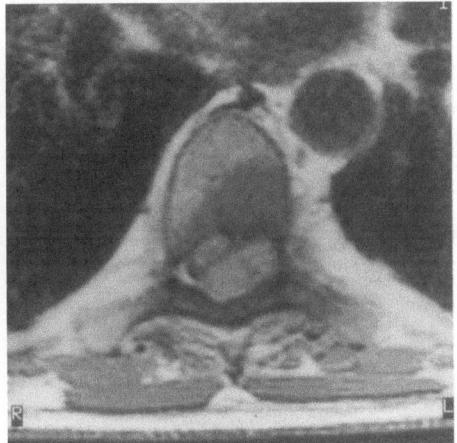

b

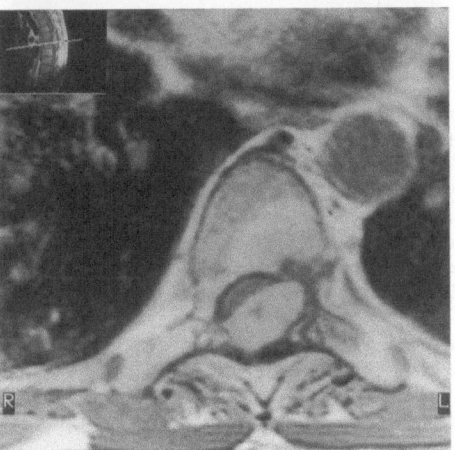

c

Fig. 5.3 a–c. Osteoblastoma in a 30-year-old man a CT image at the level of D5 after injection of intradural contrast agent. Expansile lesion originating from the posterior arch on the left side. The tumor extends into the spinal canal, and there is displacement of the dura and spinal cord to the right. There is still some intradural contrast seen around the displaced cord. b Precontrast T1-weighted transverse image at the same level as A. The tumor has an intermediate signal intensity, and the displaced myelum is easily identified. There is low signal intensity in the posterior part of the corpus due to edema. c T1-weighted transverse image after injection of Gd-DTPA. There is bright inhomogeneous contrast enhancement of the tumor. Edema enhances inhomogeneously on this image taken several minutes after contrast agent injection

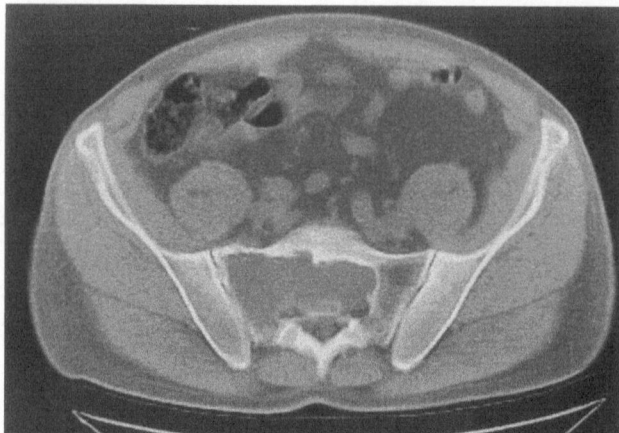

Fig. 5.4 a-c. Giant cell tumor in a 44-year-old man presenting with pain in the lower back a CT image shows large lytic lesion in the sacrum abutting the right SI joint and extending over the midline. No soft tissue is visualized. b Precontrast T1-weighted coronal image shows sacral tumor with low signal intensity. The tumor is well defined. c After injection of Gd-DTPA, T1-weighted coronal image corresponding to b shows marked enhancement of tumor

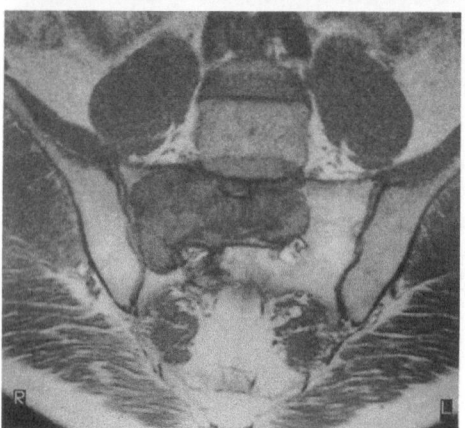

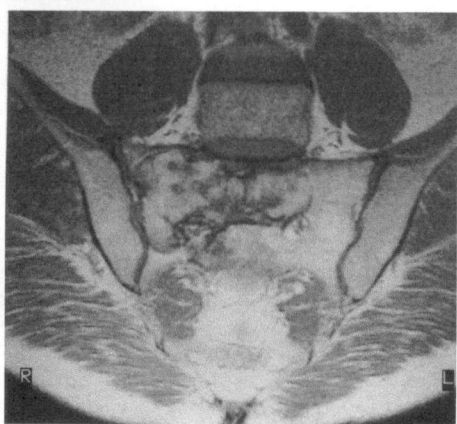

5.2.1.5
Paget's Disease

Although not a true neoplasm, Paget's disease may mimic a neoplasm, especially when located in the spine. It is characterized by extensive abnormal re-modelling of bone, and it is most prevalent in the middle-aged and elderly population of Great Britain, certain areas of continental Europe, and Australia. The disease may be asymptomatic or present with a variety of symptoms such as pain, deformity, or neu-rologic deficit.

Paget's disease frequently involves the axial skel-eton, especially the sacrum (and pelvis) and lumbar spine. Multifocal disease is not uncommon. Al-though bone resorption resulting in predominantly osteolytic lesions is characteristic early on, this is rarely appreciated on plain radiographs. Typically, Paget's disease is diagnosed in the reparative phase. Thickened and coarse trabeculation, similar to the pattern seen in hemangioma, is seen in combination with enlargement of the vertebral body and cortical thickening (Fig. 5.5). Bone remodelling may result in classic radiographic appearances such as the ivory body and the picture frame appearance.

Sarcomatous degeneration is rare, especially in the spine. Irregular destruction of bone, the presence of a soft tissue mass, rapidly progressive disease, and pain should raise suspicion of malignant degenera-tion.

Fig. 5.5. Paget's disease in a 79-year-old-woman with lower backpain. Contiguous CT images of the sacrum show diffuse osteolysis with coarse trabeculation and microfractures. Left side of the sacrum is slightly enlarged

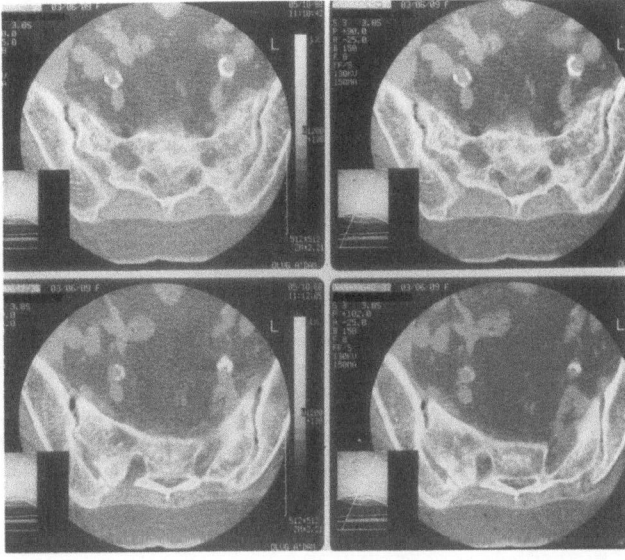

5.2.1.6
Osteosarcoma

The median age of patients with osteosarcoma in the axial skeleton is 25 years (BLOEM and KROON 1993), compared with 17 years for all patients with osteosarcoma (MULDER et al. 1993). There is a slight male predominance. Osteosarcomas comprise approximately 36% of all primary malignant bone tumors, excluding myeloma (BLOEM and KROON 1993). Approximately 6% of all primary spinal bone tumors other than hemangioma and hematologic diseases are osteosarcomas, and less than 2% of osteosarcomas are found in the spine (Table 5.3).

By definition, the tumor cells produce osteoid. The amount of osteoid, however, may be very small. The constituents of the tumor matrix vary, but in addition to osteoid, calcification and fibrous and cartilaginous tissue are often present. Osteosarcomas can be classified as intraosseous, surface, extraosseous, secondary, and multicentric. Surface osteosarcomas are further subdivided into three categories but do not occur in the spine. The intraosseous group can be subdivided into: conventional (osteoblastic, fibroblastic, chondroblastic; 75%-85% of all osteosarcomas), telangiectatic, small-cell, low-grade, and cortical types.

Patients present with pain with or without neurologic deficit. Multidisciplinary treatment combining surgery, chemotherapy, and radiation therapy is the rule. As opposed to tumors located in the appendicular skeleton, local control of osteosarcoma located in the spine may not be achieved because of technical-surgical limitations. Therefore the prognosis of spinal osteosarcomas is probably not as good as that of some types in the appendicular skeleton.

Commonly, the tumor is located in the vertebral body and posterior elements. Isolated localization in either the vertebral body or posterior column, however, is not infrequently encountered.

Typically, a combination of osteosclerosis and osteolysis is appreciated on plain radiographs. Both ends of this spectrum, however, may occur. Bone destruction is usually of the moth-eaten or permeative type, often associated with cortical destruction. The soft tissue extension is best appreciated on MRI, which is indicated in all cases to evaluate the therapeutic options.

The differential diagnosis of osteosarcoma includes osteoblastoma, lymphoma, giant cell tumor, and aneurysmal bone cyst.

5.2.1.7
Fibrous Dysplasia

The monostotic form of fibrous dysplasia is most commonly diagnosed in patients between 5 and 20 years of age. The median age at diagnosis for the polyostotic form is 8 years. Approximately 10% of patients have the polyostotic form. Fibrous dysplasia in the spine is rare: approximately 1% of spinal lesions are fibrous, and only 1% of fibrous dysplasia localizations are found in the spine. Fibrous dysplasia is a developmental disorder in which abnormal fibrous tissue and abnormal bone trabeculae and woven bone are found instead of normal bone. Patients may be asymptomatic or present with pain, deformity, neurologic deficit, abnormal skin pigmentation, or endocrine disturbances.

The vertebral bodies are more commonly involved than the posterior elements. The radiographic appearance is highly variable and may be predominantly ground glass, sclerotic, osteolytic, or even cystic.

5.2.2
Tumors of Cartilage

5.2.2.1
Enchondroma

Since enchondromas are often incidental findings, the age distribution is not well known. In our series, the median age was 35 years with a range of 3–83 years (MULDER et al. 1993). There is no gender predominance. Enchondromas are reported to comprise 12% of all primary benign bone tumors, and 3% of all primary bone tumors (MIRRA et al. 1989). The prevalence may, however, be considerably higher, since many enchondromas are asymptomatic. Approximately 4% of all primary spinal bone tumors other than hemangioma and hematologic diseases are enchondromas, and 1% of enchondromas are found in the spine (Table 5.3).

Enchondroma is a benign, lobulated, hyaline-cartilage-producing tumor surrounded by lamellar enchondral bone. The cellularity varies widely. The intercellular substance may be mucinous or chondroid. Histologic differentiation between benign enchondroma and malignant low-grade chondrosarcoma is usually difficult and depends on many parameters, of which the site of origin, the structure of the tumor, and its relationship with the surrounding normal bone are not without significance. Equally

important are the radiologic and clinical findings (MULDER et al. 1993).

The patients may present with pain, a pathologic fracture, swelling, or mechanical and cosmetic problems. Usually, an enchondroma is an incidental finding. The treatment of a symptomatic patient usually is curettage or resection. Asymptomatic lesions are best left alone. A major issue in the management of these patients is the differentiation between enchondroma and chondrosarcoma. It is virtually impossible to exclude the presence of low-grade chondrosarcoma when dealing with a benign looking enchondroma. If the patient develops symptoms, or if the lesion increases in volume or changes in radiographic appearance after closure of the growth plates, the diagnosis of chondrosarcoma has to be considered. The typical appearance of an enchondroma is that of a well-defined lobulated osteolytic lesion with punctate, flocculent, arc-or ring-like calcifications. The lesions are often expansile, cortical bone may be thinned or scalloped. Cortical destruction, soft tissue mass, a wide zone of transition, and progressive osteolytic changes are all radiographic signs of malignant transformation. The changes of malignant transformation depend on location and multiplicity. Changes of malignant degeneration are highest (30%) in axial lesions of patients with multiple enchondromas, as found in Ollier's disease and Maffucci syndrome (GIUDICI et al. 1993; see also Sect. 5.2.2.5).

The differential diagnosis includes chondrosarcoma, giant cell tumor, and aneurysmal bone cyst.

5.2.2.2
Osteochondroma

The median age of patients with osteochondromas seeking medical attention is 20 years. The vast majority of patients with osteochondromas present within the first three decades. There is a male predominance. Osteochondroma is the most common benign primary bone tumor and is estimated to account for 20%-50% of benign bone tumors (GIUDICI et al. 1993). However, osteochondroma in the axial skeleton is rare. Some 1%-8% of all primary bone tumors other than myeloma are osteochondromas. Only 1%-3% of all osteochondromas occur in the axial skeleton (KRICUN 1993). Only 7% of patients with the dominant hereditary condition of multiple exostoses, or diaphyseal aclasia, develop spinal lesions (KRICUN 1993). Like enchondroma, osteochondroma consists of hyaline cartilage. The degree of maturity is the same as that of the underlying bone and cartilage of the patient. In the growing child, the cartilage is cellular, contains binucleated chondrocytes, and grows with the child. Centrally, enchondral ossification is observed.

Although most patients do not have symptoms, they may seek medical attention because of the presence of swelling, mechanical problems (near joints), cosmetic abnormalities, pain, or even spinal cord compression.

The symptoms mentioned above may be the reason for surgical intervention. Because the possibility of malignant transformation cannot be excluded, the lesion has to be removed in one piece. If a solitary lesion exists, the chance of malignant transformation is only 1%; in the case of multiple lesions, this may be as high as 10%-25% at axial sites (JAFFE 1958). Therefore patients with multiple exostosis should be instructed to seek medical attention if pain develops or if the lesion increases in size after closure of the growth plates. Clinical or radiographic follow-up is sometimes needed. The thickness of the cartilaginous cap can be measured with ultrasound. When the thickness exceeds 2 cm, the diagnosis of malignant transformation should be considered.

When osteochondroma does occur in the spine it almost always arises from the vertebral arch, spinous process, or other posterior element, rarely from the vertebral body. The radiographic appearance is identical to that of osteochondroma elsewhere in the body. The base of the stalk, however, is not always easily localized. Marrow of the exostosis is continuous with that of the host bone. The cortex of the host bone flares into the base of the exostosis. Multiplanar MRI is needed for local staging, determination of the site of origin, and evaluation of the cartilaginous cap.

The differential diagnosis includes chondrosarcoma, osteoblastoma, if the exostosis is shallow and broad-based, and soft tissue chondroma.

5.2.2.3
Chondroblastoma

Most (87%) of the patients with chondroblastoma are between 10 and 30 years of age with a median age of 17 years (MULDER et al. 1993). There is a 2:1 male predominance. Chondroblastomas comprise approximately 3% of all primary bone tumors, excluding myeloma, and 9% of all benign primary bone tumors (MULDER 1993 et al.). Approximately 0.3% of all primary spinal bone tumors other than hemangioma and hematologic diseases are osteoblastomas, and 0.6% of osteoblastomas are found in the spine (Table 5.3).

Chondroblastoma is a highly cellular cartilaginous tumor that contains many giant cells and is associated, in 14% of cases, with secondary aneurysmal bone cyst (BLOEM and MULDER 1985, MULDER et al. 1993).

The presenting symptom is usually pain and/or fracture. Curettage is the treatment of choice. The recurrence rate, however, is high (22%). Some advocate conservative management of these patients, since chondroblastoma is probably a self-limiting disorder.

Chondroblastoma may occur anywhere in the vertebral body. Bone destruction is almost always of the geographic type. Lesions are often lobulated and have sclerotic margins. They are almost always osteolytic and contain ridges and calcifications. They are often expansile and may compromise the vertebral canal. On MRI, edema of bone marrow and soft tissue is invariably marked.

Since chondroblastoma in the spine is rare, a correct diagnosis of chondroblastoma in the spine is rarely made. Usually, well-differentiated chondrosarcoma, aneurysmal bone cyst, or osteoblastoma will be diagnosed.

5.2.2.4
Chondromyxoid Fibroma

Most (80%) of the patients with chondromyxoid fibroma are younger than 30 years; the median age is 17 years (MULDER et al. 1993). There is no gender predominance. Chondromyxoid fibroma comprises approximately 1% of all primary bone tumors, excluding myeloma, and 3.5% of all benign primary bone tumors (MULDER et al. 1993). Location in the spine is very rare (KRICUN 1993, MULDER et al. 1993).

Chondromyxoid fibroma consists of fibromyxoid tissue, and of tissue resembling hyaline cartilage. Symptoms usually consist of swelling and mild discomfort. Curettage is the treatment of choice.

Chondromyxoid fibroma is a well-defined osteolytic lesion often containing ridges. The pattern of destruction is geographic. The typical calcifications of enchondroma are not seen in chondromyxoid fibroma. Expansion of the cortex is frequently seen, the lesion may thus involve the vertebral canal. It occurs more often in the cervical than in the thoracic or lumbar spine. It usually arises from the posterior column.

Because of its rarity and atypical features, chondromyxoid fibroma is rarely diagnosed prior to biopsy.

5.2.2.5
Chondrosarcoma

In our material, 15% of all primary bone tumors and 24% of all malignant bone tumors, excluding myeloma, were chondrosarcomas (MULDER et al. 1993). Approximately 11% of all primary spinal bone tumors other than hemangioma and hematologic diseases are chondrosarcomas, and 5% of chondrosarcomas are found in the spine (Table 5.3). There is a slight male predominance. Chondrosarcomas can be sudivided into primary and secondary tumors. Secondary chondrosarcomas develop in benign cartilaginous tumors. It is estimated that in solitary enchondromas and osteochondromas, the incidence of secondary chondrosarcoma is less than 1%. In patients with multiple enchondromas or multiple osteochondromas, the incidence is estimated to be 35% and 25%, respectively. Another subdivision, according to the relationship with host bone, is into central (75% of all chondrosarcomas, arising in medullary cavity), juxtacortical (2% of all chondrosarcomas, arising from surface of bone), peripheral (15% of all chondrosarcomas, arising from cap of osteochondroma), and the rare soft tissue chondrosarcomas. Histologically, grades I (55%), II (37%), and III (8%) of the common-type (hyaline to fibromyxoid) chondrosarcoma as well as clear-cell and mesenchymal types are distinguished. The term "dedifferentiation" is reserved for chondrosarcoma changing into fibrosarcoma, malignant fibrous histiocytoma, or osteosarcoma.

Central chondrosarcomas are rarely diagnosed under the age of 10 years, the median age is 44 years for grade I, 55 years for grade II, and 26 years for grade III. The median age for peripheral chondrosarcoma is 32 years (MULDER et al. 1993).

Histologic examination of central or peripheral chondrosarcoma may show myxoid or mucoid tissue, hyaline cartilage, enchondral ossification, and undifferentiated mesenchymal tissue in the superficial layers. The lobulated architecture is fairly typical. Differentiation between benign enchondroma or osteochondroma and central or peripheral grade I chondrosarcoma is very challenging. Final diagnosis is based not only on histology, but also on radiology and clinical symptoms.

Pain with or without swelling is a reason to seek medical attention. Treatment consists of en bloc re-section. It is very important that the entire tumor is resected without spilling. The large cartilaginous tumors break apart easily during surgery when the tumor is mobilized. Borderline chondrosarcomas are often treated with curettage and local treatment (phenolization) of the wall. Prognosis is good when the entire low-grade chondrosarcoma is resected. Chances of local recurrence increase with grade III chondrosarcoma or when spilling occurs during surgery. Recurrent chondrosarcoma may have a higher grade of malignancy than the original tumor; therefore, the prognosis becomes less favorable if recurrent tumor is found.

Grade I chondrosarcoma can usually not be differentiated from enchondroma or chondrosarcoma on radiographs. At present it is not clear whether MRI can assist in differentiating the two. Typically, central chondrosarcoma is a lobulated osteolytic lesion with ring- and arc-like calcifications (Fig. 5.6a). Destruction of bone may be geographic, moth-eaten, or permeative. Cortical breakthrough with soft tissue extension and interrupted periosteal reaction is a sign of malignancy. In peripheral chondrosarcoma, the thickness of the cartilaginous cap can be an additional sign: if thickness is more than 2 cm, malignancy is considered likely. On gadolinium-enhanced MRI imaging marked serpiginous and nodular enhancement is observed in central and peripheral chondrosarcoma (GEIRNAERDT et al. 1993) (Fig. 5.6c,d).

Chondrosarcoma may arise anywhere in the vertebral body or posterior complex.

The main differential diagnosis are benign enchondroma and osteochondroma. Signs of malignancy are: malignant radiographic signs as described above, large size, marked and rapid enhancement on (dynamic) gadolinium-enhanced MRI (progressive) symptoms, spontaneous pain, progressive size of swelling, and location in the axial skeleton.

5.2.3
Tumors of Bone Marrow

5.2.3.1
Malignant Fibrous Histiocytoma/Fibrosarcoma

Although fibrosarcoma and malignant fibrous histiocytoma are two separate entities, that can be differentiated histologically, they are discussed here in the same section because the radiologic and clinical features are very similar. Prognosis and treatment are identical.

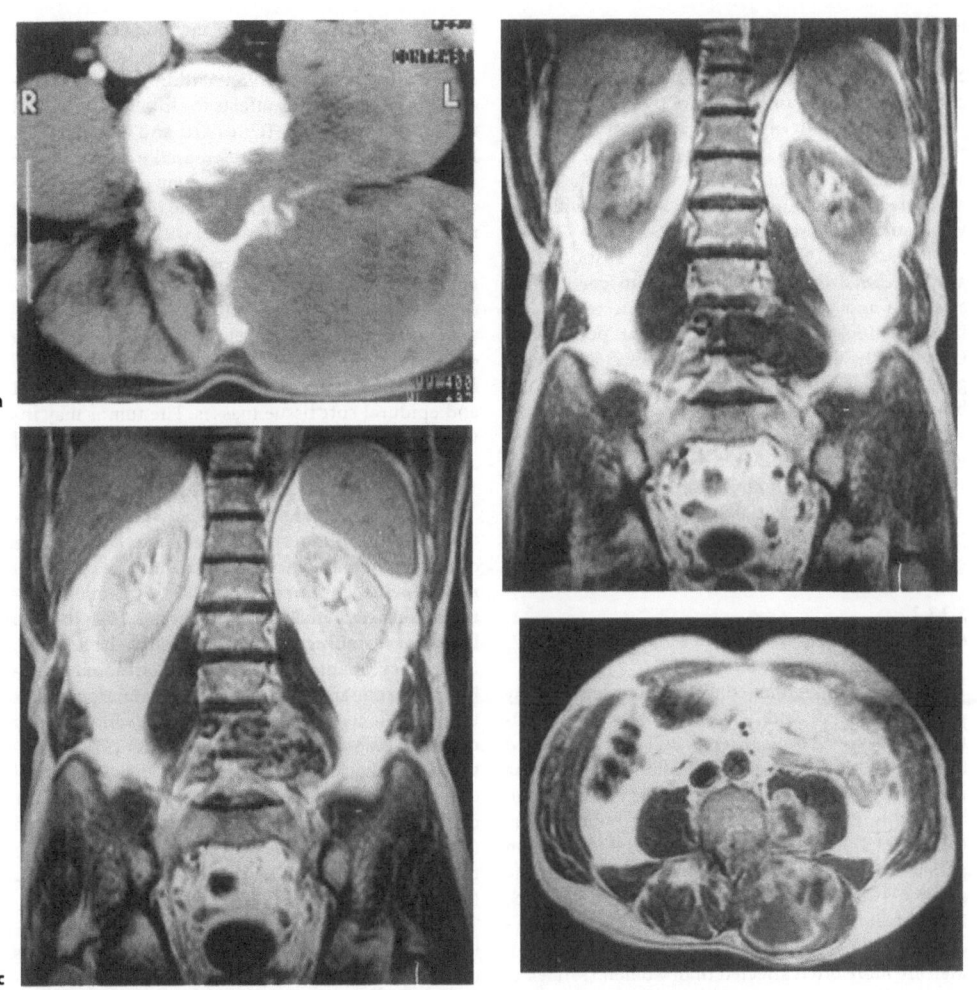

Fig. 5.6 a-d. Chondrosarcoma in a 53-year-old man with slowly progressing back pain and local swelling. **a** CT image taken at the level of L4 shows large tumor with destruction of the left side of the corpus. Substantial paravertebral extension into the psoas muscle and long back muscles. **b** Precontrast T1-weighted coronal image shows tumor with homogeneous low signal intensity in corpus L4 and left paravertebral extension. **c,d** After Gd-DTPA injection, curvilinear enhancement indicative of cartilage is visualized on **c** coronal and **d** transverse images

The occurrence of fibrosarcoma/malignant fibrous histiocytoma is evenly distributed from the second to the seventh decade with a peak incidence in the fifth decade (MULDER et al. 1993). There is a slight male predominance. The incidence is approximately 7% of all primary bone tumors, excluding myeloma, and 11% of all malignant primary bone tumors (MULDER et al. 1993). Approximately 2.5% of all primary spinal bone tumors other than hemangi-

oma and hematologic diseases are fibrosarcoma/malignant fibrous histiocytoma, and 5% of fibrosarcoma/malignant fibrous histiocytoma are found in the spine (Table 5.3).

Fibrosarcoma is characterized by tumor formation of interlacing bundles of collagen fibers without formation of osteoid or cartilage. Histologic grading from grades I to III corresponds with clinical behavior. Malignant fibrous histiocytoma is characterized by the presence of elongated spindle cells arranged in a spinning-wheel or storiform pattern and cells with histiocytic features. The tumor cells are extremely atypical, and mitotic activity is high.

Patients present with pain, and 23% of our patients presented with a pathologic fracture. Wide resection is the treatment of choice. Chemotherapy is advocated by some groups. The 5-year overall survival rate is 34% (MULDER et al. 1993).

Fibrosarcoma/malignant fibrous histiocytoma are ill-defined osteolytic tumors with cortical destruction and soft tissue extension. Destruction of bone is almost always moth-eaten or permeative. Occasionally, the tumor is well defined and shows geographic destruction. Fibrosarcoma/malignant fibrous histiocytoma is more often found in the sacrum and lumbar spine than in the thoracic or cervical spine (KRICUN 1993).

The radiologic differential diagnosis is extensive and also depends on age; it includes metastases, lymphoma, Ewing's sarcoma, osteosarcoma, and myeloma.

5.2.3.2
Myeloma

Myeloma is a malignant condition characterized by proliferation of plasma cells. Usually, such proliferation occurs in red bone marrow and is accompanied by production of monoclonal antibodies. Myeloma is the most common malignant primary bone tumor, accounting for 45% of all malignant bone tumors (MIRRA et al. 1989). The disease generally occurs in patients over 40 years of age, notably in the age group between 50 and 70 years (MIRRA et al. 1989, MULDER et al. 1993). However, we encountered myeloma in a 24-year-old patient (MULDER et al. 1993). Men are more often affected than women (MIRRA et al. 1989, MULDER et al.1993).

Myeloma usually affects the skeleton (MIRRA et al. 1989). According to the distribution of lesions over the skeleton, three types of myeloma are distinguished. The most common type is *multiple myeloma* (Kahler's disease), characterized by multifocal plasma cell proliferations. In *solitary myeloma*, the disease is limited to a single focus, and in *generalized myeloma* (myelomatosis), the disease has disseminated diffusely in bone (MIRRA et al. 1989). Especially in the spine, solitary myeloma often progresses to disseminated disease (KEMPIN and SUNDARESAN 1990). In all types of myeloma, proliferation of plasma cells preferentially occurs in red bone marrow, and consequentially myeloma occurs most of-

ten in the axial skeleton and the long bones, where red bone marrow is most abundant (MIRRA et al. 1989, MULDER et al. 1993). Within the spine, myeloma most frequently affects the lower thoracic and the lumbar vertebrae (ONOFRIO and SVIEN 1976). Initially, myeloma will preferentially occur in the vertebral body, without involvement of the posterior vertebral elements because of the lack of red bone marrow in the latter. However, with progression of the disease, red bone marrow will be present in the posterior elements due to reconversion, and consequentially, myeloma may also occur in these locations (KRICUN 1985). Myeloma may penetrate the cortical confines of the spinal canal and expand into the soft tissues. This may give rise to paravertebral and epidural soft tissue masses. The tumor may invade the dura, giving rise to cerebrospinal fluid spread, and cross the disc space (ST. AMOUR et al. 1994).

Clinical signs and symptoms in patients with myeloma result from destruction of bone, compromise of normal hematopoiesis, and production of abnormal proteins (MULDER et al. 1993). Systemic symptoms consist of malaise, fatigue, and weight loss; laboratory findings may be anemia, leukopenia, thrombocytopenia, and elevated monoclonal globulins in serum and urine. The most common symptom in patients with myeloma is pain, which usually occurs in the back (ONOFRIO and SVIEN 1976). In patients with back pain, narrowing of the spinal canal due to compression fracture of a vertebral body or epidural myeloma involvement is often encountered (RAHMOUNI et al. 1993a). After metastatic disease myeloma is the most frequent cause of paraplegia (ONOFRIO and SVIEN 1976).

Histologically, myelomatous tissue is highly cellular, and is composed of nodular to diffuse aggregates of plasma cells. Rarely, paramyloid and amyloid deposits are found.

Radiographically, several patterns are encountered in osseous myeloma: no abnormalities, osteoporosis in generalized myeloma, multiple osteolytic lesions in multiple myeloma, and a single osteolytic lesion in solitary myeloma. Infrequently, an osteosclerotic lesion is found in combination with osteolytic lesions (MULDER et al. 1993; ST. AMOUR et al. 1994). Osteoporosis in generalized myeloma cannot be distinguished from osteoporosis with other etiologies. The osteolytic lesions of myeloma typically have a "punched-out" appearance with clear, nonsclerotic borders (Fig. 5.7a). Less frequently, the borders are blurred. In general, CT or MRI are required to visualize these osteolytic lesions in the spine (MULDER et al. 1993). Destruction of cortical bone and formation of a new cortex may give rise to expansile lesions.

MRI is more sensitive than conventional imaging (plain radiography and CT) in detecting spinal myeloma. In a study by MOULOPOULOS and co-workers (1992), only 18% of the focal lesions detected by MRI were also detectable on conventional radiographs. In patients with newly diagnosed multiple myeloma, MRI detects bone marrow involvement in 69%-72% of cases (LIBSHITZ et al. 1992, MOULOPOULOS et al. 1992). Three patterns of bone marrow involvement have been described in MRI studies on multiple myeloma: focal lesions (in 45%), diffuse involvement (35%), and an inhomogeneous pattern of tiny lesions against a background of normal marrow (20%; MOULOPOULOS et al. 1992).

Focal lesions are typically hypointense relative to surrounding bone marrow on T1-weighted images and homogeneously hyperintense on T2-weighted and STIR images (MOULOPOULOS et al. 1992, RAHMOUNI et al. 1993a) (Fig. 5.7b). Less frequently, the lesions are iso- or hyperintense relative to the surrounding bone marrow (MOULOPOULOS et al. 1992, RAHMOUNI et al. 1993a). Upon administration of gadolinium focal lesions and soft tissue extensions enhance diffusely and avidly (MOULOPOULOS et al. 1992, 1994, RAHMOUNI et al. 1993a,b). More focal lesions are detected by T2-weighted spin-echo

and STIR images than by T1-weighted spin-echo and gradient-recalled-echo images (LIBSHITZ et al. 1992, MOULOPOULOS et al. 1992). When not combined with fat-suppression techniques, gadolinium masks 30% of focal lesions, because the lesions become isointense to uninvolved marrow (MOULOPOULOS et al. 1992).

The diffuse pattern reflecting total marrow replacement is characterized on T1-weighted images by homogeneously decreased signal intensity of marrow with the intervertebral discs iso- or hyperintense to the marrow (MOULOPOULOS et al. 1992). On T2-weighted images, the signal intensity of marrow is either iso- or hyperintense to muscle (LIBSHITZ et al. 1992). After administration of gadolinium, the involved marrow enhances diffusely and becomes hyperintense relative to the intervertebral discs. In normal adults, bone marrow enhancement is subtle and less intense than in the diffuse myeloma pattern (MOULOPOULOS et al. 1992). In the inhomogeneous pattern reflecting inhomogeneous marrow replacement, areas with signal characteristics as de

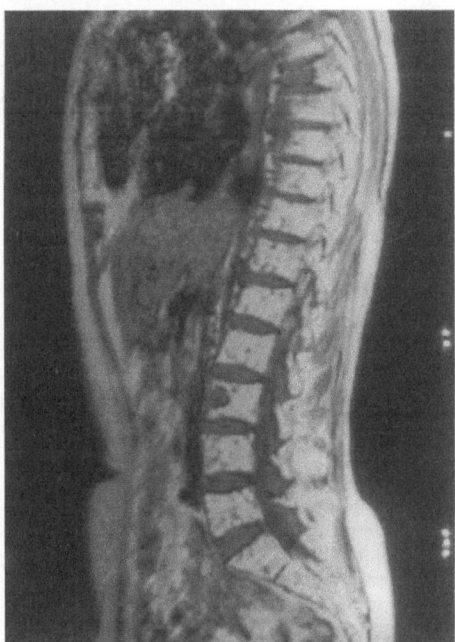

a   b

Fig. 5.7 a,b. Myeloma in 68-year-old man. a CT image at the level of L4 after injetion of intradural contrast agent. There is diffuse osteoporosis of the entire vertebra. The posterior margin of the corpus contains small punched-out lytic lesions secondary to the presence of plasmocytoma. b T1-weighted sagittal image. Throughout the entire vertebral column, small low-signal-intensity lesions representing multiple myeloma are visualized. There is a collapse of D7 with wedge deformity. The corpus of D7 has low signal intensity due to plasmocytoma. Another large lesion is seen in L3

scribed above are intermingled with areas of normal bone marrow characteristics (MOULOPOULOS et al. 1992).

The diffuse and inhomogeneous patterns are more difficult to recognize than the focal pattern, because they may be confused with normal bone marrow patterns (LIBSHITZ et al. 1992). The diffuse myeloma pattern is similar to the MRI pattern of abundant red bone marrow encountered in half of the normal population under the age of 20 (RICCI et al. 1990). The inhomogeneous pattern has to be differentiated from the MRI pattern of inhomogeneous distribution of red and yellow marrow found later in life (RICCI et al. 1990). For correct interpretation of the MRI findings in nonfocal myeloma, one should thus be aware of the bone marrow patterns in healthy subjects.

The main alternative to radiologic diagnosis of multiple myeloma lesions, notably in elder patients, is metastatic disease. In single lesions, the radiologic differential diagnosis of myeloma is: metastatic disease, chondroma, low-grade chondrosarcoma, giant cell tumor, fibrosarcoma, malignant fibrous histiocytoma, and lymphoma (MULDER et al. 1993).

Treatment for solitary myeloma consists of surgery or radiation therapy often administered in combination with systemic chemotherapy. In order to treat diffuse myeloma, radiation therapy and systemic chemotherapy may be applied (KEMPIN and SUNDARESAN 1990).

5.2.3.3
Lymphoma

Lymphomas are divided into *Hodgkin's disease* and *non-Hodgkin's lymphoma*. In both types of lymphoma, bone involvement is a common phenomenon with a frequency of 10%-25% in patients with Hodgkin's disease and an even higher frequency in non-Hodgkin's lymphoma (ST. AMOUR et al. 1994). In Hodgkin's disease, almost half of the skeletal lesions are located in the vertebrae (MULDER et al. 1993). In non-Hodgkin's lymphoma, the spine is less of a site of predilection, accounting for 7% of all skeletal lesions (MULDER et al. 1993). Apart from the osseous locations, spinal lymphoma can be located in the paravertebral and epidural soft tissues. Lymphoma constitutes 10%-30% of all spinal malignancies (GILBERT et al. 1978, RAO et al. 1982).

Several mechanisms have been described by which lymphoma involves the extradural spine. First, lymphoma may initially settle in paravertebral

lymph nodes and then invade the adjacent vertebral bodies and/or extend through the intervertebral foramina into the epidural space. Second, lymphoma may initially settle in the vertebral bone marrow; and third, lymphoma may first develop in the epidural space (LI et al. 1992; LYONS et al. 1992). At the time of diagnosis, spinal lymphoma may be limited to the initial site of occurrence or may have spread to one or more of the other spinal compartments. Within the epidural space, lymphoma may extend over long distances, covering several vertebral levels (LI et al. 1992). The dura acts as a realtive border to lymphoma spread. (ALBERTYN et al. 1992).

In Hodgkin's disease, osseous lymphoma localizations are regarded as the result of either hematogeneous spread or infiltration from the surrounding soft tissues. In addition to these mechanisms, osseous non-Hodgkin's lymphoma lesions may also be the first and only manifestation of the disease. Therefore a single osseous lesion in a patient suspected of having non-Hodgkin's lymphoma might imply stage I disease (a single primary bone lesion) or stage IV disease (secondary bone involvement). Careful examination of these patients is thus required in order to differentiate between these stages (ALBERTYN et al. 1992; ST. AMOUR et al. 1994).

The risk of spinal involvement of lymphoma is cord or cauda equina compression. Spinal cord compression is reported in 0.1%-10.2% of patients with non-Hodgkin`s lymphoma (LYONS et al. 1992). Most often, compression results from epidural lymphoma localizations, rather than from pathologic vertebral compression fractures (GOLDHAHN and GOLDHAHN 1976).

Histologically, lymphomatous tissue is highly cellular. Hemorrhage and necrosis are often present. Depending on the subtype of lymphoma, more or less fibrosis is found (MIRRA et al. 1989; MULDER et al. 1993).

On radiologic examination, spinal lymphoma is apparent in the shape of soft tissue masses and/or osseous lesions. The sensitivity of plain films to soft tissue masses in spinal lymphoma is as low as 6% and 30% to bony abnormalities (ALBERTYN et al. 1992). Paraspinal soft tissue masses, especially those at the toracic level, can be visible on plain films. However, CT and MRI are better equipped to detect paraspinal masses and masses occuring in the spinal canal. On CT, these soft tissue masses are homogeneous without any evidence of calcifications (BERES et al. 1986). In the paraspinal location, lymphoma may appear as conglomerate node masses, but also, more subtly, as "perivertebral collars" (ALBERTYN et al.

1992). The latter are characterized on CT by a smooth layer of soft tissue parallelling part or all of the anterior curvature of vertebral bodies. On MRI, the signal intensity of lymphomatous tissue on T1-weighted images is lower than or equal to that of muscle, and moderately to markedly hyperintense on T2-weighted images (LI et al. 1992; ST. AMOUR et al. 1994) (Fig. 5.8). Consequently, lymphoma locali-zations in epidural and paravertebral locations contrast with the surrounding fat.

In lymphoma, osseous lesions may be the result of pressure or invasion from adjacent lymph nodes (MULDER et al. 1993). Such lesions occur frequently on the anterior and lateral aspects of the vertebral bodies. However, osseous lesions may also arise from the bone. In Hodgkin's disease, these lesions often

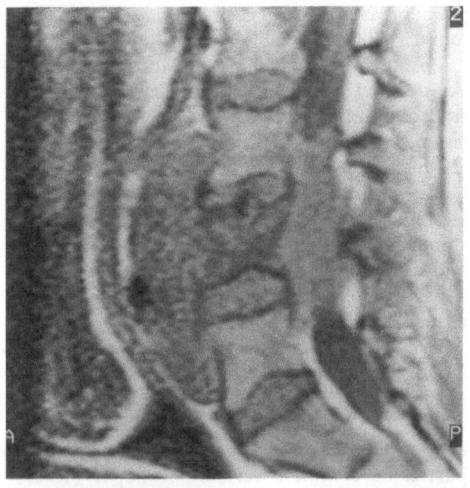

a

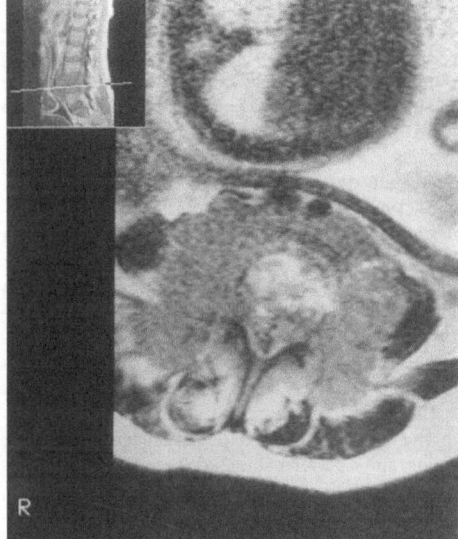

b

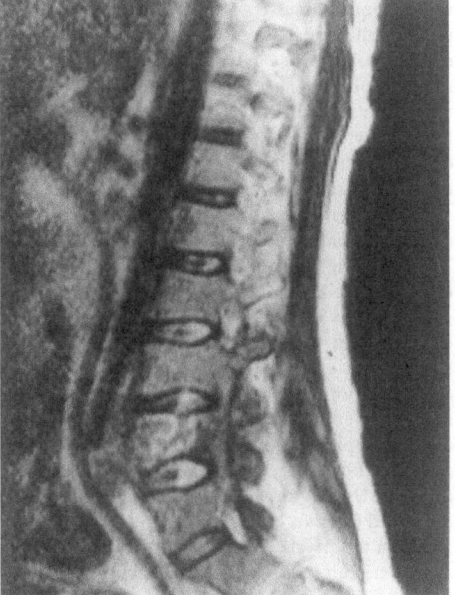

c

Fig. 5.8 a-c. Lymphoma. A 27-year-old gravida presented with severe pain secondary to a lesion in L4, allowing only short acquisition times. a Precontrast sagittal T1-weighted image shows low-signal-intensity lesion in the corpus L4. There is a marked paravertebal soft tissue mass dorsally extending into the spinal canal. b Precontrast tranverse imafe at the level of L4 shows extensive paravertebral tumor extension. c Postcontrast T1-weighted sagittal image shows inhomogeneous enhancement of the osseus part of the tumor

c

have a malignant aspect and can be purely osteolytic (30%), osteosclerotic (10%), such as in "ivory vertebra", or both lytic and sclerotic (60%). Bony changes may be apparent as multiple confluent, small lucencies or as large geographic lesions. The cortex is often eroded and may be expanded, but a periosteal reaction is mainly absent (MULDER et al. 1993). In non-Hodgkin's lymphoma, most osseous lesions also have a malignant aspect radiographically. Compared to Hodgkin's disease, fewer cases have a mixed lytic-sclerotic or purely sclerotic aspect: 78% of lesions are purely lytic. The pattern is frequently permeative or moth-eaten. Cortical bone is usually affected, and a periosteal reaction is found in two thirds of cases. In both types of lymphoma, soft tissue extension from the bone is often found, and usually does not contain calcifications (MULDER et al. 1993). On MRI examination, osseous lymphoma localizations have a lower signal intensity on T1-weighted images and a homogeneous higher or inhomogeneous high and similar signal intensity on T2-weighted images, compared to normal bone marrow (LI et al. 1992). The osseous lesions may be apparent as nodular vertebral lesions, or they may affect whole vertebrae (LI et al.1992).

The radiologic differential diagnosis of lymphoma is extensive and depends on age and specific radiographic pattern. It includes eosinophilic granuloma, metastatic disease, myeloma, Ewing's sarcoma, osteosarcoma, fibrosarcoma, malignant fibrous histiocytoma, and Paget's disease (MULDER et al. 1993).

Therapeutic options for spinal lymphoma localizations are radiation therapy and chemotherapy (HARMON 1990).

5.2.3.4
Eosinophilic Granuloma

Eosinophilic granuloma is the most common expression of a disease complex that is known as "histiocytosis X" or "Langerhans' cell histiocytosis" (MIRRA et al. 1989, MULDER et al. 1993). This disease complex is characterized by proliferation of the histiocytes of the reticuloendothelial system by unknown causes (MIRRA et al. 1989). In eosinophilic granuloma, the course of disease is benign and the lesions are usually restricted to bone, with foci in other organs rarely occurring. In the two other variants of the disease, the lesions are disseminated. Letterer-Siwe syndrome is the disseminated acute form of histiocytosis X, which often has a rapidly fatal course, and Hand-Schüller-Christian syndrome is

the disseminated chronic form (MIRRA et al. 1989).

Most patients affected by eosinophilic granuloma are 1-15 years of age, although patients as old as 62 have been described (MIRRA et al. 1989, MULDER et al. 1993). The median age is 10 years. The disease occurs twice as often in males as in females (MIRRA et al. 1989, MULDER et al. 1993). Approximately 4% of all primary spinal bone tumors other than hemangioma and hematologic diseases are eosinophilic granulomas, and 7% of eosinophilic granulomas are found in the spine (Table 5.3).

Eosinophilic granuloma mainly occurs in the skeleton and is only infrequently accompanied by lesions in other organs (TOMITA 1990). In the skeleton, lesions may be solitary or multiple. Multiple lesions are relatively frequent in the spine. In the spine, lesions are most frequently located at the thoracic level and less frequently in the lumbar and cervical spine (MULDER et al. 1993). Within a vertebra, the body is a site of predilection for eosinophilic granuloma, yet the lesion may also occur in the posterior elements (Mulder et al. 1993).

Usually, eosinophilic granuloma is a self-limited disease, and the lesions may heal spontaneously (GREENFIELD 1980, JAFFE et al. 1985). Nevertheless, during growth of the lesion complications may occur. Spinal eosinophilic granulomas often give rise to partial or complete vertebral collapse (TOMITA 1990). In children, eosinophilic granuloma is the most frequent cause of "vertebra plana", a completely collapsed, flattened vertebral corpus (MIRRA et al. 1989, MULDER et al. 1993, TOMITA 1990). Due to spontaneous regeneration of osseous structures that may occur regardless of therapy, these collapsed vertebrae may completely recover their height (NESBIT et al. 1969, VILLAS et al. 1993). This potential for healing is greatest in young children (TOMITA 1990).

Patients with eosinophilic granuloma of the spine most commonly present with localized pain (TOMITA 1990). Although vertebral collapses are frequent, neurologic deficits are rare (TOMITA 1990). Duration of symptoms is usually short with a reported median duration of 1-2 months (MULDER et al. 1993).

On gross examination, eosinophilic granulomas are soft lesions. Microscopically, the lesions contain sheets of benign histiocytes as well as eosinophilic and neutrophilic granulocytes, lymphocytes, plasma cells, and fibroblasts (MIRRA et al. 1989, MULDER et al. 1993). Usually, areas of hemorrhage and necrosis are found (MIRRA et al. 1989).

When an affected vertebra has not collapsed, the characteristic radiographic appearance of eosinophilic granuloma is one of an osteolytic lesion with clear, smooth margins (KRICUN 1993, MULDER 1993). These margins may be sclerotic. Regular destruction of cortical bone tends to be present with an uninterrupted laminated periosteal reaction (MULDER et al. 1993). In one fourth of cases, the tumor margin is ill-defined and ragged (MULDER et al. 1993). When an affected vertebra has collapsed, the adjoining intervertebral spaces typically maintain their height (KRICUN 1993, MULDER et al. 1993, NESBIT et al. 1969). Cord compression is rare, even in advanced stages of vertebral collapse (GREEN et al. 1980). Although most frequently absent, moderate epidural or paravertebral soft tissue swelling may be present (JOHNSON et al. 1993; MIRRA et al. 1989; MULDER et al. 1993). The lesion and its soft tissue extensions may enhance upon intravenous administration of contrast medium (PRENGER 1991, STULL et al. 1992). The MR appearance of eosinophilic granuloma is relatively constant (BELTRAN et al. 1993, DE SCHEPPER et al. 1993, HAGGSTROM et al. 1988, PRENGER 1991). The lesions demonstrate intermediate to high signal intensity on T1-weighted images, and high to extremely high signal intensity on T2-weighted images. Marked enhancement occurs upon administration of gadolinium (DE SCHEPPER et al. 1993, VERSTRAETE et al. 1994). This area may be surrounded by a low signal intensity rim. Outside this focal abnormality, rather diffuse, ill-defined reactive changes of the bone marrow may be visible as reduced signal intensity on T1-weighted images and increased signal intensity on T2-weighted images. The surrounding soft tissues may also show edema or involvement of the lesion. As compared to CT, MRI is superior in demonstrating bone marrow involvement, soft tissue extension, and dura mater involvement (DE SCHEPPER et al. 1993).

Since eosinophilic granuloma is a self-limited disease, once it is diagnosed, treatment may consist of bed rest followed by external immobilization (TOMITA 1990, VILLAS et al. 1993). Other therapeutic options are local injection with corticosteroids, surgical curettage, and chemotherapy (MULDER et al. 1993). In the case of progressive neural compression, low-dose irradiation might be applied (GREEN et al. 1980, TOMITA 1990).

The osseous lesions in Hand-Schüller-Christian syndrome are radiologically similar to those in eosinophilic granuloma, except that the lesions are larger and involve multiple bones (MIRRA et al. 1989). In Letterer-Siwe syndrome, all bones are affected with countless miniscule lesions that are either invisible on radiographic examination or become apparant as osteopenia or multiple osteolytic lesions and periosteal reactions (MIRRA et al. 1989).

The radiographic differential diagnosis of eosinophilic granuloma is extensive and can be better specified according to the specific radiographic aspect of the lesion and the patient's age. It includes aneurysmal bone cyst, Ewing's sarcoma, lymphoma, metastatic disease, myeloma, fibrosarcoma, and malignant fibrous histiocytoma (MULDER et al. 1993).

5.2.3.5
Ewing's Sarcoma

Ewing's sarcoma is a highly malignant primary bone tumor. Its tissue of origin is believed to be primitive skeletal mesenchyme or supporting reticular cells (MIRRA et al. 1989). The tumor usually affects children and young adults: in a series of 36 patients with primary Ewing's sarcoma of the spine, the mean age was 17 years (GRUBB et al. 1994). The tumor may be found incidentally in older patients (MULDER et al. 1993). The lesion has a predilection for male patients (M:F = 3.2; MULDER et al. 1993). Approximately 6% of Ewing's sarcoma affect the axial skeleton (Table 5.3). Ewing's sarcomas represent about 6% of spinal tumors and more than 8% of sacral tumors other than hemangioma and hematologic diseases (Table 5.3).

Ewing's sarcoma has a predilection for the lumbar spine and sacrum (BRADWAY and PRITCHARD 1990). Within the vertebrae, the tumor has a preference for the vertebral body, but it may also occur in the posterior elements (KRICUN 1993, MULDER et al. 1993).

As a primary bone tumor Ewing's sarcoma originates within the bone. The tumor rapidly spreads through the marrow spaces, initially without destruction of the trabeculae (MIRRA et al. 1989). Only rarely, the tumor extends to adjacent vertebrae (KRICUN 1993). In addition to intraosseous spread, the tumor has a propensity to extend via the cortical vascular channels into the periosseous soft tissues (BRADWAY and PRITCHARD 1990). Consequently soft tissue extension may exist without extensive cortical bone destruction (MULDER et al. 1993). Soft tissue extension has been reported in up to 90% of Ewing's sarcomas and may be of considerable size at the time of diagnosis (MIRRA et al. 1989, MULDER et al. 1993). In the spine, these soft tissue masses may be located in the epidural and/or paravertebral space, in the sacrum, the soft tissue component may extend into the pelvis (KRICUN 1993). The tumor's soft tissue component may compromise neural structures.

The average time between onset of symptoms and diagnosis in patients with spinal Ewing's sarcoma is

8 months (BRADWAY and PRITCHARD 1990). In these patients, pain near the tumor is an almost invariable finding. Other signs and symptoms are related to compromise of nerve roots and spinal cord. Fever and a palpable mass are each found in one fourth of patients (BRADWAY and PRITCHARD 1990). Constitutional findings such as weight loss, anorexia, and fatigue are also frequent (SHARAFFUDDIN et al. 1992).

On gross examination, Ewing's sarcoma of the spine is a soft tumor with a semisolid or gelatinous consistency (BRADWAY and PRITCHARD 1990). Often, these tumors are vascular and prone to bleeding (BRADWAY and PRITCHARD 1990). Areas of necrosis and hemorrhage are a frequent finding (MIRRA et al. 1989). Microscopically, the tumor is highly cellular and consists of sheets of monotonous malignant round cells (MIRRA et al. 1989). The tumor cells do not produce an intercellular matrix (MULDER et al. 1993).

On radiographic examination, the tumor usually has malignant characteristics (MULDER et al. 1993). The most common radiographic appearance of Ewing's sarcoma is an ill-defined osteolytic lesion with irregular destruction of cortical bone and interrupted periosteal new bone formation (MULDER et al. 1993). Less frequently, the lesion shows both osteolysis and osteosclerosis, or only osteosclerosis (MULDER et al. 1993). Disc space narrowing and occasionally widening of the disc space have been described (WEINSTEIN et al. 1984). The lesion may spread to adjacent vertebral bodies (WEINSTEIN et al. 1984). Usually, evidence of a soft tissue mass is found, and partial or complete vertebral collapse may occur. In general, the soft tissue mass shows no signs of calcification or ossification (MULDER et al. 1993), although exceptions to this rule may occur (WEINSTEIN et al. 1984). The most accurate assessment of the intra- and extraosseous extent of the tumor may be made by MRI. The tumor has decreased signal intensity on T1-weighted images, and increased signal intensity on T2-weighted images (BOYKO et al. 1987, ST. AMOUR et al. 1994). Enhancement of the lesion occurs after intravenous administration of gadolinium (VERSTRAETE et al. 1994).

The differential diagnosis based on the radiographic presentation includes osteosarcoma, chondrosarcoma, fibrosarcoma, malignant fibrous histiocytoma, lymphoma, bone metastases of neuroblastoma, chordoma, and eosinophilic granuloma (MULDER et al. 1993).

Treatment for spinal Ewing's sarcoma includes three modalities: surgery, radiation, and combination chemotherapy (BRADWAY and PRITCHARD 1990, GRUBB et al. 1994, SHARAFFUDDIN et al. 1992). Preoperative angiography and embolization of tumor vasculature have been advocated (SHARAFFUDDIN et al. 1992). The 5-year survival rate for primary spinal Ewing's sarcoma is 33% (GRUBB et al. 1994).

5.2.4
Tumors of Embryonal Rests

5.2.4.1
Chordoma

Chordomas are slowly growing, low-grade malignancies arising from remnants of the embryonic notochord. Chordomas may occur at any age but usually affect older patients (median age 58 years; (MULDER et al. 1993). Men are affected more often than women (BJORNSSON et al. 1993, MIRRA et al. 1989, MULDER et al. 1993). Due to their notochordal origin, chordomas are usually localized in the axial skeleton. Some 48%-60% of the lesions have been reported to occur in the sacrum, 25%-39% in the region of the clivus, and 15%-13% in the remaining spine (BJORNSSON et al. 1993, MIRRA et al. 1989, STEPHENS and SCHWARTZ 1993). Chordomas represent 8% of spinal tumors and 27% of sacral tumors other than hemangioma and hematologic diseases (Table 5.3). Occasionally, chordomas may arise in soft tissues such as the epidural space (SEBAG et al. 1993).

Due to the slow growth of chordomas, signs and symptoms develop insidiously over months or years. The clinical picture depends on the location and spread of the tumor, but may include pain, evidence of a mass lesion, and neurologic, bladder, and bowel dysfunction (MIRRA et al. 1989, STEPHENS and SCHWARTZ 1993).

Macroscopically, a chordoma is a finely encapsulated, lobulated, mucogelatinous tumor (MIRRA et al. 1989). Within the tumor, foci of hemorrhage, necrosis, cystification, and calcification may occur (MIRRA et al. 1989). Besides their cellular components, chordomas contain pools of mucinous substances and an extracellular matrix that is myxoid to chondroid. On microscopy, the tumor capsule is usually infiltrated and tumor growth is found in the surrounding tissues (MIRRA et al. 1989).

Chordomas tend to arise in the midline of the distal sacrum from S4 and S5 (HIGINBOTHAM et al. 1967). In this location, the tumor generally extends beyond the boundaries of the bone, usually anteriorly into the pelvis, and only infrequently posteriorly (MIRRA et al. 1989). Spread into the sacroiliac ligaments and compression of the nerve roots of the cauda may occur (MIRRA et al. 1989). Chordomas can occur at any level of the spine, although the cervical (48%) and the lumbar (35%) region are more often affected than the thoracic spine (17%; BJORNSSON et al. 1993). Spinal chordomas usually arise in the midline of the vertebral body and incidentally in the posterior elements (ABDELWAHAB et al. 1986, KRICUN 1993). Within the bone, expansion may occur to the posterior elements (KRICUN 1993; MULDER et al. 1993). Although the intervertebral disc is usually spared, invasion of the disc and extension to adjacent vertebrae, which is an exceptional phenomenon for bone tumors, have been reported in chordomas (DE BRUÏNE and KROON 1988, FIROOZNIA et al. 1976, KRICUN 1993; MULDER et al. 1993). Finally, the tumor often expands into the epidural space, giving rise to cord compression, and into the prevertebral soft tissues.

On roentgen examinations, most chordomas have a lytic appearance, although sclerosis may be prominent especially in vertebral chordomas (DE BRUÏNE and KROON 1988, MULDER et al. 1993). Sclerosis may occur at the periphery of the lesion as scattered foci throughout an otherwise lytic lesion, or diffusely inside the lesion (ABDELWAHAB et al. 1986, MULDER et al. 1993). The latter may even give rise to an ivory vertebra appearance (DE BRUÏNE and KROON 1988, MULDER et al. 1993). The marginal pattern of chordoma may be geographic with a sclerotic rim (KRICUN 1993), but usually the pattern is motheaten or permeative (MULDER et al. 1993). Calcification of the tumor matrix is found on plain films in 14%-50% of cases , and in up to 90% of cases on CT (KRICUN 1993 , KROL et al. 1983; SMITH et al. 1987). The soft tissue component of the lesion often has a sharply defined margin due to a fibrous pseudocapsule (MIRRA et al. 1989). On CT, the bulk of the tumor has a density similar to muscle (OOT et al. 1988). In addition, the tumor may show areas of low attenuation representing its myxoid, gelatinous, or semiliquid components (MEYER et al. 1984, MIRRA et al. 1989). Usually, enhancement occurs (OOT et al. 1988). On MRI, chordomas also tend to have a heterogeneous appearance. On T1-weighted images, signal intensity is usually low to intermediate (ROSENTHAL et al. 1985, ST. AMOUR et al. 1994, SZE et al. 1988) (Fig. 5.9a). Areas of high signal intensity on these images may represent intratumoral hemorrhage or chondroid matrix (SZE et al. 1988). On T2-weighted images, chordomas are hyperintense, re-

flecting the histologic similarity of the tumor to the nucleus pulposus (ROSENTHAL et al. 1985, SZE et al. 1988) (Fig.5.9b). Lower signal intensity on T2-weighted images and higher signal intensity on T1-weighted images may be encountered when chondroid matrix is present (MULDER et al. 1993). Low signal septations have been described in sacral chordomas on T2-weighted images (ST. AMOUR et al. 1994, SZE et al. 1988). Calcifications may be apparent as areas of low signal intensity (SZE et al. 1988). Upon administration of gadolinium, an aspecific pattern of enhancement occurs. The cellular components of the tumor enhance, in contrast to chondroid components. On angiographic examination sacral, chordomas are often avascular, whereas on other locations they may show up as vascular lesions (FIROOZNIA et al. 1976, SMITH et al. 1987, ST. AMOUR et al. 1994).

The radiologic differential diagnosis of chordoma includes metastatic disease, myeloma, lymphoma, giant cell tumor, aneurysmal bone cyst, chondroma, well-differentiated chondrosarcoma, and nerve sheath tumors (MULDER et al. 1993).

The treatment of chordomas consists primarily of surgical excision (SUNDARESAN et al. 1990). Radical excision may be curative, but due to their critical axial location and tendency to infiltrate their surroundings, radical excision of chordomas is often impossible and the recurrence rate is high. In cases where radical excision is not feasible, partial resection may be combined with radiation therapy (SUNDARESAN et al. 1990). Overall, 70%-80% of patients die within 5-10 years, usually as a consequence of recurrences (MIRRA et al. 1989). Metastases to lung, liver, muscle, bone, and skin may occur late in the course of disease, especially after recurrence (MIRRA et al. 1989, SUNDARESAN et al. 1990).

5.2.4.2
Teratoma

Teratomas consist of tissues that are foreign to the anatomic site they arise from, and they contain tissues from at least two germinal layers (KESLAR et al. 1994). Such tumors are the result of growth of a primitive totipotential cell (KESLAR et al. 1994). Most frequently, these lesions occur in the sacrococcygeal region, where they typically arise in the midline from the tissues around the tip of the coccyx. Four types of lesions that differ histologically are referred to as sacrococcygeal teratomas: (1) mature teratomas, (2) immature teratomas, containing embryonic elements, (3) mixed malignant teratomas, con-

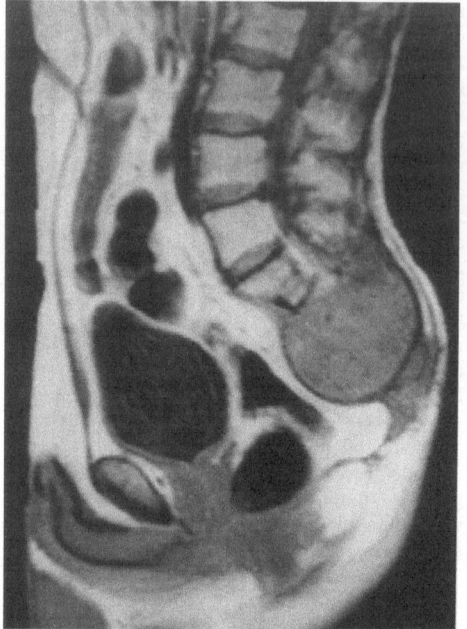
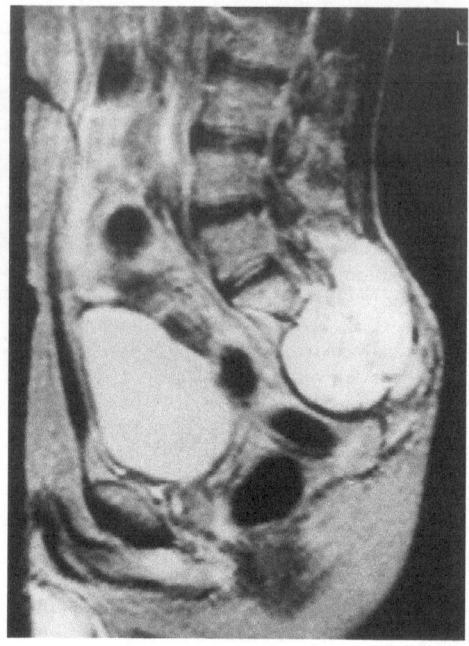

a

b

Fig. 5.9 a,b. Chordoma in a 50-year-old man with lower back pain progressing over a period of many years. **a** T1-weighted sagittal image of the sacrum shows a large, low to intermediate-signal-intensity tumor of the sacrum with significant soft tissue extension. The tumor is well delineated. **b** T2-weighted sagittal image corresponding to a shows high signal intensity, representing the mucinous character of the tumor

taining elements of endodermal sinus tumor in addition to mature or immature teratoma, and (4) pure endodermal sinus tumors. The first two are benign, the latter two malignant (KESLAR et al. 1994). Sporadically, teratomas may occur elsewhere in the spinal canal (KESLAR et al. 1994; POST and McCORMICK 1990, RUSSELL and RUBINSTEIN 1989).

Sacrococcygeal teratomas are the most frequent primary tumors of the sacrococcygeal region in children (POST and McCORMICK 1990, WERNER and TAYBI 1970). Mostly these tumors are identified at birth, although patients may present in adulthood. Females are affected four times as frequently as males. Eighteen percent of patients with sacrococcygeal teratomas have other congenital malformations, such as spinal dysraphism and sacral agenesis (KESLAR et al. 1994). Sacrococcygeal teratomas have been classified into four types according to their anatomic location. Type 1 lesions are predominantly external, type 2 lesions manifest externally but have considerable intrapelvic extension, type 3 lesions are externally apparent, but most of the lesion is located

intrapelvicly or intra-abdominally, and type 4 lesions are located completely presacrally without external manifestation (KESLAR et al. 1994). About 30% of sacrococcygeal teratomas are malignant, demonstrating infiltration into their environment (DOMELAN and SWENSON 1968). At presentation, malignant teratomas have distant metastases, to lung, liver, or bone, in 15% of cases (DOMELAN and SWENSON 1968; POST and McCORMICK 1990). Malignancy is more common in older patients, in males, and in the case of presacral expansion. The more solid the tumor, the more likely it is to be malignant (KESLAR et al. 1994; POST and McCORMICK 1990; SZE and TWOHIG 1991).

In contrast to sacrococcygeal teratomas, intraspinal teratomas may present at any age (NAIDICH et al. 1983a). The following conditions have been reported as associated anomalies: scoliosis, spina bifida, block vertebrae, and diastematomyelia (NAIDICH et al. 1983a). Spinal teratomas are most often encountered in the cervical region and at the thoracolumbar junction (SMOKER et al. 1986). Their location may be intramedullary, intradural-extra-medullary, or extradural. In all cases they tend to occur dorsally or dorsolaterally in the spinal canal (NAIDICH et al. 1983a).

Macroscopically, teratomas are encapsulated masses that contain both solid and cystic elements in 62% of cases. Mature teratomas may contain fat, cartilage, bone, hair, and other elements and tend to be more cystic. In contrast, immature teratomas generally tend to be more solid and are more prone to hemorrhage and central necrosis. Endodermal sinus tumors are usually solid lesions with cystic, mucoid, hemorrhagic, and necrotic areas. All lesions often contain calcifications and may be very vascular (KESLAR et al. 1994; POST and MCCORMICK 1990; RUSSELL and RUBINSTEIN 1989, SZE and TWOHIG 1991).

In sacrococcygeal teratomas, plain films may show an intrapelvic or external soft tissue mass. In up to 60% of cases, calcifications are seen in the solid portions of this mass (MOAZAM and TALBERT 1985). In benign teratomas, the sacrum may be eroded due to pressure, but true destruction of the sacrum is a sign of malignancy (KESLAR et al. 1994). In spinal teratomas, widening of the spinal canal may be found, which may be accompanied by a spinal block on myelography. On CT, teratomas frequently appear as heterogeneous lesions, in which cystic areas, fat, calcifications, and ossifications may be identified (KESLAR et al. 1994). Notably, the presence of combined fat and bone within the lesion is suggestive of the diagnosis (MONAJATI et al. 1986). On MRI, teratomas also have an inhomogeneous appearance. The cysts may have signal intensities similar to cerebrospinal fluid unless they are hemorrhagic or otherwise rich in proteinaceous material, which may make them appear more similar to the solid portions of the tumor (ENZMANN and DE LA PAZ 1990). Calcifications may not be visible on MRI. The presence of fat in the tumor, however, may be demonstrated by chemical shift artifact or by the effects of fat suppression techniques. On MRI, the combination of cysts and fat is suggestive of the diagnosis (ENZMANN and DE LA PAZ 1990). MRI is superior to CT in assessing of intraspinal extension of the tumor (KESLAR et al. 1994). On both CT and MRI, the solid parts of the tumor enhance after administration of contrast medium (SZE and TWOHIG 1991).

The radiographic differential diagnosis of spinal teratomas includes cavernous hemangioma, meningioma, nerve sheath tumors, lipoma, epidermoid, dermoid, other cystic epidural lesions, epidural abscess, and epidural hemorrhage. The differential di-agnosis of sacrococcygeal teratoma includes presacral sarcomas, anterior meningocele, nerve sheath tumors, and, more generally, metastatic disease, myeloma, chordoma, giant cell tumor, aneurysmal bone cyst, and osteoblastoma.

Treatment of benign and malignant teratomas consists of surgical excision. In malignant teratomas, surgery may be followed by radiation therapy and combination chemotherapy (POST and MCCORMICK 1990).

5.2.4.3
Neuroblastoma, Ganglioneuroblastoma, and Ganglioneuroma

Neuroblastoma, ganglioneuroblastoma, and ganglioneuroma are tumors that arise from the primitive neural crest cells that form the adrenal medulla and paravertebral sympathic chain in normal embryonal development. Of these tumors, neuroblastoma is the most primitive and malignant, whereas ganglioneuroma is the most mature and benign. Usually, these tumors arise in the adrenal medulla or the paravertebral tissues (RUSSELL and RUBINSTEIN 1989). Since they frequently expand to the spinal canal, they are discussed in this chapter.

Neuroblastoma is the most common solid malignancy of children, excluding CNS tumors, most often affecting children younger than 5 years of age (DIETRICH et al. 1987; SIEGEL et al. 1986). Thirteen percent of neuroblastomas have intraspinal extension, and in addition, these tumors may originate in or metastasize to the epidural space (SIEGEL et al. 1986). Consequently, neuroblastoma is the most common malignant tumor in the spinal canal in children under 4 years of age (ROVIRA 1991). Ganglioneuroblastoma and ganglioneuroma tend to occur later in childhood, predominantly affecting children between 5 and 8 years of age (HARWOOD-NASH and FITZ 1976). The paravertebral variants of these tumors also have a propensity to grow into the spinal canal through the spinal foramina and, occasionally, may be located exclusively within the spinal canal (LJUN et al. 1984).

Most frequently, spinal involvement occurs at the thoracic and lumbar spinal levels (PUNT et al. 1980). Only occasionally is the cervical level involved. Often, the paravertebral tumor expands to the epidural space through more than one neural foramen (DAVID et al. 1989; SIEGEL et al. 1986). Within the spinal canal, the tumor may spread over several spinal levels and compress the cord at a distance from the location of the paravertebral mass (HARWOOD-NASH and FITZ 1976). Extension of neuroblastoma growth through the dura has been reported (HARWOOD-NASH and FITZ 1976). The compromise of neural structures in the foramina and spinal canal may give rise to various clinical pictures.

Histologically, neuroblastomas, ganglioneuroblastomas, and ganglioneuromas are cellular lesions. In neuroblastomas, these cells are primitive and undifferentiated; ganglioneuroblastomas contain a mixture of mature and undifferentiated cell populations, whereas ganglioneuromas are composed of mature cells. Hemorrhage and necrosis as well as calcifications may be present (RUSSELL and RUBINSTEIN 1989).

Plain radiographs may display widening of vertebral foramina and the spinal canal as well as erosion of pedicles, vertebral bodies, and ribs (BALAKRISHNAN et al. 1974; PUNT et al. 1980; RESJO et al. 1979). Calcifications are found in 55% of abdominal and 25% of thoracic neuroblastomas (BOUSVAROS et al. 1986). At CT and MRI examination, the characteristic picture of a paravertebral tumor with intraspinal extension through one or more foramina is often found. On CT, neuroblastomas are often inhomogeneous lesions with soft tissue density that in most cases demonstrate calcifications (BOUSVAROS et al. 1986; DAVID et al. 1989). On MRI, neuroblastomas and ganglioneuroblastomas show low to intermediate signal intensity on T1-weighted images and high signal intensity on T2-weighted images (DAVID et al. 1989; DIETRICH and KANGARLOO 1986; DIETRICH et al. 1987; ROVIRA 1991; SIEGEL et al. 1986). These lesions may be inhomogeneous due to necrosis, hemorrhage, and the presence of calcifications. Areas of necrosis have low signal intensity on T1- weighted images and high intensity on T2-weighted images. Calcifications are depicted as areas of signal void. The signal intensity of hemorrhage varies, according to its age, from low on T1- and T2-weighted images in the acute stage via high on T1- and low on T2-weighted images in the subacute stage to high on both sequences later on (SZE and TWOHIG 1991). Upon intravenous administration of gadolinium, these tumors usually enhance.

The differential diagnosis of paraspinal tumors with spine involvement includes lymphoma, retroperitoneal sarcomas, and renal cell and lung carcinoma.

Depending on the stage of disease, treatment for neuroblastomas and ganglioneuroblastomas consists of surgery, chemotherapy, and/or radiation. In the case of ganglioneuromas, the treatment of choice is surgery (TOMITA 1990).

5.2.5
Vascular Tumors

5.2.5.1
Vertebral Hemangioma

Hemangiomas are a benign vascular proliferation of thin-walled vessels (MIRRA et al. 1989) and are considered a hamartomatous rather than a neoplastic condition. Hemangiomas are the most frequently encountered neoplasms of the spine with an estimated incidence of 11% in the general population (SCHMORL 1971). The lesions have a slight predilection for females, and although they may occur at any time of life, the incidence increases with age (SCHMORL 1971). In one third of cases, hemangiomas of the spine are multiple (SCHMORL 1971). The most common spinal locations of hemangiomas are the thoracic and lumbar levels (SCHMORL 1971). In the cervical spine, these lesions are only rarely found (KRICUN 1993). Usually, hemangiomas develop in the vertebral body, 10%-15% of them showing concomitant involvement of the posterior elements (YOCHUM et al. 1993). Rarely, the lesion is located only within the posterior elements (YOCHUM et al.1993).

Histologically, hemangiomas consist of a network of vessels lined with endothelium, filled with blood, and separated from each other by a stroma containing fibrous and adipose tissue. These vessels may have small calibers, in the capillary variant of hemangioma, or feature larger lumina of up to 1 cm, in the cavernous variant. The cellular variant has extremely high cellularity and contains relatively few conspicuous vascular lumina (MIRRA et al. 1989). Within the bone, hemangiomas replace bone marrow and erode trabecular and sometimes cortical bone. As a result, the remaining trabeculae, which are subjected to increased stress, grow thicker (MIRRA et al. 1989). Since hemangiomas follow the path of blood vessels, and blood vessels penetrate the bony boundaries, hemangiomas may expand outside the bony boundaries into the epidural space and paraspinal soft tissues (MIRRA et al. 1989). Hemangiomas may even expand into adjacent bones such as ribs (HUVOS 1991).

After initial development, most hemangiomas stabilize in growth and even regress. These lesions remain asymptomatic or are associated with non-specific low back pain, and may be revealed as an incidental finding (YOCHUM et al. 1993). However, hemangiomas may also progress (MIRRA et al. 1989) and give rise to symptoms. Signs and symptoms may result from compression of the myelum or nerve roots. These structures may be compressed in the spinal canal or a vertebral foramen due to expansion of vertebral bone, extension of hemangioma into the epidural space, pathologic compression fracture of a vertebral body, or hemorrhage (KRICUN 1993; YOCHUM et al. 1993).

On plain films, vertebral hemangiomas often have a characteristic appearance (KRICUN 1993; MULDER et al. 1993). Usually, the lesions are lytic and have a geographic pattern. The thickening of the remaining trabeculae may give rise to characteristic vertical striations, which run in a craniocaudal orientation and have been described as having the appearance of prison bars or a honeycomb (KRICUN 1993; MULDER et al. 1993; ROSS et al. 1987; YOCHUM et al. 1993). However, coarse trabeculation may be absent in hemangiomas and lesions may be entirely lytic. In extensive lesions with cortical involvement, periosteal reaction may give rise to formation of a new uninterrupted shell of cortical bone (MULDER et al. 1993). This results in expansile lesions. In contrast to Paget's disease, coarse trabeculation in hemangiomas is not accompanied by cortical thickening (KRICUN 1993). Hemangiomas may present as vertebral compression fractures.

In addition to the osseous reaction to vertebral hemangioma apparent on plain films, CT may detect the lesion itself (LAREDO et al. 1990; ROSS et al. 1987; SCHNYDER et al. 1986; YOCHUM et al. 1993). (Fig. 5.10 a). The lesion may have soft tissue or fat characteristics on CT. On CT, detection of the degree of involvement of vertebrae and involvement of soft tissues is superior as compared to plain films. Hemangiomas may enhance after intravenous administration of contrast medium (LAREDO et al. 1990). At selective angiography, the findings vary from normal to distinct hypervascularization. The latter is characterized by dense staining of the lesion during the arterial and parenchymatous phases, which may persist late into the venous phase. Feeding arteries may be dilated, and typically no early draining veins are appreciated (LAREDO et al. 1990; ROSS et al.1987).

On MRI, vertebral hemangiomas are frequently encountered. They tend to be well-circumscribed lesions with a rounded appearance when not abutting on the cortex. (Fig 5.10b, c).The lesions are often heterogeneous (LAREDO et al. 1990; ROSS et al. 1987). Areas of high signal intensity on both T1- and T2-weighted images are intermingled with spots of low signal intensity, which may give the lesions a mottled appearance (LAREDO et al. 1990; ROSS et al. 1987). The areas with low signal intensity on both sequences have been attributed to thickened trabeculae (ROSS et al. 1987). The lesions fatty contents give rise to patches of high signal intensity on T1-weighted images and intermediate signal intensity

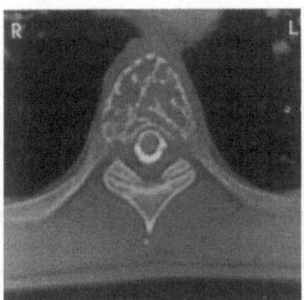 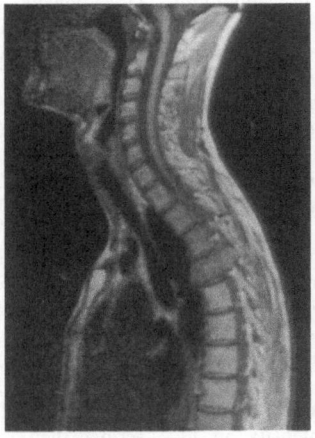 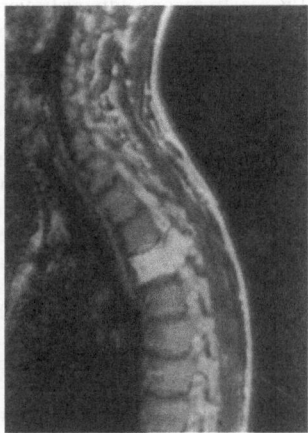

Fig. 5.10 a-c. Vertebral hemangioma in a 52-year-old asymptomatic woman. a CT image at the level of D4 after intrathecal contrast agent injection. A lytic lesion destructs the entire corpus of the vertebra. The remaining trabeculae are thickened and coarse. The hemangioma does not exist into the epidural space. b Intermediate signal intensity indicating relatively low fat content. c T2-weighted sagittal image shows high signal intensity of the corpus and posterior arch of D4.

on T2- weighted images (LAREDO et al. 1990; Ross et al. 1987). Other areas of vertebral hemangiomas typically have an inverse pattern with high signal intensity on T2-weighted images and low signal intensity on T1-weighted images (Ross et al. 1987). An explanation for the latter MR characteristics is still lacking. Hemangiomas enhance after intravenous administration of gadolinium (VERSTRAETE et al. 1994). The MR appearance of extraosseous extensions of hemangiomas differ from that of the osseous component due to a lack of fat content. On T1-weighted images these soft tissue extensions have intermediate rather than high signal intensity, on T2-weighted images, their appearance is similar to that of the osseous component (ROSS et al. 1987).

On T1-weighted images, the appearance of vertebral hemangiomas is similar to that of vertebral focal fat collections. This similarity, the high frequency of focal fat collections, and insufficient awareness of the fact that the diagnosis of hemangioma requires high signal on T2-weighted images as well as high signal on T1-weighted images has led to overdiagnosis of vertebral hemangiomas (HACKNEY 1992). The increased signal intensity of fat on T2-weighted fast-spinecho images has led to further confusion. However, differentiation between hemangiomas and focal fat collections may be facilitated in several ways. First, this may be done by employing frequency-selective chemical shift techniques to suppress the fat signal. Using this technique in T2-weighted images, focal fat collections vanish, while hemangiomas continue to have high signal intensity. Upon intravenous administration of gadolinium, fat-suppressed T1-weighted images show enhancement in hemangiomas, and again no abnormalities in focal fat deposition. Finally, CT may reveal the characteristic bony abnormalities in hemangiomas, whereas focal fat depositions are not accompanied by abnormalities in trabecular structure.

Apart from giving rise to confusion, the fat content of vertebral hemangiomas may also provide prognostic information. In a series of 32 vertebral hemangiomas, asymptomatic hemangiomas showed complete fatty stroma at CT and increased signal intensity on T1-weighted images, which were associated with normal or slightly increased vascularization at angiography and contrast-enhanced CT (LAREDO et al. 1990). In contrast, compressive hemangiomas demonstrated soft tissue attenuation on CT and intermediate signal intensity on T1-weighted images, as well as hypervascularization on angiography and contrast-enhanced CT. Consequently, the investigators suggested that fatty verte-

bral hemangiomas represent inactive forms of hemangiomas, whereas a lack of adipose characteristics indicates a more active vascular lesion with potential to compress the spinal cord (LAREDO et al. 1990).

As mentioned above spinal hemangiomas are often multiple and of no clinical significance. However, sporadically multiple hemangiomatous lesions, i.e., hemangiomatosis, may be part of a more complex syndrome. Syndromes associated with osseous hemangiomatosis are Maffucci's disease, Kasabach-Merritt syndrome, Klippel-Trenaunay syndrome, Parkes-Weber syndrome, and Osler-Weber-Rendu disease (MIRRA et al. 1989).

Apart from focal fat depositions, the radiologic differential diagnosis of vertebral hemangiomas includes myeloma, metastatic disease, eosinophilic granuloma, and Paget's disease (MULDER et al. 1993).

Asymptomatic vertebral hemangiomas do not require further analysis or treatment. In symptomatic lesions, the radiologic diagnosis should be confirmed by fine needle biopsy, and further treatment may be performed. Therapy may be conservative or consist of embolization, radiation treatment, surgery, or a combination of these procedures. (BARTELS et al. 1991; DAGI and SCHMIDEK 1990, MENEI et al. 1994; YOCHUM et al. 1993).

5.2.5.2
Epidural Cavernous Hemangioma

Most spinal hemangiomas arise from the bone. Occassionally, however, cavernous hemangiomas originating from the epidural space may be encountered (ENOMATA and GOTO 1991, FEIDER and YUILLE 1991, GOLWYN 1992, HAINES and KROL 1991, SALOMON and FREILICH 1988). These lesions are estimated to account for 4% of spinal epidural masses and most often are located in the thoracic and lumbar regions (FEIDER and YUILLE 1991). Epidural cavernous hemangiomas have a rounded or elongated appearance, or, when expanding through the intervertebral foramina to the paravertebral tissues, may be dumbbell-shaped. The lesions may extend into multiple foramina (GOLWYN et al. 1992). A myelogram may reveal an epidural mass or block (FEIDER and YUILLE 1991). On CT, the lesion may be apparent as a homogeneous mass isodense with muscle. On MRI, these lesions are well circumscribed; they are hypo- to isointense on T1-weighted images and hyperintense on T2-weighted images. On T2-weighted images the lesions may be surrounded by a hypointense rim, and upon intravenous administration of gadolinium, peripheral enhancement has been described (FEIDER and YUILLE 1991, GOLWYN et al. 1992). These hemangiomas may calcify, which may be apparent on both CT and MRI (SALOMON and FREILICH 1988). Epidural hemangiomas may expand into the surrounding osseous structures, although vertebral hemangiomas more often expand into the epidural space (FEIDER and YUILLE 1991).

5.2.5.3
Aneurysmal Bone Cyst

An aneurysmal bone cyst is a benign condition characterized by cyst-like structures filled with unclotted blood (MIRRA et al. 1989). The cyst's origin is not yet fully understood, but it has been postulated that the initial event is a disruption of subperiosteal or intraosseous blood vessels due to the presence of a benign or malignant tumor or a blunt traumatic episode (MIRRA et al. 1989). The disruption of intraosseous blood vessels results in a rapidly enlarging anomalous vascular lesion (MIRRA et al. 1989). The bone reacts to this vascular lesion with a reparative process, creating tissues partially similar to those found in callus and myositis ossificans (MIRRA et al. 1989). The final result is a lesion containing cyst-like spaces filled with liquid, unclotted blood that is surrounded by aberrant injury tissue and contains fibroblasts, myofibroblasts, osteoid, woven bone, occassional chondroid, hemorrhage, focal hemosiderin deposits, and clusters of osteoclast-like giant cells (MIRRA et al. 1989). Although this theory is hard to prove, it has been demonstrated that about onethird of aneurysmal bone cysts are accompanied by other bone lesions (BIESECKER et al. 1970, BONAKDARPOUR et al. 1978, MARTINEZ and SISSONS 1988).

Aneurysmal bone cysts represent more than 13% of the primary bone tumors of the spine and sacrum other than hemangioma and hematologic diseases, and more than 10% of aneurysmal bone cysts are found in the spine (> 6%) and sacrum (> 4% Table 5.3). Seventy-five percent of patients are under 20 years and 90% under 30 years of age (DAHLIN and McLEOD 1982, MIRRA et al. 1989, MULDER et al. 1993). Females and males are almost equally affected (MIRRA et al. 1989, MULDER et al. 1993). Within the spine, aneurysmal bone cysts may be found at any level, although only one coccygeal location has been described (KRICUN 1993 LIFESO and YOUNGE 1985). In twothirds of cases, aneurysmal bone cysts involve both vertebral body and arch, in one fourth of cases only the arch is involved, and in the remaining cases the lesion is confined to the vertebral body (MULDER et al. 1993). Aneurysmal bone cysts have an expansile growth pattern (DAHLIN and McLEOD 1982, MULDER et al. 1993). Unlike other benign bone lesions (apart from osteomyelitis), aneurysmal bone cysts may extend into intervertebral discs as well as into neighboring vertebrae and ribs (DAHLIN and McLEOD 1982).

In spinal aneurysmal bone cysts, compression of nerve roots or the spinal cord may occur due to expansion of the lesion or collapse of a vertebral body. This may cause pain and neurologic deficits. Swelling may also be apparent, and sometimes the lesions grows at an alarming rate, suggesting malignancy (MULDER et al. 1993). The duration of symptoms prior to diagnosis is typically 6-8 months (AMELI et al. 1985, HAY et al. 1978).

On plain films and CT, the majority of aneurysmal bone cysts present as smooth or lobulated purely lytic lesions (DAHLIN and McLEOD 1982, MULDER et al. 1993) (Fig.5.11 a). Infrequently, lesions show bony septa and ridges (MULDER et al. 1993). In 94% of cases the destruction pattern is geographic and in 6% of cases moth-eaten (MULDER et al. 1993). Often, the lesion is surrounded by a sclerotic rim (DAHLIN and McLEOD 1982, MULDER et al. 1993). The cortex is eroded in 94% of cases (MULDER et al. 1993). Displacement of periosteum and periosteal bone formation give rise to a bony shell that surrounds the extraosseous part of the tumor (DAHLIN and McLEOD 1982, MULDER et al. 1993). This shell may be very thin and may only be rendered visible by CT (DAHLIN and McLEOD 1982, MULDER et al. 1993). Such expansion of bone is apparent in 80% of cases. Incidentally, the growth rate does not allow the time necessary for a bony shell to develop (MULDER et al. 1993). Even in such cases, the boundary between the lesion and the surrounding soft tissues is distinct, smooth, and clear (HUDSON 1984). When the patient is kept in the same position before scanning for at least 10 min, layering of the fluid content in the cystic parts of the lesion may give rise to fluid-fluid levels on CT (HUDSON 1984). In these cases, the dependent layer tends to have a higher density than the supernatant. Aneurysmal bone cysts not demonstrating fluid-fluid levels may be either inhomogeneous or rather homogeneous. Upon intravenous administration of contrast medium, aneurysmal bone cysts may or may not enhance (BRET et al. 1982, HUDSON 1984, JANSEN et al. 1990, WANG et al. 1984). The angiographic appearance of aneurysmal bone cysts is aspecific, with many feeding vessels, a dense tumor stain, an arteriovenous shunt, or contrast pooling in the capillary phase (DISCH et al. 1986). Myelography may demonstrate an extradural mass.

On MRI aneurysmal bone cysts are clearly delineated rounded or lobulated lesions (BELTRAN et al. 1986, CARO et al. 1991, HUDSON 1984, MUNK et al. 1989) (Fig. 5.11b, c). Their appearance is usually heterogeneous on T1-weighted images and more homogeneous on T2-weighted images. The signal intensities of the various cysts of a lesion tend to differ (MUNK et al. 1989). Within the cysts, fluid-fluid levels may be apparent (BELTRAN et al. 1986, HUDSON 1984, MUNK et al. 1989). In general, the dependent layer has a higher signal intensity on T1-weighted images than the supernatant, but the opposite may also be true (MUNK et al. 1989). Fluid-fluid levels are more often encountered on T1- than on

T2-weighted images. Sometimes, the solid components of the lesion, the septa, may be seen as structures of low signal intensity on T2-weighted images (BELTRAN et al. 1986, MUNK et al. 1989). These septa enhance upon administration of gadolinium (CARO et al. 1991). Aneurysmal bone cysts are surrounded by a thin, well-circumscribed rim that has a low signal intensity on both T1- and T2-weighted images due to fibrous and osseous tissues (MUNK et al. 1989).

Radiologic appearance of the lesion is often characteristic. Nevertheless, the radiographic appearance of aneurysmal bone cyst may include giant cell tumor, fibrous dysplasia, chondroma, chondroblastoma, or osteoblastoma (MULDER et al. 1993). Therefore the diagnosis should be confirmed histologically before treatment is undertaken (MULDER et al. 1993). For this purpose, needle biopsy has been advo-

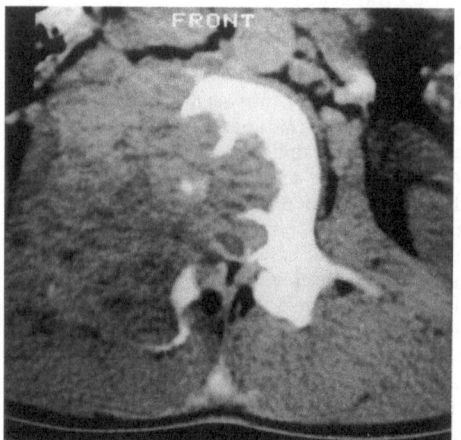

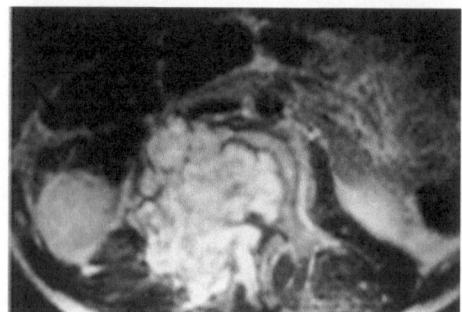

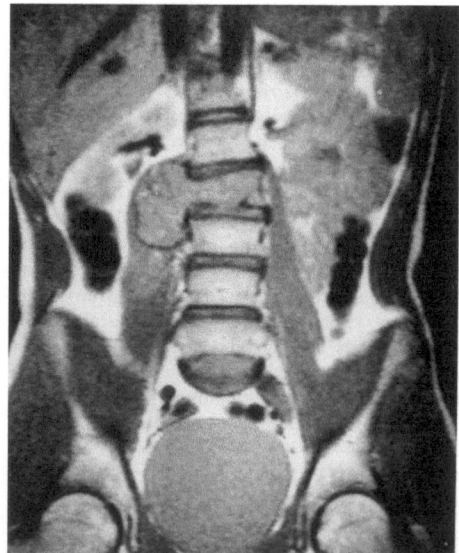

Fig. 5.11a-c. Aneurysmal bone cyst in a 25-year-old patient. a CT image at the level of L2. Destruction of the right side of corpus and arch by tumor with slight heterogeneous attenuation equal to muscle. Major right vertebral extension of the tumor mass is appreciated. Posteriorly, a thin shell of cortical bone surrounds the tumor. b T1-weighted coronal image shows intermediate signal intensity of L2 due to tumor with right paravertebral extension. The paravertebral tumor is surrounded by a rim of low signal intensity due to thin cortex. Inside the lesion, small hyperintense foci representing blood are seen. c T2-weighted transverse image at the level of L2 shows large tumor mass inside corpus and arch with paravertebral extension. Low signal rim around the tumor inside the corpus is caused by sclerotic margin of the tumor

cated (MULDER et al. 1993). The subsequent treatment of choice is surgical curettage of the lesion (TOMITA 1990). In order to limit blood loss during this procedure, preoperative embolization might be considered. The recurrence rate of aneurysmal bone cysts after treatment is as high as 25% (TOMITA 1990).

5.2.5.4
Hemangioblastoma

The majority of spinal hemangioblastomas occurs within the dural sac (see Chap. 3). However, 8% of spinal hemangioblastomas are located extradurally (BROWNE et al.1976). The best imaging technique for these lesions is contrast-enhanced MRI (CHOYKE et al. 1995). With this technique, hemangioblastomas appear as diffusely and avidly enhancing lesions. On T1-weighted images the signal intensity of the lesions may be higher or lower than, or similar to, that of the cord, whereas on T2-weighted images the lesions are hyperintense (ST. AMOUR et al. 1994). If lesions are symptomatic, treatment consists of surgical removal. When encountering a spinal hemangioblastoma, von Hippel-Lindau disease should be suspected, since 80% percent of spinal hemangioblastomas are associated with this disease (CHOYKE et al. 1995).

5.2.5.5
Angiosarcoma and Hemangioendothelioma

Angiosarcoma and *hemangioendothelioma* are conditions characterized by malignant proliferation of endothelial cells. The lesions of both conditions consist of a network of irregular anastomosing vascular channels that are lined by one or more layers of abnormally organized endothelial cells (MIRRA et al. 1989). Compared to angiosarcomas, hemangioendotheliomas are better differentiated and metastasize less avidly (MULDER et al. 1993). Within bone, both tumors are rare, and about 12.5% of them occur in the osseous spine (MULDER et al. 1993). Angiosarcomas and hemangioendotheliomas represent about 2% of spinal tumors other than hemangioma and hematologic diseases (Table 5.3). The lesions may be solitary or multifocal. In the multifocal variants, the lesions tend to cluster in a single anatomic region and even in a single bone (DAGI and SCHMIDEK 1990, MIRRA et al. 1989).

On radiologic examination, angiosarcomas often have a highly malignant, yet aspecific appearance (MIRRA et al. 1989, MULDER et al. 1993). On radio-

graphs, the lesions are osteolytic (DAGI and SCHMIDEK 1990, MIRRA et al. 1989, MULDER et al. 1993). They are smooth or lobulated, and their borders vary from welldemarcated to indistinct and occassionally exhibit a sclerotic rim (DAGI and SCHMIDEK 1990, MULDER et al. 1993). Usually, the cortex is locally destroyed and a periosteal reaction is present (MULDER et al. 1993). Soft tissue extension may occur. On angiography, the lesion's rich vascularity is apparent (DAGI and SCHMIDEK 1990).

The radiographic features of hemangioendotheliomas are less predictable than those of angiosarcomas (MULDER et al. 1993). Radiographic appearance may vary from unequivocally benign to malignant. Lesions are purely osteolytic or show coarse trabeculation (ABRAHAMS et al. 1992, MULDER et al. 1993). In general, the lesions have clear lobulated or smooth borders with a sclerotic rim. The cortex may be eroded, mostly in a regular way. Soft tissue mass is a frequent finding, but periosteal reactions are uncommon (ABRAHAMS et al. 1992). Angiograms show a vascular blush and feeding vessels (ABRAHAMS et al. 1992). On MR examination, the lesions are very heterogeneous (ABRAHAMS et al. 1992). On T1-weighted images, most of the tumor has either a lower signal intensity than the surrounding bone marrow, or a high signal intensity. The latter has been attributed to slow flowing blood, thrombus, and fatty contents. On T2-weighted images, most of the lesion has a high signal intensity. Areas of low signal intensity on both sequences may be seen throughout the lesions, presumably due to bone, fibrous elements, calcifications, or fast flow.

The radiographic differential diagnosis of angiosarcoma includes fibrosarcoma, malignant fibrous histiocytoma, lymphoma, and chondrosarcoma (MULDER et al. 1993). When the radiographic appearance of hemangioendothelioma is mainly benign, aneurysmal bone cyst, giant cell tumor, chondroblastoma, fibrous dysplasia, and hemangioma should be considered. In hemangioendothelioma with a radiographically more malignant aspect, differential diagnosis includes myeloma and metastatic disease (MULDER et al. 1993). Therapy consists of a combination of surgical resection and irradiation (DAGI and SCHMIDEK 1990).

5.2.5.6
Hemangiopericytoma

Hemangiopericytoma is a malignant vascular tumor derived from pericytes, the smooth muscle cells that surround small blood vessels (ENZINGER and WEISS 1988, MIRRA et al. 1989). Microscopically, these tumors contain branching vascular channels lined by a single layer of endothelium and surrounded by a proliferation of pericytes (ENZINGER and WEISS 1988, MIRRA 1989). Such tumors may occur anywhere in the body but predominate in the soft tissues. In bone, these tumors are extremely rare and usually result from expansion of a soft tissue tumor. In the spine, hemangiopericytomas have been described in the epidural space and in bone (MCMASTER et al. 1975, MIRRA et al. 1989, MURASZKO et al. 1982, RADLEY and MCDONALD 1992). Hemangiopericytomas represent 0.6% of the primary bone tumors of the spine and sacrum other than hemangioma and hematologic diseases (Table 5.3).

Osseous hemangiopericytomas have an atypical radiologic appearance (MIRRA et al. 1989, MULDER et al. 1993). The lesions are rounded and osteolytic, and may contain osseous ridges and septa. The aspect of the lesion may vary from well delineated and modestly aggressive to indistinct and aggressive. Cortical destruction and periosteal reactions may occur, and the tumor may expand into the soft tissues. Epidural hemangiopericytomas may appear as rounded, well-circumscribed lesions (RADLEY and MCDONALD 1992). On angiography, contrast-enhanced CT, and MRI examination, the hypervascular nature of the tumor may be apparent (CIZNELI et al. 1992, DAGI and SCHMIDEK 1990, Muraszko et al. 1982). The radiologic differential diagnosis of hemangiopericytoma includes metastatic disease, myeloma, chordoma, eosinophilic granuloma, and aneurysmal bone cyst (MULDER et al. 1993).

The malignant nature of hemangiopericytomas is apparent from the high incidence of recurrence and the ability to give rise to distant metastases (MULDER et al. 1993). Treatment is primarily surgical, and due to the vascular nature of the lesion, presurgical embolization might be considered (CIZNELI et al. 1992, DAGI and SCHMIDEK 1990, MURASZKO et al. 1982).

5.2.6
Tumors of Nerve Sheaths

Nerve sheath tumors arise from Schwann cells, the cells that envelope axons of the peripheral nervous system (RUSSELL and RUBINSTEIN 1989). Two types of benign nerve sheath tumors are discernible: *schwannomas* and *neurofibromas*. Malignant schwannomas and malignant neurofibromas are virtually indistinguishable and often considered as one group, referred to as *malignant nerve sheath tumors*. In the spine, about 70% of nerve sheath tumors are located entirely within the dural sac, and therefore these lesions are described in detail in Chap. 3. However, 15% of spinal nerve sheath tumors have both an intradural and an extradural component, and another 15% are entirely extradural in location (NITTNER 1976, ST. AMOUR et al. 1994).

Since axons lose their myelin sheath when entering bony structures, extradural nerve sheath tumors primarily involve the soft tissues of the spine (MIRRA et al. 1989). The tumors may occur in the epidural space, in the foramina, paravertebrally, or in all of these locations at the same time. Within the epidural space, the tumors are often located posterolaterally, since they usually arise from a dorsal nerve root (MIRRA et al. 1989). In this location, schwannomas tend to be round when small but ovoid, elongated, or lobulated when larger. Neurofibromas tend to be round or fusiform in appearance, or may grow in a plexiform fashion when multiple nerves are involved. Nerve sheath tumors with an extradural component are prone to grow in a dumbbell fashion with extension both within and without the spinal canal. Multiple intervertebral foramina may be involved in this growth pattern. Growth of nerve sheath tumors may cause erosion of the surrounding bony structures and compression of neural structures. In addition, compromise of the vertebral artery may occur in the cervical spine (MIRRA et al. 1989, RUSSELL and RUBINSTEIN 1989, ST. AMOUR et al. 1994).

As in their intradural location, extradural benign nerve sheath tumors are well-circumscribed, smoothly delineated lesions. These tumors can erode adjacent osseous structures, which may be apparent radiographically as scalloping of the vertebrae and widening of the spinal canal and intervertebral foramina (Fig. 5.12a). Such erosions are typically osteolytic, sharply demarcated, and may have a sclerotic margin (MULDER et al. 1993). On CT examination, nerve sheath tumors are usually isodense to the spinal cord and generally have no calcifications. On MRI examination, neurilemmomas as compared to the myelum varies from hypo- to isointense on T1-weighted images, and are variably hyperintense on T2-weighted images (FRIEDMAN 1992) (Fig. 5.12b,c). Diffuse hypointensity on T2-weighted images has

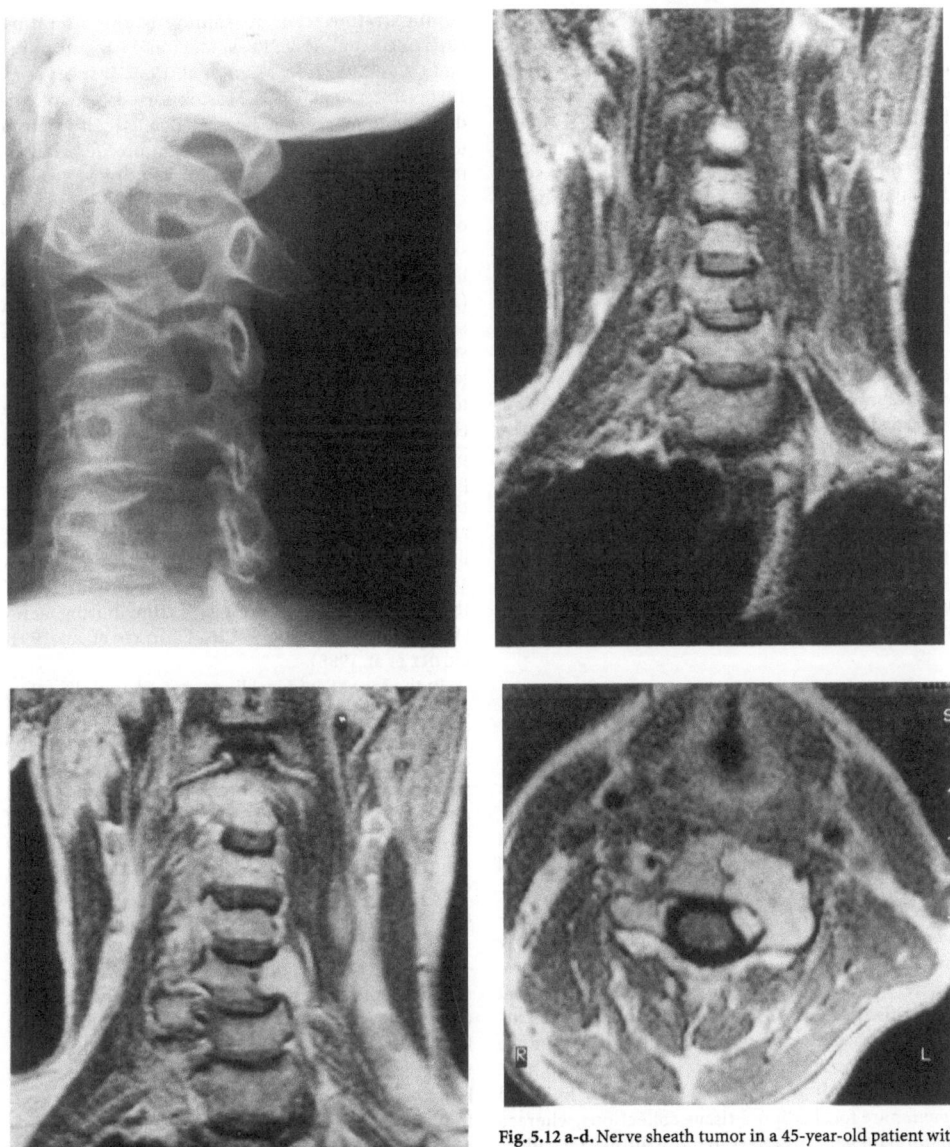

Fig. 5.12 a-d. Nerve sheath tumor in a 45-year-old patient with radiculopathy in the left arm. **a** Oblique radiograph of the cervical spine. Widening of intervertebral foramina is observed. **b** Coronal T1-weighted image shows a low-signal-intensity lesion extending into the left side of the corpus. **c** Coronal postcontrast T1-weighted image demonstrates homogeneous enhancement of the well-defined mass. **d** Postcontrast T1-weighted axial image shows enhancing mass on the left side of the corpus and arch of C5. There is intradural, extramedullary extension of the lesion without cord displacement

also been described (FRIEDMAN 1992). Neurilem-momas demonstrate heterogeneous enhancement upon administration of contrast medium, with the enhancement typically involving the periphery of the lesion (FRIEDMAN 1992) (Fig. 5.12d). Neuro-fibromas are more uniform than neurilemmomas both on unenhanced and enhanced MR scans (FRIEDMAN 1992). Neurofibromas have a slightly higher signal intensity than muscle on T1-weighted images and a markedly increased signal intensity on T2-weighted images. On T2-weighted images, neurofibromas characteristically show a central area of decreased signal intensity (BURK et al. 1987).

Extradural nerve sheath tumors located in an in-tervertebral foramen may simulate a herniated in-tervertebral disc. In such cases, confusion may be in-creased after intravenous administration of contrast material, since cystic nerve sheath tumors may dem-onstrate rim enhancement in the same way as herni-ated discs. In addition, cystic nerve sheath tumors may simulate other extradural cystic lesions such as synovial cysts (ST. AMOUR et al. 1994). The differen-tial diagnosis of dumbbell-shaped lesions includes neuroblastoma, lymphoma, retroperitoneal sarco-mas, metastases, and hemangioblastoma.

5.2.7
Tumors of Adipose Tissue

Lipomas not associated with dysraphism account for about 1% of primary spinal tumors in several series (EHNI and LOVE 1945; NITTNER 1976). Forty percent of these lipomas were extradural and 60% intradural (EHNI and LOVE 1945). The vast majority of extra-dural lipomas occur in the epidural space. In the os-seous spine, lipomas are exceedingly rare (CHOW and LEE 1992; MIRRA et al. 1989). In the epidural space, lipomas may be associated with spinal dysraphism. In such cases, other abnormalities at-tributable to abnormal closure of the neural tube are usually present, and these lesions often have extraspinal and/or intradural extensions. Epidural *lipomas* are focal adipose tissue collections, whereas epidural *lipomatosis* refers to more diffuse fat collec-tion. *Angiolipoma* differs from lipoma or lipomato-sis by the presence of an extensive vascular network within the fatty tissues. *Angiomyolipomas* are com-posed of sheets and bundles of smooth muscle tissue in addition to the adipose and vascular components (ENZINGER and WEISS 1988).

Strong evidence for a causal relationship between the occurrence of epidural lipomatosis and steroid

administration can be found in the literature (BUTHIAU et al. 1988; FESSLER et al. 1992; JUNGREIS and COHEN 1987; KAPLAN et al. 1989; LIPSON et al. 1980; QUINT et al. 1988). Most reported cases of epi-dural lipomatosis have been associated with steroid use, and reversal of the epidural fat proliferation af-ter tapering of steroids has been described (KAPLAN et al. 1989; MAEHARA et al. 1991). Although one case of lipomatosis in a patient with Cushing's syndrome secondary to an adrenal tumor has been described, lipomatosis usually results from exogenous steroids (NOËL et al. 1992). In general, epidural lipomatosis is associated with prolonged regimens of high-dose steroid, and the extent of lipomatosis seems to corre-late with steroid dosage, with the fat collection ex-tending over more spinal levels the higher the dose (KAPLAN et al. 1989; ROY-CAMILLE et al. 1991). Nevertheless, lipomatosis has been observed with prednisone dosages as low as 15 mg daily and in treatment durations as short as 4 months (ARCHER and SMITH 1982; KAPLAN et al. 1989). Rarely, lipomatosis develops in patients not consuming high amounts of steroids, and in a high proportion of these cases obesity seems to be a contributing factor (BADAMI and HINCK 1982; HADDAD et al. 1991; QUINT et al. 1988).

In the case of epidural lipomas and angiolipomas, a relationship with steroid use has not been estab-lished. Extradural lipomas may occur at any age, and occur equally in both sexes (GIUFFRÈ 1976). Eighty percent of angiolipomas occur in the fifth and sixth decade (ST. AMOUR et al. 1994). The occurrence of both endothelium and lipocytes in angiolipomas suggests that the tumor is derived from persistent fetal peridural mesenchyme, since both endothelium and adipose tissue arise from this tissue in the nor-mal development (GIUFFRÈ 1976).

Lipomas and angiolipomas are soft, well-circum-scribed, thinly encapsulated, rounded masses (ENZINGER and WEISS 1988). Histologically, epidural lipomatosis and lipomas consist of normal adipose tissue and blood vessels. These lesions may erode bony structures but always remain within the con-founds of the epidural space. Angiolipomas consist of mature fat cells separated from each other by an extensive branching network of small vessels (ENZINGER and WEISS 1988). Angiolipomas may (1) be encapsulated, (2) lack a capsule and remain con-fined to the extradural space, and (3) infiltrate into the surrounding osseous structures (HADDAD et al.1986; MASCALCHI et al. 1991; VON HANWEHR et al. 1985). The infiltrative subset of angiolipomas are slow-growing nonmalignant lesions that may infiltrate the vertebral body and pedicles (KURODA et al. 1990; VON HANWEHR et al. 1985).

Lipomatosis, lipomas, and angiolipomas all have a preference for the thoracic spinal level and all predominantly occur posteriorly to the thecal sac (ST. AMOUR et al. 1994). In twothirds of cases lipomatosis occurs at the thoracic level, and in the remaining cases at the lumbar level. One case of lipomatosis in the sacral canal has been described (CHAPMAN et al. 1981), but lipomatosis at the cervical level has never been mentioned in the literature. At the thoracic level lipomatosis tends to be located posterior to the cord, whereas at the lumbar level, although it is again most prominent posteriorly, the proliferation of fat may extend all around the thecal sac (ST. AMOUR et al. 1994). In a series of 40 extradural lipomas and angiolipomas reported by GIUFFRE (1976), 80% of the lesions were located at the thoracic level. In this series, other lesions were found at the craniospinal, cervical, lumbar, and lumbosacral levels. Like lipomatosis, lipomas and angiolipomas are predominantly located posteriorly in the spinal canal, although exceptions occur (PAGNI and CANAVERO 1992). In their typical posterior location, lipomas and angiolipomas are often spindle-shaped elongated lesions. Occasionally, lipomas may extend from the spinal canal to form paravertebral masses (GIUFFRÈ 1976).

Lipomatosis, lipomas, and angiolipomas may give rise to clinical signs and symptoms due to compression of the neural contents of the spinal canal (GIUFFRÈ 1976; KAPLAN et al. 1989; PAGNI and CANAVERO 1992). Depending on the location of the lesion, cord compression or radiculopathy may occur. The severity of the clinical picture may vary from mild symptoms to complete paraplegia. In lipomatosis, the clinical course is usually characterized by slow progression of symptoms, although courses as brief as 2 weeks have been described (HEALY et al. 1987). In lipomas and angiolipomas, the duration of symptoms is less than 1 year in twothirds of cases (GIUFFRÈ 1976). In these cases, the short duration of symptoms may contrast with the remarkable size of the lesions at the time of diagnosis (GIUFFRÈ 1976). Presumably, acute clinical deterioration is the result of impairment of blood supply to the spinal cord which occurs when the tumor has reached a critical size (GIUFFRÈ 1976).

On MRI, epidural lipomatosis and lipomas have the same signal intensity as normal epidural fat on all sequences (Fig. 5.13).In case of doubt, the fatty content of the lesion might be confirmed by fat-suppression techniques. The only visible difference between these lesions and normal epidural fat is the amount of local adipose tissue. When the distance between the posterior aspect of the thecal sac and the dorsal confines of the spinal canal in the midthoracic region is greater than 6 mm, epidural lipomatosis should be suspected (QUINT et al. 1988). Epidural lipomatous lesions may extend over several vertebral levels and taper gradually cranially, caudally, and laterally. At the thoracic level, the thecal sac is often displaced anteriorly, whereas it remains in the normal position at the lumbar level (ST. AMOUR et al. 1994).

Angiolipomas may have distinguishing characteristics on MRI (MASCALCHI et al. 1991; MATSUSHIMA et al. 1987; WEILL et al. 1991). On T2-weighted images, the signal intensity of these tumors is variable. The lesions may have a higher signal intensity than epidural fat on T2-weighted images and may contain areas with a lower signal intensity on T1-weighted images. Upon intravenous administration of gadolinium, the low-intensity areas on T1-weighted images may show enhancement. In addition, extension into the surrounding osseous structures may be encountered.

Infrequently, lipomatous lesions in the epidural space induce abnormalities visible on plain radiographs. Long-standing lesions may give rise to erosion of the bony surroundings of the spinal canal, and erosion of vertebral body and pedicles may be found in infiltrating angiolipomas (KURODA et al. 1990; VON HANWEHR et al. 1985). In lipomatosis and lipomas, CT findings may be similar to those described for MRI (ARCHER and SMITH 1982; BUTHIAU et al. 1988; FESSLER et al. 1992; HADDAD et al. 1991; JUNGREIS and COHEN 1987; LIPSON et al. 1980; NOËL et al. 1992; QUINT et al. 1988; ROY-CAMILLE et al. 1991; WEILL et al. 1991). On CT, these lesions are homogeneous and have attenuation values characteristic for adipose tissue. However, apart from having fat characteristics, angiolipomas may be entirely of soft tissue density on CT examination, or may be inhomogeneous with areas of soft tissue density in an otherwise fatty lesion (MASCALCHI et al. 1991; MATSUSHIMA et al. 1987; VON HANWEHR et al. 1985; WEILL et al. 1991). Enhancement after administration of intravenous contrast medium has been described in these angiomatous adipose lesions (MATSUSHIMA et al. 1987; WEILL et al. 1991). Intravertebral extensions of infiltrating angiolipomas may give rise to a pattern of osseous erosion that is similar to that of primary osseous hemangiomas (ST. AMOUR et al. 1994).In contrast to hemangiomas, these osseous extensions of angiolipomas tend to demonstrate poor contrast enhancement (VON HANWEHR

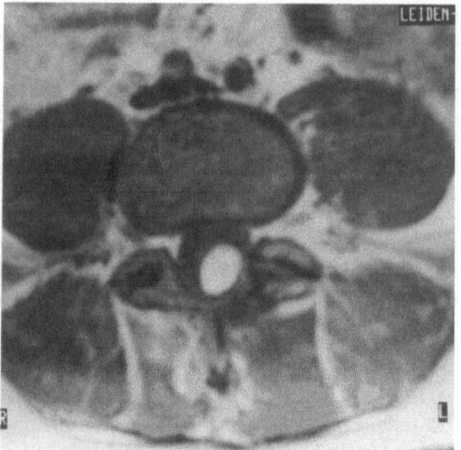

Fig. 5.13. Epidural lipoma in a 44-year-old asymptomatic woman. T1- weighted transverse image at the level of L4 shows a well-defined high-signal-intensity lesion in the epidural space. No other abnormalities were observed in this patient

et al. 1985). On myelography, symmetric complete or partial blocks are almost invariably found in symptomatic lipomatosis. Asymmetric extradural defects may represent lipomas or angiolipomas instead. At the lumbar level, lipomatosis may simulate spinal stenosis (St. Amour et al. 1994).

Symptomatic epidural lipomatosis requires treatment. This may be conservative: tapering of steroid therapy, or weight loss in obese patients. When conservative treatment fails or the clinical picture rapidly progresses, surgical decompression may even be indicated. If extradural lipomas or angiolipomas require treatment, surgery is the therapy of choice (St. Amour et al. 1994).

5.2.8
Extramedullary Hematopoiesis

Medullary hematopoiesis may become insufficient due to an increased breakdown of blood, such as in beta-thalassemia or other chronic hemolytic anemias, or due to replacement of hematopoietic bone marrow, such as in myelofibrosis or other myeloproliferative disorders. Under such circumstances, hematopoiesis may shift to other areas in order to maintain sufficient erythrogenesis (Chaljub et al. 1991; Shaver and Clore 1981). One of the sites where the resulting extramedullary hematopoiesis may occur is within the spinal canal. Intraspinal extramedullary hematopoiesis may give

rise to spinal cord compression (Buetow et al. 1990; Chaljub et al. 1991; Kalina and Hillstrom 1992; Price and Bell 1985; Shaver and Clore 1981).

On CT and MR examination, extramedullary hematopoiesis presents as one or several elongated masses in the epidural space. Most frequently, these masses occur at the thoracic level and may be located both anterior and posterior from the cord (Kalina and Hillstrom 1992; Papavasiliou et al. 1990). On CT examination, the masses are denser than epidural fat. Myelography shows constriction of the thecal sac. On MRI, both T1- and T2-weighted images demonstrate slightly higher signal intensity in the mass than in the bone marrow of adjacent vertebral bodies (Pantongrag-Brown and Suwanwela 1992). Upon intravenous administration of gadolinium, the lesions show avid enhancement (Buetow et al. 1990). Often, the diagnosis may be suggested by additional observations made during radiologic examination, such as evidence of bone marrow changes or other sites of extramedullary hematopoiesis. The differential diagnosis includes lymphoma, chloroma, neuroblastoma, sarcoma, meningioma, hemangioblastoma, angioblastoma, and epidural abscess and hemorrhage. Symptomatic intraspinal extramedullary hematopoiesis may be treated by low-dose irradiation.

5.2.9
Epidural Tumor-like Conditions

5.2.9.1
Neurenteric Cyst

In normal fetal development there is a transient communication between the ventrally located yolk sac and the dorsal ectodermal surface of the embryo. When this communication, the neurenteric canal, fails to close, a fistula may persist between the intestinal lumen and the dorsal skin. This fistula is located in the midline and traverses the mesentery, prevertebral soft tissues, vertebral body, thecal sac, myelum, vertebral arch, and subcutaneous fat. Such a fistula is extremely rare, and more frequently only parts of the canal persist. A part of the canal may persist as a neurenteric cyst. Such cysts may occur at any site along the trajectory of the duct (Naidich et al. 1991).

Although most neurenteric cysts of the spine are located within the dura, extradural lesions do occur. The cysts typically occur in the midline, in general ventral or ventrolateral to the cord. They tend to be located in the cervicothoracic junction or close to the conus medullaris (NAIDICH et al. 1991). The cyst may have an extraspinal component in the preverte-bral tissues,with which it communicates through a vertebral defect. Often, the cyst is accompanied by anomalies such as scoliosis, hemivertebrae, anterior or posterior spina bifida, and myelomeningoceles (ARAI et al. 1992; GLEESON and STOVIN 1961; NAIDICH et al. 1991). On MRI and CT examination, the cysts are smoothly delineated, circumscribed le-sions with a homogeneous appearance. On CT, these lesions are hypodense or isodense to the cord and do not show contrast enhancement. On T1-weighted images, the lesions have a signal intensity similar to cerebrospinal fluid, although signal intensity may be higher due to higher protein content (GLEESON and STOVIN 1961). On T2-weighted images, signal inten-sity is higher than that of cerebrospinal fluid (GEREMIA et al. 1988). Intraspinal neurenteric cysts may give rise to progressive cord compression in adults (D'ALMEIDA and STEWARD 1981). The radio-logic differential diagnosis of neurenteric cysts in-cludes synovial/ganglion cyst, dermoid, epidermoid teratoma, arachnoideal cyst, cystic neurofibroma, and a free intervertebral disc fragment.

5.2.9.2
Epidermoid and Dermoid Cysts

Epidermoid and *dermoid cysts* result from inclusion of ectodermal elements under the skin. Inclusion may occur during the embryonic period at the time of closure of the neural tube. Furthermore, epider-moid cysts may have an iatrogenic origin, resulting from displacement of skin tissue by lumbar punc-ture or myelomeningocele repair. Epidermoid cysts consist of a wall of simple squamous epithelium sup-ported by a layer of collagen, enveloping a collection of desquamated keratin. In addition to these com-ponents, dermoids also contain skin appendages, such as hair follicles, sebaceous glands and possibly sweat glands, and occasionally bone and cartilage (RUSSELL and RUBINSTEIN 1989).

Although most epidermoid and dermoid cysts oc-cur within the thecal sac, they may also be localized in the epidural space (ST. AMOUR et al. 1994). Most frequently, lesions are located in the lumbar region (LIST 1941). In the epidural space, they occur in the midline and, contrary to neurenteric cysts, posterior to the thecal sac. They are smoothly marginated and tend to have a heterogeneous appearance on MRI (DE PENA et al. 1989; HATFIELD et al. 1989, PHILLIPS and CHIU 1987; VISCIANI et al. 1989). The signal in-

tensity of epidermoids and dermoids on T1- and T2-weighted images varies and may be similar to or higher than that of cerebro-spinal fluid. Moreover, on T1-weighted images areas of high signal intensity may be found in dermoid cysts; these areas have fat characteristics on CT. The walls of epidermoid and dermoid cysts tend to be visible on MR examination. The wall of epidermoid cysts may be hyperintense to the remainder of the lesion on T1-weighted images, and hypointense on T2-weighted images. Epider-moid and dermoid cysts usually show no contrast enhancement. Their association with spina bifida, diastomatomyelia, myelomeningocele, hemiverte-brae, block vertebrae, and notably dermal sinus may be of help in differentiating them from other lesions (BARKOVICH et al. 1991; LIST 1941). In the case of epidermoids, the patient's medical history often in-cludes past lumbar punctures. Based on their radio-graphic appearance, the differential diagnosis of dermoids and epidermoids includes other cystic epi-dural lesions, such as synovial/ganglion cyst, neu-renteric cyst, arachnoideal cyst, cystic nerve sheath tumors, and other epidural lesions with high signal intensity on T1-weighted images, e.g., teratoma, lipo-mas, cavernous hemangioma, and epidural abscess and hemorrhage. Finally, meningioma should be considered.

5.2.9.3
Arachnoideal Cyst

Arachnoideal cysts are cystic lesions, filled with cerebrospinal fluid, that communicate with the sub-arachnoideal space (ST. AMOUR et al. 1994). These le-sions may occur within the dural sac, although they are more frequently located in the extradural com-partment. Most extradural arachnoideal cysts tend to be either outpouchings of arachnoidea through a dural defect or diverticula lined by both dura and arachnoidea. Sometimes, these cysts have no arach-noideal lining and are delineated by connective tis-sue. Most often the cysts are congenital or of un-known origin; less frequently they are post-trau-matic. Once present, arachnoideal cysts have a ten-dency to enlarge due to cerebrospinal fluid pulsa-tions and may compromise neural structures. Ac-cording to their location and content, NABORS and coworkers (1988) discriminated three types of arach-noideal cysts. *Type I* cysts are extradural out-pouchings of the dural sac that do not contain neural tissue. *Type II* lesions are also extradural, but contain nerve root fibers. Type II lesions may be either diverticula of the nerve root sheath proximal to the posterior root ganglion that contain nerve roots or are known as Tarlov cysts, arising at or distal to the posterior nerve root ganglion and containing neural tissue in the wall. Finally, *type III* lesions are intra-dural arachnoideal cysts.

Tarlov cysts may occur at any level, but are most prevalent and symptomatic in the sacrum (NABORS et al. 1988). Two thirds of the other extradural arachnoideal cysts are located at the thoracic level: 10% are thoracolumbar, 20% lumbosacral, and 5% cervical. Eighty-five percent of these lesions are situated posterior or posterolateral to the thecal sac, and 15% lateral to it (NAIDICH et al. 1983b). Anterior lo-cations of arachnoideal cysts are seldom and have a cervical predilection. Half of the extradural arachnoideal cysts expand through an intervertebral foramen. Within the spinal canal, cysts may extend over several vertebral levels and compress the thecal sac. The connection with the subarachnoideal space is usually located in the cranial aspect of the cyst. Extradural arachnoideal cysts may be multiple. The lesions affect males more often than females, have been described in all age groups, and may give rise to signs and symptoms (NAIDICH et al. 1983b). The treatment of choice for extradural arachnoideal cysts is surgery.

On plain films, enlargement of the spinal canal or a vertebral foramen may be evident (NABORS et al. 1988, NAIDICH et al. 1983b). Myelography may show an extradural mass or a block. The cyst may or may not fill up with contrast medium on conventional myelography. On CT, filling of the cyst is almost always detected, although delayed CT examination may be required (NABORS et al. 1988; NAIDICH et al. 1983b). On MRI, the cysts are smoothly delineated, homogeneous lesions (COLE et al. 1989; CONGIA et al. 1992; ROBINSON et al. 1989, SUNDARAM and AWWAD 1986; (Fig.5.14) VERSTRAETE et al. 1989). Signal intensities are similar to those of cerebrospi-nal fluid on all sequences. On T2-weighted images the signal intensity may be slightly higher than that of cerebrospinal fluid due to decreased pulsation of cerebrospinal fluid in the cyst. Following gadolinium administration, enhancement should be absent (NORTH et al. 1990). Intraspinal cysts may displace the epidural fat and compress the thecal sac (NAIDICH et al. 1983b). Although the presence of nerve roots in a type II lesion may be evident on ra-diologic examination, type I and II lesions can often not be distinguished on images (ST. AMOUR et al. 1994). Large extradural arachnoideal cysts in the sacrum may be confused with meningoceles. Al-though arachnoideal cysts may erode the spinal ca-nal, they are distinguishable because, in contrast to meningoceles, they are not accompanied by closure defects of the osseous spine (ST. AMOUR et al. 1994). Arachnoideal cysts in the neural foramina may be discriminated from lateral meningoceles, because the latter have a wide communication with the subarachnoideal space and tend to be associated with neurofibromatosis (ST. AMOUR et al. 1994). Fur-thermore, the radiographic differential diagnosis in-cludes other epidural cystic lesions, such as synovial/ ganglion cysts, neurenteric cysts, dermoid, epider-moid teratoma, and cystic nerve sheath tumors.

5.2.9.4
Synovial Cysts and Ganglion Cysts

Synovial cysts and *ganglion cysts* consist of a wall of fibrous connective tissue surrounding a collection of myxoid, proteinaceous material which may con-tain blood products and gas (AWWAD et al. 1990, FARDON and SIMMONS 1989, JACKSON et al. 1989, SILBERGLEIT et al. 1990). The cystic wall may be cal-cified and contain hemosiderin and vascular foci. Unlike ganglion cysts, by histologic definition, syno-vial cysts are lined by a synovial membrane and communicate with a synovial joint (YUH et al. 1991). Discrimination of these lesions based on histology is often difficult, and it is impossible on radiologic grounds. Therefore the names of the lesions are of-ten used interchangeably (MULDER et al. 1993). The lesions have been ascribed to degeneration and trauma and have also been considered congenital (KJERULF et al. 1986; RHOTON et al. 1976; YUH et al. 1991).

In the spine, the cysts are located extradurally in the proximity of an apophyseal joint. Usually the le-sions occur posterolaterally in the epidural space and anteromedial to a facet joint (RHOTON et al. 1976; ST. AMOUR et al. 1994). Other possible epidural locations are dorsal to the cord in the midline and adjacent to the ligamentum flavum (ABDULLAH et al. 1984; KJERULF et al. 1986). From an epidural origin the cysts may also expand through the interverte-bral foramen into the paravertebral soft tissues (ST. AMOUR et al. 1994). Cysts tend to occur at the lumbar level: in more than twothirds of cases at the L4-5 level, less frequently at L3-4 and L5-S1, and only rarely at other spinal levels (JACKSON et al. 1989; LIU et al. 1990; RHOTON et al. 1976). Plain films and CT may show evidence of degenerative changes at a facet joint, and myelography may demonstrate an

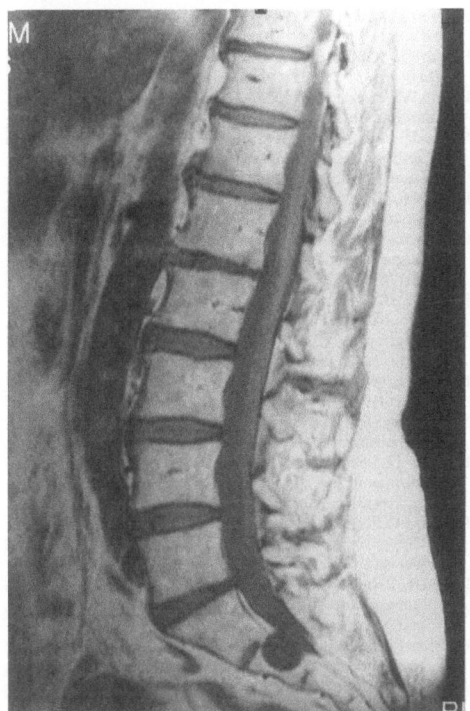
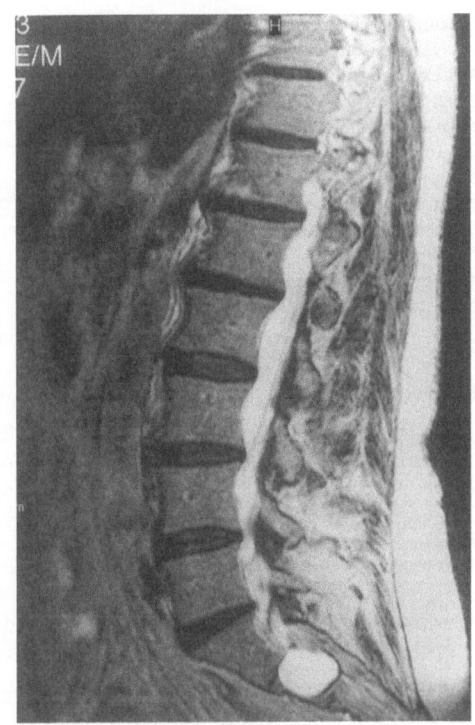

a   b

Fig. 5.14 a,b. Arachnoideal cyst in a 45-year-old asymptomatic man. a T1-weighted sagittal image of lumbosacral vertebral column shows well-defined low-signal-intensity lesion in S2 extending into the spinal canal. b On T2-weighted image the lesion has a high signal intensity identical to that of CSF. The lesion is characteristic of a cyst

extradural defect (RHOTON et al. 1976). Centrally, cysts show fluid attenuation on CT examination or, in the case of prior hemorrhage, high attenuation, and they may have a calcified rim (MUNDAY et al. 1994). In addition, low attenuation due to the presence of gas may be found in the cysts, in association with a vacuum phenomenon in the adjacent joint (MUNDAY et al. 1994). On MR examination, the cysts are clearly delineated, rounded lesions located in the epidural space adjacent to an apophyseal joint (DAVIS et al. 1990; JACKSON et al. 1989; SILBERGLEIT et al. 1990; YUH et al. 1991). On both T1- and T2-weighted images, signal intensity of the cystic content is similar to or higher than that of cerebrospinal fluid. The cystic wall tends to be hypointense, notably on T2-weighted images. Flow voids may be present due to calcifications or gas in the cyst. Upon gadolinium administration, the cystic capsule and other solid components of the cyst may show enhancement (SILBERGLEIT et al. 1990; YUH et al.

1991). The adjoining joint often shows degenerative changes and may also demonstrate gadolinium enhancement (YUH et al. 1991). The radiologic differential diagnosis of synovial and ganglion cysts includes other epidural cystic lesions, such as neurenteric cysts, dermoid, epidermoid, teratoma, and arachnoideal cyst, cystic nerve sheath tumors, and also free intervertebral disc fragments. Synovial and ganglion cysts are generally accompanied by chronic low back pain (RHOTON et al. 1976). Therapeutic measures may be conservative, or consist of steroid injections or surgical excision (RHOTON et al. 1976; ST. AMOUR et al. 1994).

5.2.9.5
Ossification of Spinal Ligaments

Ossification of the posterior longitudinal ligament and the less frequent ossification of the ligamentum flavum may give rise to compression of the cord and nerve roots and may simulate epidural tumors on MR examination (MUNDAY et al. 1994; OTAKE et al. 1992; SUGIMURA et al. 1992; YAMASHITA et al. 1990). Most often, these lesions demonstrate a flow void due to the presence of thick calcification or compact bone, and such a picture seldom presents a diagnostic problem. However, the appearance of high signal intensity in these lesions, due to the presence of fatty bone marrow, may be confusing. Under such circumstances, CT may unequivocally demonstrate the bony nature of the lesion.

References

Abdelwahab IF, O'Leary PF, Steiner GC, et al (1986) Case report 357. Skeletal Radiol 15:242-246

Abdullah AF, Chambers RW, Daut DP (1984) Lumbar nerve root compression by synovial cysts of the ligamentum flavum. Report of four cases. Neurosurg 60: 617-620

Abrahams TG, Wolodymyr B, Jones M (1992) Epitheloid hemangioendothelioma of bone. A report of two cases and review of the literature. Skeletal Radiol 21:509-513

Albertyn LE, Croft G, Kuss B, Dale B (1992) The perivertebral collar - a new sign in lymphoproliferative malignancies. Australas Radiol 36:214-218

Ameli NO, Abbassioun K, Saleh H, Eslamdoost A (1985) Aneurysmal bone cysts of the spine: report of 17 cases. Neurosurg 63:685-690

Arai Y, Yamauchi Y, Tsuji, T, et al (1992) Spinal neurenteric cyst. Report of two cases and review of forty-one cases reported in Japan. Spine 17:1421-1424

Archer CR, Smith KR (1982) Extradural lipomatosis simulating an acute heriated nucleus pulposus. Neurosurg 57:559-562

Awwad EE, Martin DS, Smith KR, Bucholz RD (1990) MR imaging of lumbar juxtaarticular cysts. Comput Assist Tomogr 14:415-417

Badami JP, Hinck VC (1982) Symptomatic deposition of epidural fat in a morbidly obese woman. Am J Neuroradiol 3:664-665

Balakrishnan V, Rice MS, Simpson DA (1974) Spinal neuroblastomas: diagnosis, treatment, and prognosis. J Neurosurg 40:431-438

Barkovich AJ, Edwards MSB, Cogen PH (1991) MR evaluation of spinal dermal sinus tracts in children. Am J Neuroradiol 12:123-129

Bartels RH, Grotenhuis JA, van der Spek JA (1991) Symptomatic vertebral hemangiomas. J Neurosurg 35:187-192

Beltran J, Simon DC, Levy M, et al (1986) Aneurysmal bone cysts: MR imaging at 1.5 T. Radiology 158:689-690

Beltran J, Aparisi F, Bonmati LM, et al (1993) Eosinophilic granuloma: MRI manifestations. Skeletal Radiol 22:157-161

Beres J, Pech P, Berns TF, et al (1986) Spinal epidural lymphomas: CT features in seven patients. Am J Neuroradiol 7: 327-328

Biesecker JL, Marcove RC, Huvos AG, Mike V (1970) Aneurysmal bone cysts: a clinicopathologic study of 66 cases. Cancer 26:615-625

Bjornsson J, Wold LE, Ebersold MJ, et al (1993) Chordoma of the mobile spine: a clinicopathologic analysis of 40 patients. Cancer 71:735-740

Bloem JL, Mulder JD (1985) Chondroblastoma: a clinical and radiological study of 104 cases. Skeletal Radiol 14:1-9

Bloem JL, Kroon HM (1993) Osseous lesions. Radiol Clin North Am 31:261-278

Bloem W, Fawcett DW (1994) Textbook of histology, 12th edn. Chapman and Hall, New York

Bonakdarpour A, Levy WM, Aegerter E (1978) Primary and secondary aneurysmal bone cyst: a radiological study of 75 cases. Radiology 126:75-83

Bousvaros A, Kirks DR, Grossman H (1986) Imaging of neuroblastoma: an overview. Pediatr Radiol 16:89-106

Boyko OB, Cory DA, Cohen MD, et al (1987) MR imaging of osteogenic and Ewing's sarcoma. AJR Am J Roentgenol 148:317-322

Bradway JK, Pritchard DJ (1990) Ewing's sarcoma of the spine. In: Sundaresan N, Schmidek HH, Schiller AL, Rosenthal DI (eds) Tumors of the spine - diagnosis and clinical management. Saunders, Philadelphia, pp 235-239

Bret P, Confavreux C, Thouard H, Pialat J (1982) Aneurysmal bone cyst of the cervical spine: report of a case investigated by CT and treated by a two-stage surgical procedure. Neurosurgery 10:111-115

Browne TR, Adams RD, Robertson GH (1976) Hemangioblastoma of the spinal cord. Review and report of five cases. Arch Neurol 33:435-441

Buetow PC, Perry JJ, Geyer CA (1990) Gd-DTPA enhancement in CNS extramedullary hematopoiesis. Am J Neuroradiol 11:411-412

Burk DL, Brunberg JA, Kanal E, Latchaw RE, Wolf GL (1987) Spinal and paraspinal neurofibromatosis: surface coil MR imaging at 1.5 T. Radiology 162:797-801

Buthiau D, Piette JC, Ducerveau MN, et al (1988) Steroid-induced spinal epidural lipomatosis: CT survey. J Comput Assist Tomogr 12:501-503

Caro PA, Mandell GA, Stanton RP (1991) Aneurysmal bone cyst of the spine in children. Pediatr Radiol 21:114-116

Chaljub G, Guinto FC, Crow WN, Kumar R (1991) MRI diagnosis of spinal cord compression in beta-thalassemia. Spine 16:583-584

Chapman PH, Martuza RL, Poletti CE, Karchner AW (1981) Symptomatic spinal epidural lipomatosis associated with Cushing's syndrome. Neurosurgery 8:724-727

Chow LT, Lee KC (1992) Intraosseous lipoma. A clinicopathologic study of nine cases. Am J Surg Pathol 16:401-410

Choyke PL, Glenn GM, Walther MM, et al (1995) Von Hippel-Linday disease: genetic, clinical, and imaging features. Radiology 194:629-642

Cizneli MO, Ilgit ET, Ulug H, Erdogan A (1992) A giant paraspinal hemangiopericytoma and its preoperative embolization. Neuroradiology 34:81-83

Cole GP, Flannery AM, Gulati AK (1989) Intrasacral meningocele. Case report and review of the literature. Spine 14:1418-1420

Congia S, Coraddu M, Tronci S, et al (1992) Myelographic and MRI appearances of a thoracic spinal extradural arachnoid cyst of the spine with extra- and intraspinal extension. Neuroradiology 34:444-446

d'Almeida AC, Steward DJ (1981) Neurenteric cyst: case report and literature review. Neurosurgery 8:596-599

Dagi TF, Schmidek HH (1990) Vascular tumors of the spine. In: Sundaresan N, Schmidek HH, Schiller AL, Rosenthal DE (eds) Tumors of the spine - diagnosis and clinical managment. Saunders, Philadelphia, pp 181-191

Dahlin DC, McLeod RA (1982) Aneurysmal bone cyst and other non-neoplastic conditions. Skeletal Radiol 8:243-250

David R, Lamki N, Fan S, et al (1989) The many faces of neuroblastoma. Radiographics 9:859-882

Davis R, Iliya A, Roque C, Pampati M (1990) The advantage of magnetic resonance imaging in diagnosis of a lumbar synovial cyst. Spine 15:244-246

de Bruïne FT, Kroon HM (1988) Spinal chordoma: radiologic features in 14 cases. AJR Am J Roentgenol 150:861-863

De Pena CA, Lee Y-Y, Tassel PV, et al (1989) MR appearance of acquired spinal epidermoid tumor. Am J Neuroradiol 10:97

De Schepper AMA, Ramon F, Van Marck E (1993) MR imaging of eosinophilic granuloma: report of 11 cases. Skeletal Radiol 22:163-166

Dietrich RB, Kangarloo H (1986) Retriperitoneal mass with intradural extension: value of magnetic resonance imaging in neuroblastoma. AJR Am J Roentgenol 146:251-254

Dietrich RB, Kangarloo H, Lenarsky C, Feig SA (1987) Neuroblastoma: the role of MR imaging. AJR Am Roentgenol 148:937-942

Disch S, Grubb RL, Gado MH, et al (1986) Aneurysmal bone cyst of the cervico-thoracic spine: CT evaluation of the value a preoperative embolization. Neurosurgery 19:290-293

Domelan WA, Swenson O (1968) Benign and malignant sacrococcygeal teratomas. Surgery 64:834-846

Ehni G, Love JG (1945) Intraspinal lipomas. Report of cases, review of the literature, and clinical and pathologic study. Arch Neurol and Psychiatry 53:1-28

Enneking WF, Spanier SS, Goodman MA (1980) A system for the surgical staging of musculo-skeletal sarcoma. Clin Orthop 153:106

Enneking WF (1985) Staging of musculoskeletal neoplasms, from the Musculoskeletal Tumor Society. Skeletal Radiol 13:183-194

Enneking WF (1990) Staging of musculoskeletal neoplasms. In: Sundaresan N, Schmidek HH, Schiller AL, Rosenthal DI (eds) Tumors of the spine – diagnosis and clinical management. Saunders, Philadelphia, pp 22-45

Enomata H, Goto H (1991) Spinal epidural cavernous angioma: MRI findings. Neuroradiology 33:462

Enzinger FM, Weiss SW (1988) Soft tissue tumors, 2nd edn. Mosby, St. Louis

Enzmann DR, de la Paz RL (1990) Tumors. In: Enzmann DR, de la Paz RL, Rubin JB, (eds) Magnetic resonance of the spine. Mosby, St. Louis, pp 352-354

Fardon DF, Simmons JD (1989) Gas-filled intraspinal synovial cyst. Spine 14:127-129

Feider HK, Yuille DL (1991) An epidural cavernous hemangioma of the spine. Am J Neuroradiol 12:243-244

Fessler RG, Johnson DL, Brown FD et al. (1992) Epidural lipomatosis in steroid-treated patients. Spine 17:183-188

Firooznia H, Pinto RS, Lin JP, et al (1976) Chordoma: radiologic evaluation in 20 cases. AJr Am J Roentgenol 127:797-805

Friedman DP (1992) Intradural schwannomas of the spine: MR findings with emphasis on contrast-enhancement characteristics. AJR Am J Roentgenol 158:1347-1350

Geirnaerdt MJA, Bloem JL, Eulderink F, et al (1993) Gd-DTPA enhanced MR imaging of cartilaginous tumors. Radiology 186:813-817

Geremia GK, Russell EJ, Clasen RA (1988) MRI characteristics of a neurenteric cyst. Am J Neuroradiol 9:978-980

Gilbert RW, Kim JH, Posner JB (1978) Epidural spinal cord compression from metastatic tumor: diagnosis and treatment. Ann Neurol 3:40-51

Giudici MA, Moser RP, Kransdorf MJ (1993) Cartilaginous tumors. Radiol Clin North Am 31:237-260

Giuffrè R (1976) Spinal lipomas. In: Vinken PJ, Bruyn GW (eds) Tumours of the spine and spinal cord, part II. Elsevier, New York, pp 389-414 (Handbook of clinical neurology, vol 20)

Gleeson JA, Stovin PGI (1961) Mediastinal enterogenous cysts associated with vertebral anomalies. Clin radiol 12:41-48

Goldhahn W-E, Goldhahn G (1976) Neoplasms of the spinal epidural space, with special reference to lymphogranulomatosis. In: Vinken PJ, Bruyn GW (eds) Tumours of the spine and spinal cord, part I. Elsevier, New York, pp 103-135 (Handbook of clinical neurology, vol 19)

Golwyn DH, Cardenas CA, Murtagh FR, et al (1992) MRI of a cervical extradural cavernous hemangioma. Neuroradiology 34:68-69

Green NE, Robertson WE, Kilroy AW (1980) Eosinophilic granuloma of the spine with associated neural deficit. J Bone Joint Surg [Am] 62:1198-1202

Greenfield GB (1980) Radiology of bone diseases. Lippincott, Philadelphia

Grubb MR, Currier BL, Pritchard DJ, Ebersold MJ (1994) Primary Ewing's sarcoma of the spine. Spine 19:309-313

Hackney DB (1992) Neoplasms and related disorders. Top Magn Reson Imaging 4:37-61

Haddad FS, Abla A, Allam CK (1986) Extradural spinal angiolipoma. Surg Neurol 26:473-486

Haddad SF, Hitchon PW, Godersky JC (1991) Idiopathic and glucocorticoid-induced spinal epidural lipomatosis. J Neurosurg 74:38-42

Haggstrom JA, Brown JC, Marsh PW (1988) Eosinophilic granuloma of the spine: MR demonstration. J Comput Assist Tomogr 12:344-345

Haines AB, Krol G (1991) Dumbbell shaped spinal cavernous hemangioma: a case report. Am J Neuroradiol 12:1021-1022

Harmon DC (1990) Chemotherapy. In: Sundaresan N, Schmidek HH, Schiller AL, Rosenthal DI (eds) Tumors of the spine – diagnosis and clinical managment. Saunders, Philadelphia, pp 92-95

Harwood-Nash D, Fitz CR (1976) Neuroradiology in infants and children. Mosby, St. Louis

Hatfield MK, Udesky RH, Struiling AM, et al (1989) MR imaging of a spinal epidermoid tumor. Am J Neuroradiol 10:95

Hay MC, Paterson D, Taylor TKF (1978) Aneurysmal bone cysts of the spine. J Bone Joint Surg [Br] 60:406-411

Healy ME, Hesselink JR, Ostrup RC, Alksne JF (1987) Demonstration by magnetic resonance of symptomatic spinal epidural lipomatosis. Neurosurgery 21:414-415

Higinbotham NL, Philips RF, Harr HW, et al (1967) Chordoma. Thirty-five-year study at Memorial Hospital. Cancer 20:1841-1850

Horner NB, Pinto RS (1989) The fat-cap sign: an aid to MR evaluation of extradural spinal tumors. Am J Neuroradiol 10:93

Hudson TM (1984) Fluid levels in aneurysmal bone cysts: a CT feature. AJR Am J Roentgenol 142:1001-1004

Huvos AG (1991) Bone tumors. Diagnosis, treatment, and prognosis. Saunders, Philadelphia

Jackson DE, Atlas SW, Main JR, Norman D (1989) Intraspinal synovial cysts: MR imaging. Radiology 170:527-530

Jaffe HL (1958) Tumors and tumorous conditions of the bones and joints. Lea and Febiger, Philadelphia

Jaffe N, Robertson R, Takane Y, et al (1985) Control of primary osteosarcoma with chemotherapy. Cancer 56:461-466

Jansen J, Terwey B, Markakis E (1990) MRI diagnosis of aneurysmal bone cysts. Neurosurg Rev 13:161-166

Johnson S, Klostermeier T, Weinstein A (1993) Case report 768. Skeletal Radiol 22:63-65

Jungreis CA, Cohen WA (1987) Spinal cord compression induced by steroid therapy: CT findings. J Comput Assist Tomogr 11:245-247

Kalina P, Hillstrom MM (1992) MR of extramedullary hematopoiesis causing cord compression in beta-thalassemia. Am J Neuroradiol 13:1407-1409

Kaplan JG, Barasch E, Hirschfield A, et al (1989) Spinal epidural lipomatosis: a serious complication of iatrogenic Cushing's syndrome. Neurology 39:1031-1034

Kempin S, Sundaresan N (1990) Disorders of the spine related to plasma cell dyscrasias. In: Sundaresan N, Schmidek HH, Schiller AL, Rosenthal DI (eds) Tumors of the spine – diagnosis and clinical management. Saunders, Philadelphia, pp 214-225

Keslar PJ, Buck JL, Suarez ES (1994) From the archives of the AFIP. Germ cell tumors of the sacrococcygeal region: radiologic-pathologic correlation. Radiographics 14:607-620

Kjerulf TD, Terry DW, Boubelik RJ (1986) Lumbar synovial or ganglion cysts. Neurosurgery 19:415-420

Kricun ME (1985) Red-yellow marrow conversion: its effect on the location of some solitary bone lesions. Skeletal Radiol 14:10-19

Kricun (1993) Imaging of bone tumors. Saunders, Philadelphia

Krol G, Sundaresan N, Deck M (1983) Computed tomography of axial chordomas. J Comput Assist Tomogr 7:286-289

Kuroda S, Abe H, Akino M, et al (1990) Infiltrating spinal angiolipoma causing myelopathy: case report. Neurosurgery 27:315-318

Laredo JD, Assouline E, Gelbert F, et al (1990) Vertebral hemangiomas: fat content as a sign of aggressiveness. Radiology 177:467-472

Li MH, Holtas S, Larsson E-M (1992) MR imaging of spinal lymphoma. Acta Radiol 33:338-342

Libshitz HI, Malthouse SR, Cunningham D, et al (1992) Multiple myeloma: appearance at MR imaging. Radiol 182:833-837

Lifeso RM, Younge D (1985) Aneurysmal bone cysts of the spine. Int Orthop 8:281-285

Lipson SJ, Neheedy MH, Kaplan MM, Bienfang DC (1980) Spinal stenosis caused by epidural lipomatosis in Cushing's syndrome. N Eng J Med 302:36

List CF (1941) Intraspinal epidermoids, dermoids, and dermal sinuses. Surg Gynecol Obstet 73:525-538

Liu SS, Williams KD, Drayer BP, et al (1990) Synovial cysts of the lumbo-sacral spine: diagnosis by MR imaging. Am J Neuroradiol 10:1239-1242

Ljung F, Helin I, Stromblad LG (1984) Ganglioneuroma with an uncommon location in a six-year-old girl. Acta Paediatr Scand 73:411-413

Lodwick GS, Wilson AJ, Farrell C, et al (1980) Determining growth rates of focal lesions of bone from radiographs. Radiology 134:577-583

Lyons MK, O'Neill BP, Marsh WR, Kurtin PJ (1992) Primary spinal epidural non-Hodgkin's lymphoma: report of eight patients and review of the literature. Neurosurgery 30:675-680

Macdonald DR (1990) Clinical manifestations. In: Sundaresan N, Schmidek HH, Schiller AL, Rosenthal DI (eds) Tumors of the spine – diagnosis and clinical management. Saunders, Philadelphia, pp 6-21

Madewell JE, Moser RP (1988) Radiologic evaluation of soft tissue tumors. In: Enzinger FM, Weiss SW (eds) Soft tissue tumors. Mosby, St Louis, pp 43-82

Maehara T, Tanohata K, Noda M, Nakayama D (1991) Medically treated steroid-induced spinal epidural lipomatosis. J Neurosurg 74:38-42

Martinez V, Sissons HA (1988) Aneurysmal bone cyst: a review of 123 cases including m primary lesions and those secondary to other bone pathology. Cancer 61:2291-2304

Mascalchi M, Arnetoli G, Pazzo GD et al. (1991) MR of spinal angiolipoma. Am J Neuroradiol 12:744-745

Matsushima K, Shinohara Y, Yamamoto M, et al (1987) Spinal extradural angiolipoma: MR and CT diagnosis. J Comput Assist Tomogr 11:1104-1106

McMaster MJ, Soule EH, Ivins JC (1975) Hemangiopericytoma: a clinicopathological study and long-term follow-up of 60 patients. Cancer 36:2232-2244

Menei P, Rickeh A, Favier T, et al (1994) Vertebral hemangioma. Spontaneous spinal canal remodeling after fracture. Spine 19:849-851

Meyer JE, Lepke RA, Lindfors KK, et al (1984) Chordomas: their CT appearance in the cervical, thoracic, and lumbar spine. Radiology 153:693-696

Mirra JM, Picci P, Gold RH (1989) Bone tumors – clinical, radiologic, and pathologic correlations. Lea and Febiger, Philadelphia

Moazam F, Talbert JL (1985) Congenital anorectal malformations. Arch Surg 120:856-859

Monajati A, Spitzer RM, Wiley JL, Heggeness L (1986) MR imaging of a spinal teratoma. J of Comput Assist Tomogr 10:307-310

Moulopoulos LA, Dimopoulos MA, Alexanian R, et al (1994) Multiple myeloma: MR patterns of response to treatment. Radiology 193: 441-446

Moulopoulos LA, Varma DGK, Dimopoulos MA, et al (1992) Multiple myeloma: spinal imaging in patients with untreated newly diagnosed disease. Radiology 185:833-840

Mulder JD, Schütte HE, Kroon HM, Taconis WK (1993) Radiologic atlas of bone tumors. Elsevier, Amsterdam

Munday TL, Johnson MH, Hayes CW, et al (1994) Musculoskeletal causes of spinal axis compromise: beyond the usual suspects. Radiographics 14:1225-1245

Munk P, Helms CA, Johnston J, et al (1989) MR imaging of aneurysmal bone cysts. AJR Am J Roentgenol 153:99-101

Muraszko KM, Antunes JL, Hilal SK, Michelsen WJ (1982) Hemangiopericytoma of the spine. Neurosurgery 10:473-479

Nabors MW, Pait TG, Byrd EB, et al (1988) Updated assessment and current classification of spinal meningeal cysts. J Neurosurg 68:366-377

Naidich TP, McLone DG, Harwood Nash DC (1983a) Spinal dysraphism. In: Newton TH, Potts DG (eds) Computed tomography of the spine and spinal cord. Clavadel, San Anselmo, pp 336-340

Naidich TP, McLone DG, Harwood-Nash DC (1983b) Arachnoid cysts, paravertebral meningoceles, and perineural cysts. In: Newton TH, Potts DG (eds) Computed tomography of the spine and spinal cord. Clavadel, San Anselmo, pp 383-396

Naidich TP, Zimmerman RA, McLone DG, Raybaud CA, Altman NR (1991) Congenital anomalies of the spine and spinal cord. In: Atlas SW (ed) Magnetic resonance imaging of the brain and spine. Raven, New York, pp 865-919

Nesbit ME, Kieffer B, d'Angio GJ (1969) Reconstitution of vertebral height in histiocytosis: a long-term follow-up. J Bone Joint Surg [Am]51:1360-1368

Nittner K (1976) Spinal meningiomas, neurinomas, and neurofibromas and hourglass tumours. In: Vinken PJ, Bruyn GW (eds) Tumours of the spine and spinal cord, part II. Elsevier, New York, pp 177-322 (Handbook of clinical neurology, vol 20)

Noël P, Pepersack T, Vanbinst A, Allé J-L (1992) Spinal epidural lipomatosis in Cushing's syndrome secondary to an adrenal tumor. Neurology 42:1250-1251

North RB, Kidd DH, Wang H (1990) Occult, bilateral anterior sacral and intrasacral meningeal and perineural cysts: case report and review of the literature. Neurosurgery 27:981-986

Onofrio BM, Svien HJ (1976) Solitary and multiple vertebral myelomas. In: Vinken PJ, Bruyn GW (eds) Tumours of the spine and spinal cord, part II. Elsevier, New York, pp 9-18 (Handbook of clinical neurology, vol 20)

Oot RF, Melville GE, New PFJ, et al (1988) The role of MR and CT in evaluating clival chordomas and chondrosarcomas. Am J Neuroradiol 9:715-723

Otake S, Matsuo M, Nishizawa S, et al (1992) Ossification of the posterior longitudinal ligament: MR evaluation. Am J Neuroradiol 13:1059-1067

Pagni CA, Canavero S (1992) Spinal epidural angiolipoma: rare or unreported? Neurosurgery 31:758-764

Pantongrag-Brown L, Suwanwela N (1992) Case report: chronic spinal cord compression from extramedullary hematopoiesis in thalassaemia - MRI findings. Clin Radiol 46:281-283

Papavasiliou C, Gouliamos A, Vlakos L, et al. (1990) CT and MRI of symptomatic involvement by extramedullary hematopoiesis. Clin Radiol 42:91-92

Phillips J, Chiu L (1987) Magnetic resonance of intraspinal epidermoid cyst: a case report. J Comput Assist Tomogr 11:181-183

Post KD, McCormick PC (1990) Surgical considerations in pelvic tumors with intraspinal extension. In: Sundaresan N, Schmidek HH, Schiller AL, Rosenthal DI (eds) Tumors of the spine - diagnosis and clinical management. Saunders, Philadelphia, pp 391-410

Prenger EC (1991) Magnetic resonance imaging of the pediatric spine. Semin Ultrasound CT MR 12:410-428

Price F, Bell H (1985) Spinal cord compression due to extramedullary hematopoiesis: successful treatment in a patient with long-standing myelofibrosis. J Am Med Assoc 253:2876-2877

Punt F, Pritchard J, Pincott JR, Till K (1980) Neuroblastoma: a review of 21 cases presenting with cord compression. Cancer 45:3095-3101

Quint DJ, Boulos RS, Sanders WP, et al (1988) Epidural lipomatosis. Radiology 169:485-490

Radley MG, McDonald JV (1992) Meningeal hemangiopericytoma of the posterior fossa and thoracic spinal epidural space: case report. Neurosurgery 30:446-452

Rahmouni A, Divine M, Mathieu D, et al (1993a) Detection of multiple myeloma involving the spine: efficacy of fat-suppression and contrast-enhanced MR imaging. AJR Am J Roentgenol 160:1049-1052

Rahmouni A, Divine M, Mathieu D, et al (1993b) MR appearance of multiple myeloma of the spine before and after treatment. AJR Am J Roentgenol 160:1053-1057

Rao TV, Narayanaswamy KS, Shankar SK (1982) "Primary" spinal epidural lymphomas. A clinico-pathological study. Acta Neurochir (Wien) 62:307-317

Rasmussen TB, Kernohan JW, Adson AW (1940) Pathologic classification, with surgical consideration, of intraspinal tumors. Ann Surg 111:513-530

Resjo IM, Harwood-Nash D, Fitz CR, Chuang S (1979) CT metrizamide myelography for intraspinal and paraspinal neoplasms in infants and children. AJR Am J Roentgenol 132:367-372

Resnick D, Niwayama G (1988) Diagnosis of bone and joint tumors, 2nd edn. Saunders, Philadelphia

Rhoton AL, Kao CC, Uihlein A (1976) Extradural ganglion cyst. In: Vinken PJ, Bruyn GW (eds) Tumours of the spine and spinal cord, part II. Elsevier, New York, pp 605-609 (Handbook of clinical neurology, vol 20)

Ricci C, Cova M, Kang YS, et al (1990) Normal age related patterns of cellular and fatty bone marrow distribution in the axial skeleton: MR imaging study. Radiology 177:83-88

Robinson L, Dominguez R, Cabrera J, et al (1989) Multiple meningeal cysts in Marfan's syndrome. Am J Neuroradiol 10:1275-1276

Rosenberg AE, Schiller AL (1990) Tumorous lesions of the spine: an overview. In: Sundaresan N, Schmidek HH, Schiller AL, Rosenthal DI (eds) Tumors of the spine - diagnosis and clinical management. Saunders, Philadelphia, pp 82-85

Rosenthal DI, Scott JA, Marcove RC (1985) Sacrococcygeal chordoma: magnetic resonance imaging and computed tomography. AJR Am J Roentgenol 145:143-147

Ross JS, Masaryk TJ, Modic MT, et al (1987) Vertebral hemangiomas: MR imaging. Radiology 165:165-169

Rovira M (1991) Intraspinal neuroblastoma. In: Quencer RM (ed) MRI of the spine. Raven, New York, pp 150-151

Roy-Camille R, Mazel CH, Husson JL, Saillant G (1991) Symptomatic spinal epidural lipomatosis induced by long-term steroid treatment. Review of the literature and report of two additional cases. Spine 16:1365-1371

Russell DS, Rubinstein LJ (1989) Pathology of tumours of the nervous system, 5th edn. Williams and Wilkins, Baltimore

Salomon Q, Freilich MD (1988) Calcified hemangioma of the spinal canal: unusual CT and MR presentation. Am J Neuroradiol 9:799-802

Schäfer E-R (1976) The spinal compression syndrome - a review of differential diagnosis. In: Vinken PJ, Bruyn GW (eds) Tumours of the spine and spinal cord, part II. Elsevier, New York, pp 347-386 (Handbook of clinical neurology, vol 20)

Schmidek HH, Schiller AL (1990) Premalignant lesions of the osseous spine and classification of primary tumors. In: Sundaresan N, Schmidek HH, Schiller AL, Rosenthal DI (eds) Tumors of the spine - diagnosis and clinical management. Saunders, Philadelphia, pp 3-5

Schmorl G (1971) The human spine in health and disease, 2nd edn. Grune and Stratton, New York

Schnyder P, Fankhauser H, Mausouri B (1986) Computed tomography in spinal hemangioma with cord compression. Skeletal Radiol 15:372-375

Sebag G, Dubois J, Beniaminowitz A, et al (1993) Extraosseous spinal chordoma: radiographic appearance. Am J Neuroradiol 14:205-207

Sharaffuddin MJA, Haddad FS, Hitchon PW, et al (1992) Treatment options in primary Ewing's sarcoma of the spine: report of 7 cases and review of the literature. Neurosurgery 30:610-619

Shaver RW, Clore FR (1981) Extramedullary hematopoiesis in myeloid dysplasia. AJR Am J Roentgenol 137:874-876

Siegel MJ, Jamroz GA, Glazer HS, Abramson CL (1986) MR imaging of intraspinal extension of neuroblastoma. J Comput Assist Tomogr 10:593-595

Silbergleit R, Gebarski SS, Brungerg JA, et al (1990) Lumbar synovial cysts: correlation of myelographic, CT, MR and pathologic findings. AJR Am J Roentgenol 11:777-779

Smith J, Ludwig RL, Marcove RC (1987) Sacrococcygeal chordoma: a clinicoradiological study of 60 patients. Skeletal Radiol 16:37-44

Smoker WRK, Biller J, Moore SA, et al (1986) Intradural spinal teratoma: case report and review of the literature. Am J Neuroradiol 7:905-910

St. Amour TE, Hodges SC, Laakman RW, Tamas DE (1994) MRI of the spine. Raven, New York

Stephens GC, Schwartz HS (1993) Lumbosacral chordoma resection: image integration and surgical planning. J Surg Oncol 54:226-232

Stull MA, Kransdorf MJ, Devaney KO (1992) Langerhans cell histiocytosis of bone. Radiographics 12:801-823

Sugimura H, Kakitsubata Y, Suzuki Y, et al (1992) MRI of ossification of ligamentum flavum. J Comput Assist Tomogr 16:73-76

Sundaram M, Awwad EE (1986) Magnetic resonance imaging of arachnoid cysts destroying the sacrum. AJR Am J Roentgenol 146:359-360

Sundaresan N, Rosenthal DI, Schiller AL, Krol G (1990) Chordomas. In: Sundaresan N, Schmidek HH, Schiller AL, Rosenthal DI (eds) Tumors of the spine – diagnosis and clinical management. Saunders, Philadelphia, pp 192-213

Sze G, Uichanco LS, Brant-Zawadski MN, et al (1988) Chordomas: MR imaging. Radiology 166:187-191

Sze G, Twohig M (1991) Neoplastic disease of the spine and spinal cord. In: Atlas SW (ed) Magnetic resonance imaging of the brain and spine. Raven, New York, pp 921-965

Takemoto K, Matsumura Y, Hashimoto H, et al (1988) MR imaging of intraspinal tumors – capability in histological differentiation and compartmentalization of extramedullary tumors. Neuroradiology 30:303-309

Tomita T (1990) Special considerations in surgery of pediatric spine tumors. In: Sundaresan N, Schiller AL, Rosenthal DI (eds) Tumors of the spine–diagnosis and clinical management. Saunders, Philadelphia, pp 258-271

Verstraete KL, Martens F, Smeets, P, et al (1989) Traumatic lumbosacral nerve root meningoceles. The value of myelography, CT, and MRI in the assessment of nerve root continuity. Neuroradiology 31:425-429

Verstraete KL, De Deene Y, Roels H, et al (1994) Benign and malignant musculoskeletal lesions: dynamic contrast-enhanced MR imaging – parametric "first-pass" images depict tissue vascularization and perfusion. Radiology 192:835-843

Villas C, Martinez-Peric R, Barrios RH, Beguiristain JL (1993) Eosinophilic granuloma of the spine with and without vertebra plana: long-term follow-up of six cases. J Spinal Disord 6:260-268

Visciani A, Savoiardo M, Balestrini MR, Solero CL (1989) Iatrogenic intraspinal epidermoid tumor: myelo CT and MRI diagnosis. Neuroradiology 31:273-275

von Hanwehr R, Apuzzo MLJ, Ahmadi J, Chandrasoma P (1985) Thoracic spinal angiomyolipoma: case report and literature review. Neurosurgery 16:406-411

Wang AY, Lipson SJ, Haykal HA, et al (1984) CT of aneurysmal bone cyst of the L1 vertebral body. J Comput Assist Tomogr 8:1186-1189

Weill A, del Carpio-O'Donovan R, Tampieri D, et al (1991) Spinal angiolipomas: CT and MR characteristics. J Comput Assist Tomogr 15:83-85

Weinstein JB, Siegel MJ, Griffith RC (1984) Spinal Ewing's sarcoma: misleading appearances. Skeletal Radiol 11:262-265

Werner JL, Taybi H (1970) Presacral masses in childhood. AJR Am J Roentgenol 109:403-409

Yamashita Y, Takahashi M, Matsuno Y, et al (1990) Spinal cord compression due to ossification of ligaments: MR imaging. Radiology 175:843-848

Yochum TR, Lile RL, Schultz GD, et al (1993) Acquired spinal stenosis secondary to an expanding thoracic vertebral hemangioma. Spine 18:299-305

Yuh WTC, Drew JM, Weinstein JN, et al (1991) Intraspinal synovial cysts. Magnetic resonance evaluation. Spine 16:740-745

6 Imaging of Extradural Tumours: Secondary Tumours in Childhood

J. RATCLIFFE

6.1 Introduction and Pathology

Neoplasms are relatively rare in childhood compared to the incidence of neoplasms in adult life. In the USA, the estimated number of new cancers in 1992 was 1130000 for patients of all ages (BORING et al. 1992), but approximately only 6000 (0.5%) children are diagnosed with cancer each year (MILLER 1989), of which fewer than 3000 die. The metastases of the commonest neoplasms in adult life–breast, lung and prostatic carcinomas–have a predilection to involve bone, and spinal metastases are far commoner in adults than in children. Epidural metastases causing cord compression were observed in only 5% of 2259 children with solid malignant tumours (KLEIN et al. 1991). As a result the generalist will only rarely see a child with spinal extradural tumour, which is characteristically protean in its clini-

J. RATCLIFFE, FRCS(E), FRCR, FRACR Department of Radiological Sciences, Royal Children's Hospital Herston, Queensland 4029, Australia

cal manifestation, and it is likely that the paediatric radiologist will have had more experience of this condition than the referring physician.

Tumours of childhood which involve the spine secondarily either by metastasis or by direct spread are typically the leukaemias, neuroblastoma, Ewing's tumour, primitive neuroectodermal tumours (PNET), other small round cell tumours of childhood, the various forms of lymphoma and disseminated rhabdomyosarcoma (Table 6.1; KLEIN et al. 1991). Any malignant tumour, however, may be the primary source for secondary involvement of the spine.

Table 6.1. Childhood tumours metastasising to spine causing compression of the spinal cord (after KLEIN et al 1991)

Pathology	Number	Percent
Neuroblastoma	32	28
Ewing's sarcoma	30	26
Osteosarcoma	16	14
Rhabdomyosarcoma	14	12
Hodgkin's disease	8	7
Germ cell tumour	4	4
Others	3	3
Total	113	

Histiocytosis X is not a true neoplastic process but is the most common destructive process found in the paediatric spine and must be considered in the differential diagnosis of extradural spinal tumour. Histiocytic lesions may be multiple or in older children may be single. Diagnosis will often be by biopsy because the lesions in the early stages mimic neoplastic deposits except that histiocytic lesions are usually "cold" on scintiscan.

Paediatric tumour can be confused clinically with infection because many paediatric tumours can be associated with fever and leucocytosis. Chemotherapy for neoplasm suppresses host defences, which may confuse the clinical distinction between spinal secondary tumour and infection. Analysis of the results of imaging investigations in the light of anatomical knowledge can often help to confirm the presence of infection (RATCLIFFE 1985). However, no amount of imaging can absolutely establish a histological or microbiological diagnosis, and the paediatric radiologist must be prepared to perform biopsies frequently in many equivocal cases.

6.2
Presentation

Secondary tumour of the spine may be found in three different ways, and the purpose and process of imaging management differ according to how and when the spinal secondary is found. Children may present for medical attention because of the symptoms and signs of their spinal secondary tumour, the spinal tumour may be found in the work-up after discovery of the primary tumour, or the spinal secondary tumour may be discovered after treatment of the primary has started, no spinal secondary tumour having been suspected initially.

When a child presents because of spinal symptoms, imaging is directed at establishing whether the symptoms are due to inflammatory, mechanical or neoplastic causes and, if neoplastic, whether the tumour is primary or secondary. If secondary, then the primary tumour must be identified. Imaging must be extensive, thorough and urgent.

In the child who has presented with other symptoms and the primary tumour has been identified as of a type which may commonly spread to the skeleton and in which treatment is modified by the presence of secondary spread, then the secondaries must be sought in order to stage the disease and to help monitor the response to treatment. In the absence of spinal symptoms, however, investigation can be limited. If the neoplasm is one in which treatment is not modified by the presence of non-symptomatic spinal secondaries such as in leukaemia, which constitutes approximately 30% of all childhood neoplasia, then the identification of spinal secondaries is not usually performed.

If the primary tumour is one which does not usually metastasise to bone, such as CNS tumours or nephroblastoma (except the rare clear cell form), which between them constitute another 25% of childhood neoplasms, then spinal and bone investigations are not necessary.

If the symptoms or signs of the extradural spinal secondary tumour are first identified after treatment of the primary tumour has started, investigation must again be thorough and urgent to confirm that the symptoms are due to a neoplastic process and not to a mechanical or inflammatory complication of treatment. If the interval between commencing apparently successful treatment and the identification of the spinal secondary tumour is more than 6 months, then the possibility of a second primary tumour should be considered. Second primary tumours must be distinguished from radiation induced sarcomas which can also occur in children. A number of syndromes and conditions found in children, such as sporadic aniridia, Beckwith-Wiedemann syndrome and neurofibromatosis type I, are associated with neoplasms, and second primary tumours are not uncommon. Radiation-induced sarcomas can occur, but the interval, by definition, must be at least 4 years and the average interval is about 11 years (WIKLUND et al. 1991)

6.3
Symptomatology

Articulate older children with symptomatic extradural spinal tumours are able to describe and localise their symptoms with the same clarity and precision as adults. Sadly, lack of awareness on the part of parents and attending physicians will often result in a significant delay before a correct diagnosis is made. A useful adage is that any child thought to have a prolapsed intervertebral disc has a spinal tumour until proven otherwise (and even in the absence of tumour prolapsed intervertebral disc is probably not the correct diagnosis).

Spinal tumours in infants and younger children who cannot articulate well are much more difficult to identify. Pain may be expressed as irritability and ascribed to teething or reflux oesophagitis, especially as food refusal often accompanies chronic pain in childhood.

Neurological deficit in the infant may present as developmental stasis in caudal motor development, such as a refusal or inability to advance to crawling from sitting, or as caudal motor regression, such as an inability to walk after walking has been established. Changes in bowel or bladder function which in the adult will result in urgent investigation are often not recognised in the infant, and in the older child will usually be ascribed initially to almost any cause except spinal tumour.

The net result is that spinal tumours in children are recognised later in their course than are spinal tumours in adults.

6.4
Imaging Investigations

In the investigation of spinal symptoms in childhood there is no substitute for an awareness of the possible diagnosis of spinal tumour combined with a good clinical history and examination by a sympathetic and experienced physician. The paediatric radiologist must be prepared to take on this role, as he or she is likely to have more experience in the diagnosis of spinal tumours in children than the primary physician. The paediatric radiologist can urgently focus investigations to an appropriate minimum for proper management by the paediatric oncology or surgical team.

The planning and interpretation of imaging by the paediatric radiologist must take into account the purpose for which imaging is being performed and recognise that the developing paediatric spine, although superficially similar to the adult spinal column, has significant anatomical differences (Table 6.2).

Table 6.2. Anatomical differences between infant and adult vertebrae

Feature	Infant	Adult
Vertebra	Three jointed parts	Single bone
Arterial supply	Three layers in centrum, two metaphyseal and one equatorial; free intraosseous anastomosis; relatively avascular	Also has peripheral supply from secondary periosteal arteries; intraosseous arteries are end arteries; very well vascularised

6.5
Anatomy of the Paediatric Spine

Secondary tumour spread to the spinal column is either by direct spread from adjacent soft tissue or through metastasis via the blood stream or lymphatics. Comprehensive understanding of the anatomy of the spinal column and its blood supply helps explain some of the phenomena imaged. Recognition of the changes during maturation are particularly important for the paediatric radiologist.

6.5.1
Ossification Centres

It is conventional in the adult to think of the spinal column as consisting of 24 mobile bones (7 cervical, 12 thoracic and 5 lumbar vertebrae), a single mass of sacrum formed from 5 sacral segments and a few mobile coccygeal segments. The ventral half of the majority of each spinal bone is a solid cylinder attached to its cephalad and caudal neighbours by a fibrocartilaginous synchondrosis, the intervertebral disc. The dorsal half of each spinal bone, is a hollow cylinder attached firmly anteriorly to the ventral half of the spinal bone, articulating with its cephalad and caudal neighbours through two pairs of synovial joints. From this dorsal hollow cylinder arise three spikes which are the lateral and midline spinous processes. In the adult this is a single bone.

In the infant each vertebra consists of at least three separate bones, a centrum and paired bones for the neural arch. Each has its own blood supply and is joined to its neighbour within the same vertebra by an avascular cartilaginous synchondrosis which allows growth to proceed (KNUTSON 1961).

During the first 2 years of life the ossification centres of the neural arch fuse together (KNUTSON 1961). The ossification centres forming the pedicle of the neural arch do not fuse to the centrum until much later, starting at about 3 years in the upper spine and completing the process in the lower lumbar spine at about 7-9 years of age.

6.5.2
Blood Supply

The blood supply of the human paediatric and adult spinal column has been described in some detail (Table 6.3). The reader is referred to these papers for details, and only a composite summary is presented here in text and in Fig. 6.1-6.3.

6.5.2.1
Arterial Supply of Vertebral Body

At birth the spinal column is covered by a regular network of perichondrial (later periosteal) anastomosing arteries, the primary periosteal arteries, which arise from the segmental arteries. When ossification of the vertebral body is complete in adulthood, new and irregularly placed arteries arise from the primary periosteal vessels and the new periosteal arteries are called the secondary periosteal arteries. The secondary periosteal arteries increase in number as age advances (WILEY and TRUETA 1959; RATCLIFFE 1986).

In infancy and early childhood the interior of the vertebral body is supplied by primary intraosseous arteries which lie in three horizontal planes, one at

Table 6.3. Works on the blood supply of the vertebral column

Author(s)	Date	Subject
BOHMIG	1930	Arterial and venous supply of intervertebral disc
WAGONER and PRENDERGRASS	1932	Arterial and venous supply of vertebral body
BATSON	1940	Venous plexus of adult spine
FERGUSON	1950	Arterial and venous supply of fetal and infant spine
HARRIS and JONES	1956	Arterial supply to adult cervical spine
BATSON	1957	Venous plexus of adult spine
WILEY and TRUETA	1959	Arterial and venous supply of adult vertebral bodies
MINEIRO	1965	Arterial and venous supply of infant and adult spine
CROCK et al.	1973	Venous drainage of adult vertebral body
CROCK and YOSHIZAWA	1976	Arterial and venous supply of lumbar vertebrae
JAMIOLKOWSKA	1979	Arterial supply to adult lumbar neural arch
RATCLIFFE	1980	Arterial supply to adult lumbar vertebrae
RATCLIFFE	1981	Arterial supply to juvenile spine
RATCLIFFE	1982	Intraosseous arterial anastomoses in spine
RATCLIFFE	1986	Changes with age of arterial supply of spine

the equator and one near each metaphysis (RATCLIFFE 1981). These anastomose one with another and, as the vertebral body increases in size, the primary periosteal arteries increase in length in a radial fashion because the vertebra increase in diameter by the surface accretion of avascular cartilage. The ossification centre increases in diameter in a centrifugal manner following the expanding cartilaginous anlage (Fig 6.3). This results in the nutrient branches of the primary intraosseous arteries being directed centrifugally. The primary intraosseous arteries have a characteristic appearance (Fig 6.4).

At some time near adolescence the intraosseous anastomoses involute and the primary intraosseous arteries become end arteries (RATCLIFFE 1982). When ossification of the vertebral body is complete in late adolescence, the ossification centre comes in contact with the periosteum and a number of arteries arise from the secondary periosteal arteries and enter the bone, and are called secondary intraosseous arteries. These are morphologically quite different from the primary intraosseous arteries; they are short, supplying only the outer third of the vertebral body, have a smaller diameter, and have centripetally directed terminal branches (RATCLIFFE 1982, 1986; Fig. 6.5).

During childhood, adult life and senescence there can be no increase in the number of primary intraosseous arteries; there may be a reduction because of atheroma and embolism. In adult life the primary intraosseous arteries continue to grow in length, and in order to accommodate this increase in length, the arteries become increasingly coiled in the marrow cavity (Fig 6.6; RATCLIFFE 1986).

The secondary intraosseous arteries, however, do increase in number as age advances (RATCLIFFE 1986). The vertebral body in old age is a very well vascularised structure (WILEY and TRUETA 1959).

6.5.2.2
The Venous Drainage of the Vertebral Body

The venous system of the vertebral body is also arranged in three horizontal layers (CROCK et al. 1973, CROCK and YOSHIZAWA 1976) which correspond to the primary intraosseous arteries. The basivertebral veins correspond to the equatorial arteries and the horizontal subarticular collecting veins correspond to the metaphyseal arteries. These veins are large, similar in size, and thin-walled within the marrow and are reported to have numerous vertical anastomoses with one another even in adult life. The intraosseous veins of the vertebral body are dissimilar to most other venous systems in that myriads of minute venules drain into much larger venous sinuses without any uniform transition in calibre; CROCK and coworkers (1973) compared their appearance to that of the fibrous root system of some plants in which many of the roots are of similar size with clusters of fine radicles called root hairs. It has been noted that it is easy to inject barium suspensions into the intraosseous larger vertebral veins in post-mortem specimens but difficult to opacify the small radicles (WILEY and TRUETA 1959).

The basivertebral veins drain posteriorly into the anterior internal venous plexus which lies within the spinal canal anterior to the dura of the spinal cord and forms part of Batson's plexus. The anterior inter-

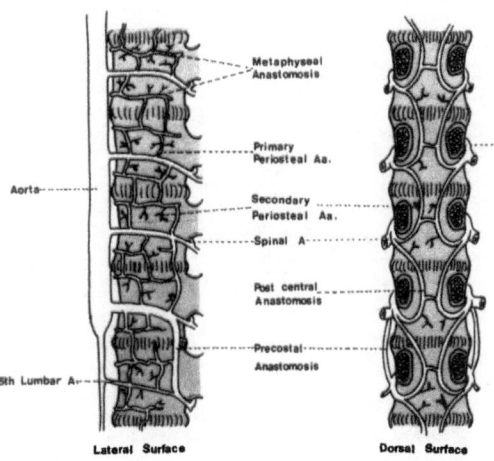

Figure 6.1

Fig. 6.1. Extraosseous arteries of the adult human lumbar vertebral bodies showing the antero-lateral surface and posterior surface of the lumbar spine with pedicles removed. See text for details.(from RATCLIFFE 1980 with permission from the *Journal of Anatomy*, Cambridge University Press)

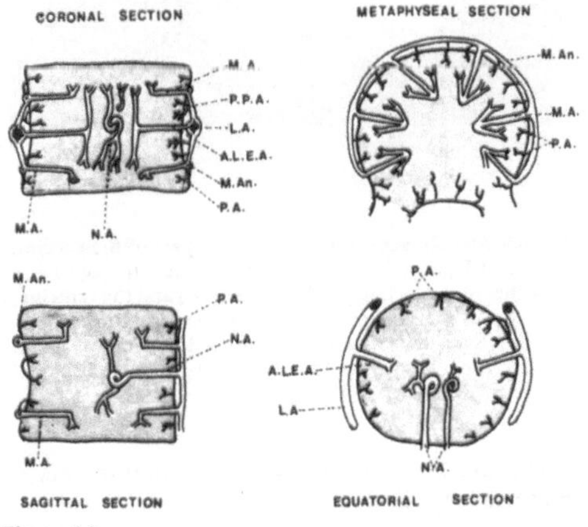

Figure 6.2.

Fig. 6.2. Intraosseous arteries of the adult human lumbar vertebra. The secondary periosteal arteries are not shown, in order to keep the diagram simple.Note that the fairly regular spacing of the secondary periosteal arteries on the vertebral surface results in clustering at the origin of the pedicle. (from RATCLIFFE 1980 with permission from the *Journal of Anatomy*, Cambridge University Press)

Name of artery	Arterial species
LA lumbar artery	Segmental artery
NA "nutrient" artery or, more properly, posterior equatorial artery	Primary intraosseous arteries
ALEA antero-lateral equatorial artery	
MA metaphyseal artery	
MAn metaphyseal anastomosis	Primary perichondral and periosteal extraosseous
PPA primary periosteal artery	anastomosis
PA peripheral artery	Secondary intraosseous artery

Fig. 6.3. Arterial supply to the vertebral body during development. The half-tone areas represent the cartilage of the developing vertebral body. The *left-hand column* represents axial sections in the metaphysis; *the second column* represents axial sections at the equator; the *third column* represents coronal sections; and the *fourth column* represents sagittal sections with the posterior surface of the vertebra to the right. The row *at top* represents the findings in the late foetus or neonate; the *second row* represents the findings in the late infancy; the *third row* represents the findings in childhood; and the *fourth row* represents the findings in a teenager. (From RATCLIFFE 1981 with permission from the *Journal of Anatomy*, Cambridge University Press)

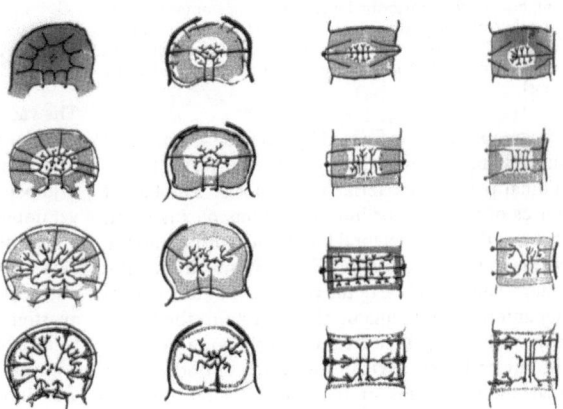

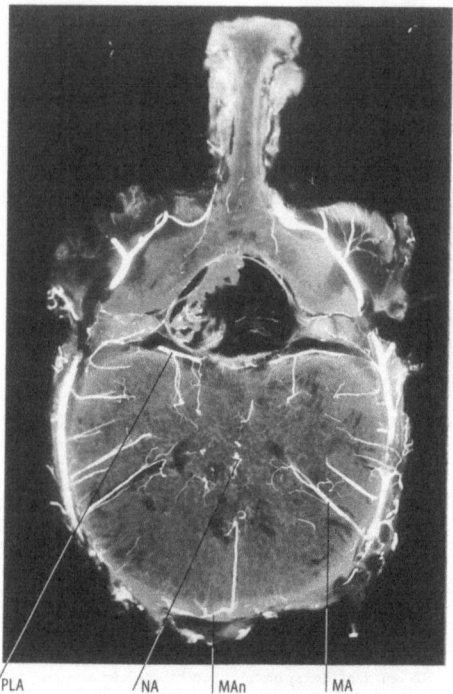

PLA   NA   MAn   MA

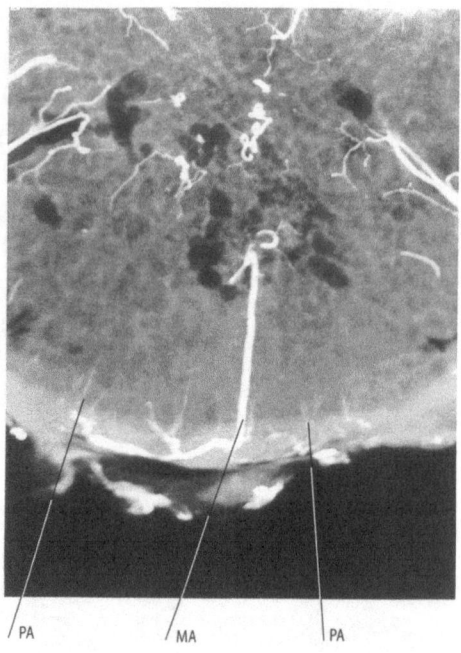

/ PA   / MA | PA

Fig. 6.5. An enlargement of the anterior part of the specimen shown in Fig. 6.4. This better demonstrates the centrifugal branches of the metaphyseal arteries (*MA*) and the centripetal branches of the smaller peripheral or secondary intraosseous arteries (*PA*). This arterial dimorphism is development and age-related.(From RATCLIFFE 1978, 1980 with permission from the *Journal of Anatomy*, Cambridge University Press)

Fig. 6.4. Radiograph of a horizontal section 3 mm thick from the second lumbar vertebra of a man aged 56 years after post - mortem injection of the aorta with a suspension of barium sulphate in gelatin. This shows the lower metaphyseal radial arteries (MA) which converge towards the centre and give off many centrifugal branches that have supplied the expanding ossification centre during growth. Behind the midpoint of the centrum the discally directed branches of the posterior equatorial arteries are shown: these used sometimes to be called "nutrient" arteries as are some arteries that supply the shaft of long bones. *PLA*, posterior longitudinal anastomosis; *MAn*, anterolateral metaphyseal anastomosis; *NA*, branches of the "nutrient" arteries. (From RATCLIFFE 1978, 1980 with permission from the *Journal of Anatomy*, Cambridge University Press)

nal venous plexus is formed by a series of rhomboid shaped anastomoses similar to the posterior longitudinal periosteal arterial anastomosis. The lateral apices of the anterior internal venous plexus drain through the intervertebral foramina to drain into the segmental veins. A network of veins drains the antero-lateral surface of the vertebral bodies, including antero-lateral equatorial arteries and the metaphyseal horizontal subarticular collecting veins of the antero-lateral parts of the vertebral bodies. The anastomosing veins of the antero-lateral surfaces

drain into the segmental veins and into the azygos and hemiazygos systems.

6.5.2.3
The Arterial Supply and Venous Drainage of the Neural Arch

The vascular supply of the neural arch has been less documented than the vascular supply of the vertebral body, and the following section is a composite synopsis of some published papers and of some as yet unpublished material of the author's.

The neural arch has a complex arterial anastomosis both on its internal and external surface from which also arise the arteries to the muscles of the back. These anastomoses communicate with each other at the intervertebral foramina and in the spaces between neighbouring laminae. From these arterial anastomoses arise intraosseous branches which supply the bone of

Fig. 6.6. Radiograph of a horizontal slice 20 mm thick from a lumbar vertebral body of a man aged 69 years after injection with a suspension of barium sulphate and gelatin. The periosteum and its vessels have been dissected off the left side. This image shows the right lumbar artery (*LA*), metaphyseal anastomosis (*MAn*), part of posterior longitudinal anastomosis (*PLA*), posterior equatorial arteries (*NA*), Antero-lateral equatorial arteries (*ALEA*) and metaphyseal arteries (*MA*). Only a few secondary intraosseous or peripheral arteries (*PA*) are seen in the reproduction.Notice in this figure and in Fig. 6.4 the crowding of arteries in the postero-lateral "corners" of the vertebral bodies where the pedicles arise and the nerve root passes through the intervertebral foramen. (From RATCLIFFE 1978, 1980 with permission from the *Journal of Anatomy*, Cambridge University Press)

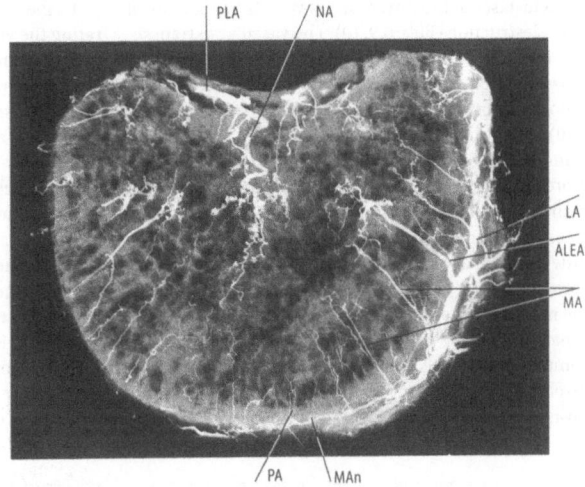

the neural arch. The intraosseous arteries are simpler morphologically than those of the vertebral body, do not seem to coil to the same extent as age advances, and the presence of intraosseous arterial anastomoses within the neural arch has not been explored.

The extraosseous venous system parallels the extraosseous arterial system and forms part of Batson's plexus, but the intraosseous veins of the neural arch have yet to be described.

The very extensive venous plexus which is now known as Batson's plexus was described as early as 1685 by VIESSENS and in the early 19th century by BRESCHET (1819; cited by BATSON 1957).

These earlier works were acknowledged by Batson, but it is to Batson himself that credit must go for recognising the function of the vertebral venous plexus.

He pointed out that it is an extracavity route for venous return, a storage space for reserve blood volume and has potential as a means for the spread of blood-borne metastatic disease from one systemic site to another without passing through the filter bed of the pulmonary capillaries. The elegant animal experiments of COMAN and DE LONG (1951) confirmed this potential. Batson's plexus is a complex reticulum of valveless periosteal veins on the surface of the vertebral bodies and neural arches and within the spinal canal extending from the venae vasorum of the thigh to the diploic veins of the cranium. Veins from the entire trunk drain into this plexus; of particular significance are veins from the prostatic, uterine and vesical plexuses and the chest wall including breast.

6.5.3
Relevance of Anatomy to the Appearance of Spinal Secondary Tumours

6.5.3.1
Growth Cartilage

Cartilage is a good but not perfect barrier to the spread of neoplasm yet a very poor barrier to the spread of infection. It follows that a destructive process identified on CT or MRI crossing these cartilaginous barriers in infancy is much more likely to be an infective than a neoplastic process because the barrier effect of the cartilage would tend to contain neoplasm. In older children, although the neoplasm may breach the bony plate between arch and centrum, focally this plate remains relatively intact with destruction of cancellous bone on both sides of the plate, whether the deposit occurred in the body (Fig. 6.7) or in the neural arch (Fig. 6.8).

6.5.3.2
Vascular Supply

The metastasis of tumour to the spine is presumed to be both arterial and venous. The importance of Batson's plexus in the metastasis of tumour has been adequately discussed in the chapter on extramedullary tumours in adults (Chap.4).

Metastases in the intraosseous vessels produce local bone destruction (Figs. 6.9, 10). The vascular extraosseous anastomoses may be involved by the centrifugal growth of tumour along vascular lumina (arterial or venous) from the site of intraosseous metastasis (Fig. 6.10) or by primary metastasis in the extraosseous anastomoses (Fig 6.8). One would conjecture that this is more likely in the slower flowing venous anastomoses than in the arterial anastomoses. Metastases in the extraosseous anastomoses may be greatly exophytic with little evidence of bone invasion across the cartilaginous vertebral anlage or cortex. The exophytic component of the metastasis is of particular interest within the spinal canal, where these extradural secondary tumours cause compression of the spinal contents with evidence of displacement and compression of the pedicle without invasion or destructive invasion of the cortex.

In the adult vertebral body there are no septa separating the very vascular vertebral body from the neural arch, nor are there many intraosseous arterial anastomoses. It could be inferred that tumor embolism could result in a small area of bone necrosis. Tumour deposited in the adult vertebral body can permeate rapidly into the root of the neural arch, destroying the outline of the pedicle. In addition, the adult vertebra is supplied with secondary periosteal arteries which increase in number as age advances. These are particularly densely clustered near the "corners" of the vertebral bodies, which is where the antero-lateral and posterior surfaces meet near the intervertebral foramen. Particularly in the adult and elderly the density of vessels entering the vertebral body is greater here than elsewhere in the vertebral body (Figs. 6.2, 6.6). Increased frequency of deposition of metastases at this site will result not only in

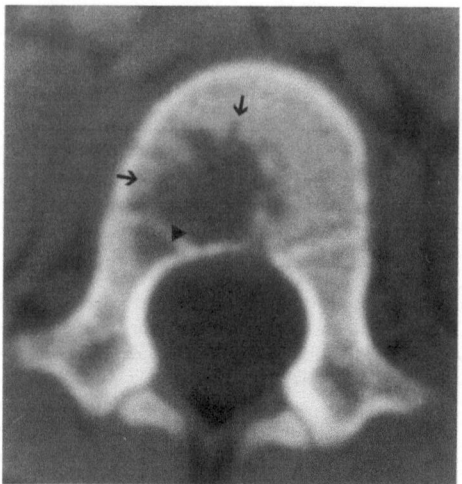

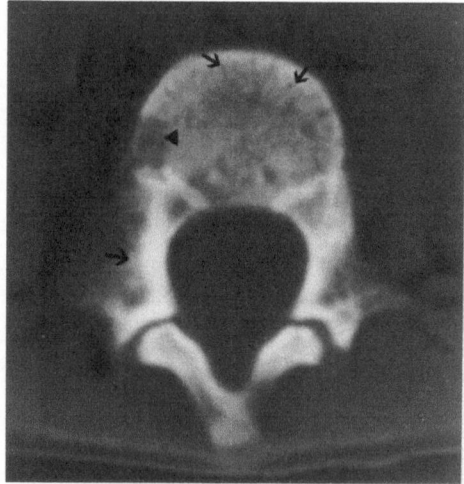

Fig. 6.7. A5-mm CT section of upper lumbar vertebra of a 5-year-old boy with neuroblastoma. This image shows a lytic focus due to metastasis in the upper metaphyseal region of an upper lumbar vertebral body. The tumour cell embolus may have impacted in the right nutrient artery. The metastasis expands in finger-like projections (*arrows*) which may correspond to the channels in the bone formed by the metaphyseal vessels. Whether the tumour is spreading along arteries or veins or the perivascular space is uncertain. The tumour seems to have breached the cartilage and calcific end plate between the right pedicle and centrum but the endplate appears relatively intact (*arrowhead*). Less clearly seen on the bone window is tumour which lies on the anterior wall of the spinal canal, probably deep to the posterior longitudinal ligament

Fig. 6.8. A5-mm CT section of upper lumbar vertebra of a 4.5-year-old boy with neuroblastoma. This image shows a metastasis which has embolised in perichondrial vessels of the right neural arch (*long arrow*) and has spread anteriorly crossing the cartilagino-calcific end plate of the centro-neural joint extraosseously and has begun to invade the centrum (*arrowhead*) from the surface. The end plate is well preserved, being relatively resistant to destruction by tumour. Normal vascular channels for metaphyseal vessels are shown (*short arrows*). In the adult this process would have produced ischaemia or infarction of the bone subjacent to the spreading neoplasm because the intraosseous arteries are end arteries. In the child the intraosseous arteries are anastomotic, and it is unlikely that this process mechanically devitalises bone. The result of this anatomical difference between adults and children may influence the spread of tumor in vertebral body and the effectiveness of the distribution to tumour of blood-borne chemotherapeutic agents and intrinsic host defence systems

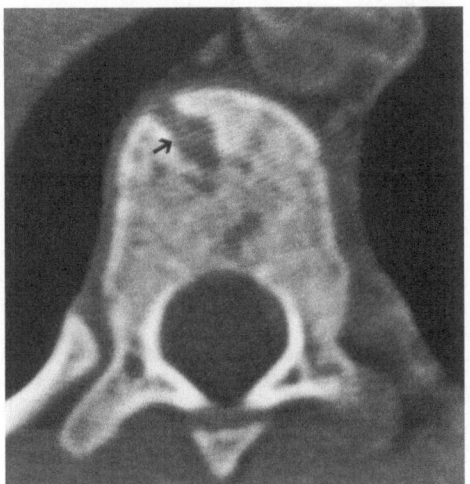

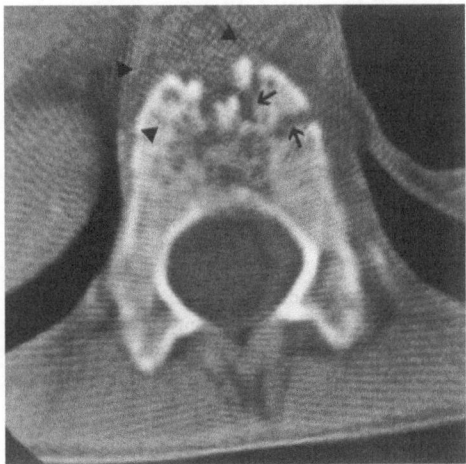

Fig. 6.9. A 3-mm CT section of thoracic vertebra of a 9-year-old girl with ganglioneuroblastoma. Metastasis in the vertebral body has expanded the normal channel of a metaphyseal or antero-lateral equatorial vessel, showing the radial spread of tumour parallel to the vessel (*arrow*) similar to the tumour spread shown in Fig. 6.7

Fig. 6.10. A 3-mm CT section of a different thoracic vertebra from the same patient as shown in Fig. 6.9. Metastases are shown in the upper metaphysis of the vertebral body. This image shows tumour expanding the radial vascular channels (*arrows*) of metaphyseal vessels. Anteriorly there is exophytic tumour (*arrowheads*), which is not well shown on bone window. There may also be some central bone destruction. Whether the tumour cell embolus was originally superficial with tumour spread down the vascular channels to the centrum, or whether the tumour embolus was in one of the metaphyseal vessels and spread centrifugally and centripetally, is conjectural. Some normal metaphyseal vascular channels are shown on the right (*open arrowhead*)

the common loss of the pedicle but also in single nerve root compression, which is relatively uncommon in childhood.

6.6
Imaging in Childhood Extradural Secondary Neoplasms

In the infant or child with symptoms referrable to the spine or spinal cord, the plan of investigation described below and summarised in Table 6.4 is appropriate.

Neurological symptoms and signs constitute an emergency, and we arrange, in consultation with the neurosurgical team, for urgent MRI. In institutions where access to MRI is limited, sufficient information for acute surgical management can be obtained from myelography followed by CT. In patients without neurological symptoms or signs the rate of investigation is more leisurely and investigation takes the directions indicated by clinical and pathological findings.

6.6.1
Plain Spinal Radiographs

Plain spinal radiographs in AP and lateral projection are still useful investigations and unsurpassed by any more modern modality in providing significant information rapidly, painlessly, and cheaply in many children with spinal disease. It is our practice, at presentation of a child with possible spinal tumour, to arrange for a radionuclide scan using a bone-seeking radiopharmaceutical and to request colleagues to undertake a clinical and biochemical search for primary tumour, infection and histiocytosis.

If at the time of presentation there is clinical or radiological suspicion that a spinal lesion exists which may be either neoplastic or tuberculous, it is our practice to perform a plain chest radiograph.

A slowly expanding lesion within the spinal canal will cause separation of the pedicles, which will also be narrowed. On the frontal projection of the spine, each pair of pedicles must be compared with the pairs above and below to assess (a) the width of the spinal canal and (b) the size of the pedicle (Fig. 6.11). On the lateral projection, comparison must be made with neighbouring vertebrae of (a) the AP diameter of the spinal canal of each vertebra, (b) the size of the intervertebral foramen and (c) the size of each pedicle in both horizontal length and vertical height.

A rapidly growing tumour will produce paraparesis without identifiable abnormality on the plain radiograph.

Absence of a pedicle may be due to complete destruction by compression from an intraspinal tumour, invasion by an epidural tumour, metastasis to the bone of the neural arch or a congenital anomaly. In the latter two cases, its counterpart will not be attenuated or displaced from the midline, and in the case of congenital anomaly it may be denser than normal.

Sclerotic spinal secondary tumour of the spine in childhood is rare but can occur in lymphoma. The dense flattened vertebral body of vertebra plana, which used to be called Calvé's disease, is characteristic of histiocytosis.

6.6.2
Nuclear Medicine Studies

A bone seeking radiopharmaceutical is used to demonstrate an abnormal increase in turnover of cal- cium (hot spots) in the skeleton and whether the hot spot is single or multiple. Hot spots will be identified in discitis and other types of infection which are of more than 24 h duration, in nearly all neoplasms of bone in childhood and in traumatic lesions. Photopenic areas (cold spots) may be found in histiocytosis and bone cysts if there has not been pathologic fracture and attempt at repair. Tumours of the spinal cord, meninges or epidural space without bone involvement will produce no change in the gamma camera images unless the pressure of an expanding lesion has produced a reactive change in the neural arch.

The gamma camera images show the number and location of hot spots and will help direct investigations with better anatomical resolution such as CT. If there is calcium metabolism in tissues other than skeleton, these too will be identified by the gamma camera. Of particular relevance are the calcium metabolism in a proportion of neuroblastomas (Fig. 6.12) and new bone formation in osteosarcoma secondaries which can be demonstrated by the bone scan.

The bone scan is a generally reliable screening procedure for significant bone pathology (GOSFIELD et al. 1993). It should be noted that some patients with spinal metastases shown on MRI have had negative or equivocal bone scans (KATTAPURAM et al. 1990; AITCHISON et al. 1992), and the negative bone scan should not be regarded as absolute refutation of the presence of neoplasm.

Table 6.4. Indications for imaging investigations in children suspected of having spinal extradural tumour

Indication		Investigation
Clinical condition	Imaging finding	
Back pain, no known neoplasm: ? Tumour ? Histiocytosis ? Infection		(1) AP and lateral radiography, (2) bone scintiscan; if either abnormal, go to MRI
Known neoplasm: ? Stage 1		Bone scintiscan; if abnormal, go to MRI
Paraparesis or other neurological abnormality	Abnormal radio- graphs or scintiscan	MRI (if not immediately available, myelography followed by CT)
Back pain, known neoplasm, no known secondary tumour		(1) Radiography, (2) bone scintiscan, (3) MRI
	Spinal lesion found on MRI, nature unknown	CT-guided biopsy

The scintiscan will almost always show uptake of radiotracer in peridiscal areas in discitis and vertebral osteomyelitis.

Metiodobenzylguanidine (MIBG) in which the iodine is a radioactive isotope may be used to identify the primary and secondary deposits of biochemically active tumours of adrenal medullary and related cell origin (GERRARD et al. 1987; MOYES et al. 1989; JACOBS et al. 1990). The commonest by far in childhood is neuroblastoma, but phaeochromocytoma and carcinoid tumour may also take up this radiopharmaceutical. When positive, this is a useful and fairly specific test, but not all neuroblastomas take up MIBG and its value is equivocal (BOULIERE-NAJEAN et al. 1992).

Gallium-67 is a radioactive isotope taken up by lymphomas of some histological types but not by others. It accumulates in sites of infection and in the large bowel. Its value is controversial (COHEN 1992).

6.6.3
Planar Tomography

Linear or complex geometric planar tomography is now of historical interest in the investigation of spinal tumours. Prior to CT, tomography was extensively used both on its own and in conjunction with myelography in identifying the position of tumours and spinal compression. There is still probably a small niche for linear tomography in the planning or monitoring of reconstructive surgery after spinal tumour has been successfully treated.

6.6.4
Ultrasound

We have found no place for ultrasound in the detection or management of spinal tumour.

Many of the tumours which give rise to spinal secondary deposits are of intra-abdominal solid organ or lymphatic tissue origin, and ultrasonic examination of the abdomen is invaluable in providing rapid, painless and accurate information concerning the intra-abdominal solid organs. In addition the status of the bladder should be recorded; as stated above, spinal compromise of bladder function may not be recognised in an infant with a spinal tumour, and the paediatric radiologist should seek to confirm that the bladder can be emptied.

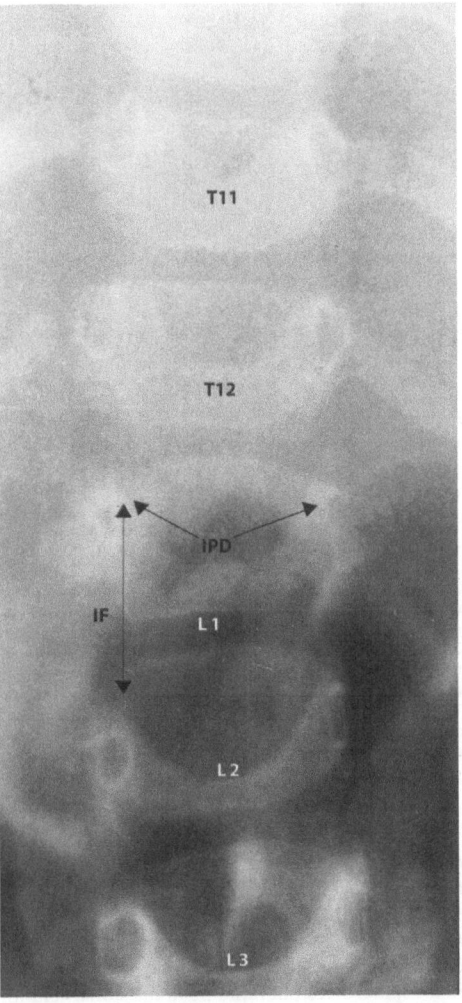

Fig. 6.11. AP radiograph of thoraco-lumbar junction of a 7-year-old girl with increasing weakness in both legs. School phobia was originally thought to be responsible but subsequent investigations revealed a dumbbell-shaped ganglioneuroblastoma. The pedicles of the 12th thoracic and third lumbar vertebrae are within normal limits. The pedicles of first and second lumbar vertebrae are smaller than normal, and the interpedicular distance (*IPD*) is wider than the interpedicular distance above and below. This is a common radiological sign of both extradural and intradural tumour in childhood. The height of the right intervertebral foramen (*IF*) between the first and second lumbar vertebra is greater than normal at the waist of the dumbbell tumour. This shows that it was an extradural tumour, because intradural tumours do not usually herniate through the intervertebral foramina. The cortex of the abnormal pedicle is clearly visible, whereas in the adult the absent pedicle is a useful sign (one not often found in children)

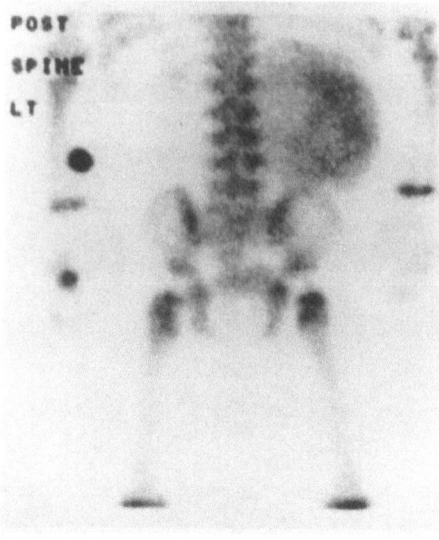

Fig. 6.12. Posterior view of a scintiscan of an infant of 14 months with a huge neuroblastoma on the right. The radiopharmaceutical used was technetium-99 phosphonate. It has been taken up in the tumour which on plain abdominal film had shown extensive calcification most marked in its lateral part. There is also increased uptake of radiotracer in the proximal femora. The increased photon density over the right side of the lumbar spine is largely due to overlap from the abdominal tumour-although there was marrow involvement and widespread bony metastases became more evident later

6.6.5
Myelography

Myelography in the past was invaluable for the localisation of masses impinging upon or arising within the spinal theca but tumours in the spinal column which do not impinge on the spinal theca cannot be visualised by myelography alone. In institutions where MRI is not readily available myelography is still useful both on its own or, better, prior to CT. CT myelography is discussed below (Sect. 6.6.7.1).

6.6.6
Magnetic Resonance Imaging

MRI is probably the most useful imaging modality for spinal secondary tumours (Sze 1991; Godersky et al. 1987; Sarpel et al. 1987) and generally more sensitive than plain radiographs, CT or radionuclide

scan (Avrihami et al. 1989). Like any other investigation, however, a few false negatives do occur (Helweg-Larsen et al. 1992). MRI does suffer from being expensive. It is also time-consuming because care must be taken to prevent the images from being degraded by motion artefact.

MRI is indicated if there is evidence of spinal cord compression, surgery on the spine is contemplated or diagnosis is in doubt. It is our practice to centre attention and imaging on those sections of the spine where a lesion causing neurological compromise may be located and on any section in which radionuclide studies indicate a hot spot. In all patients in whom neoplasm, infection or histiocytosis is suspected we perform T1- and T2- weighted scans in the sagittal plane (Fig. 6.13) and the axial plane. After intravenous gadolinium DPTA, which we administer in all such patients, we perform T1-weighted scans in sagittal and axial planes. Even when using 1.5 -T machines this can be a prolonged procedure, and we will often use general anaesthesia for young children so that there is no movement artefact. In order to reduce the time of investigation, the axial plane scans can be limited to areas of interest already identified on plain radiographs, radionuclide scans, clinical examination and sagittal MRI images.

Multiple spinal deposits can be identified on MRI, but MRI should not be used for screening to identify or exclude vertebral secondary tumours; that should be done in advance by the radionuclide scan with a bone-seeking radiopharmaceutical, because this is much cheaper, easily accessible and generally – not absolutely – reliable.

The normal maturation of the marrow from a low signal intensity to moderate signal intensity during the first year of life (Sebag et al. 1993) should not cause confusion. Residues rests of red marrow in vertebral bodies which may hypertrophy in rebound response after chemotherapy (Fig. 6.14) may cause confusion which will only be resolved by biopsy or repeat MRI after an interval.

MRI can produce excellent anatomical detail of the contents of the spinal canal and the vertebral column, but the histological diagnosis remains conjectural even after MRI.

6.6.7
Computerised Tomography

Abdominal and chest CT may be indicated for the investigation of the primary tumour or for staging a lymphoma. Spinal secondary deposits may be ob-

Fig. 6.13a,b. Sagittal MRI sections, 4.5 mm thick, of the spine of a 9-year-old girl with disseminated ganglioneuroblastoma. a TR 660, TE 16; b TR 2200, TE multiple. These images show the importance of both T1-weighted and T2-weighted sequences in identifying tumour in the spine in which conversion from red to yellow marrow is taking place. The largest metastases of this neuroblastoma were in the neural arches of the 12th thoracic and first lumbar vertebrae (*arrowheads*). Metastases are shown in thoracic vertebrae 8 and 9 (*arrows*) as low signal on T1-weighted and high signal on T2-weighted images with high conspicuity on the T2-weighted images. Using both sequences helps to differentiate tumour from "fat islands" and other normal fat which is often noticeable in the perivascular regions

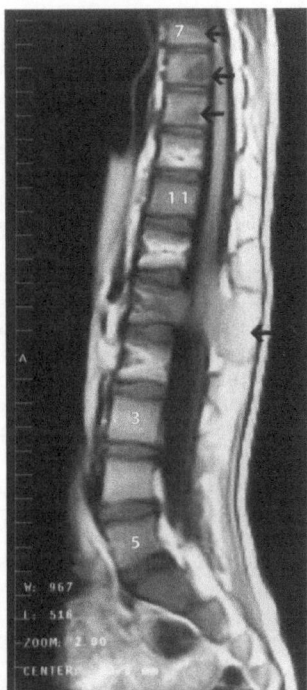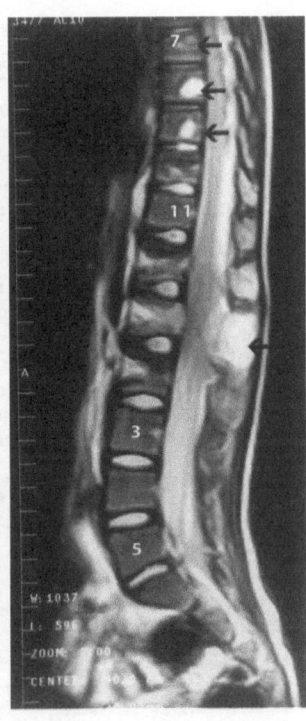

served during the course of these scans. Prior radionuclide scan is likely to have indicated their presence, and in the absence of neurological signs we document their presence by making images using appropriate window settings but do not specifically image them. MRI will be available to us in children who have neurological compromise, and CT will be used to further define the anatomy of bony destruction in order to assist in the monitoring of chemotherapy and in the planning of surgery to stabilise or reconstruct the vertebral column. Spiral CT is likely to be invaluable in this context, but as yet we have no experience of this modality in children with spinal secondary deposits.

6.6.7.1
CT Myelography

Prior to the availability of MRI, CT myelography was essential in demonstrating the relationship of intradural structures with intradural space-occupying lesions and extradural lesions compressing the dural sac. Myelography alone only reveals the shape of the dural

sac and its contents, whereas CT reveals the relationship of the sac and its contents with lesions in vertebral bodies, neural arches and paraspinal regions (Figs. 6.15, 6.16). It is still of immense value if MRI is not immediately available, and in some patients may be superior to MRI (HELWEG-LARSEN et al. 1992). CT should be performed after the myelogram, and in most instances the upper margin of an apparently complete block can be visualised (BOESEN et al. 1991).

6.6.7.2
CT with Biopsy

The main purpose of CT in extradural spinal secondary tumour in our institution at present is to guide percutaneous biopsy. This is indicated firstly in the child in whom an extradural spinal tumour is found and a primary tumour or a more easily accessible secondary tumour is not identified, and secondly in the child in whom malignancy has been recognised and who has a spinal lesion which may be a secondary tumour or some other pathology such as infection.

Histologists require biopsy cores of tissue for the diagnosis of childhood tumours, most of which are histologically complex. Fine needle aspiration may be adequate for the cytological recognition of carcinoma, but this is not appropriate in paediatric practice. We will biopsy tumours greater than 1 cm in diameter in the vertebral body of thoracic or lumbar spine, in any neural arch and in the extradural spinal canal below the level of the conus medullaris. The thoracic vertebral bodies can be biopsied without having to enter the pleural space (BRUGIERES et al. 1990). Although CT guided biopsy of cervical vertebral body has been performed elsewhere successfully (BRUGIERES et al. 1992), we are reluctant to perform biopsy of the cervical vertebral body in children because of the small size of the vertebral body relative to the size of a biopsiable lesion and the size

of an end cutting biopsy needle. We are also anxious about the possible damage to the vertebral arteries using a postero-lateral access. These lesions can be biopsied relatively easily transorally, but at our institution this is done by the orthopaedic surgeons and we have no experience of anterior biopsy approach. Our reluctance to biopsy extradural tumours above the level of the conus medullaris is due to the risk of acute cord compression should haemorrhage occur into the tumour at biopsy; we argue that if this occurs in a tumour compressing the cauda equina, there will be less risk of residual neurological deficit after urgent laminectomy than if the spinal cord were to be compressed.

We use end-cutting biopsy needles, either of the Ackermann type (Cook, Bloomington, Indiana, USA) for well- calcified tissue or 16-gauge Franseen

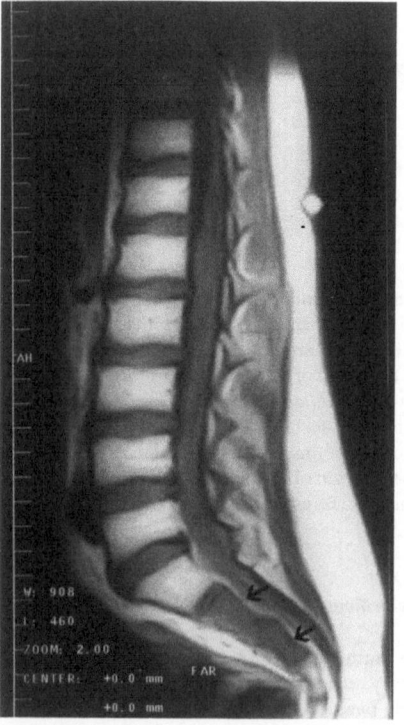

Fig. 6.14. Sagittal T1-weighted MRI section, 4.5 mm thick, of the spine of an 11-year-old boy recovering from chemotherapy for pelvic Ewing's tumour. TR 660, TE 16. This image shows extensive fat in the marrow of most of the vertebrae but with low signal from the bodies of two sacral sections (*arrows*), which was thought at another institution to be due to neoplasm (no T2-weighted images had been obtained). CT-guided needle biopsies proved the low signal material was healthy red bone marrow

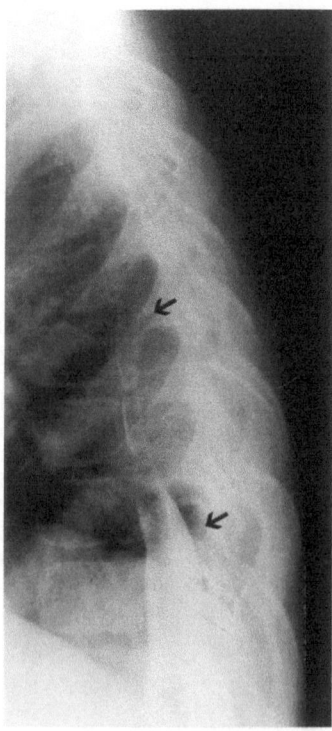

Fig. 6.15. Thoracic myelogram in a boy aged 11 years with weakness in his legs. This clearly shows the lower and, on this occasion, the upper limits (*arrows*) of a large extradural tumour which was a metastasis from a previously unrecognised huge pelvic Ewing's tumor. This investigation gives little indication of the lateral extent of tumour.

needle (Cook) for tumour which has breached the cortical surface or lies deep to eggshell thickness of bone. On one occasion we have done co-axial biopsy using the Ackermann needle to perforate the cortex of a lumbar vertebra and then obtained several cores of tumour using a Franseen needle.

We perform the biopsy under general anaesthetic because it is common for other invasive procedures such as lumbar puncture for CSF cytology and marrow aspiration to be performed at the same time. In younger children we perform the chest CT to look for pulmonary secondaries or mediastinal masses, if indicated, under the same anaesthetic because of the improved resolution obtained with controlled respiration.

We perform the spinal biopsy with the patient prone and will do planning CT scan of the vertebra to be biopsied as well as the vertebra above and below it in the prone position to verify the anatomy. It is our practice to make a CT image with the needle at the near edge of the tumour and a second image when the tumour has been transfixed by the needle before the core and needle are withdrawn to confirm that the lesion has been biopsied (Fig. 6.17). If doubt exists, another pass is made with CT confirmation. We send the specimen directly to the laboratory unfixed so that microbiological, genetic and immunological tests can be performed as well as histology.

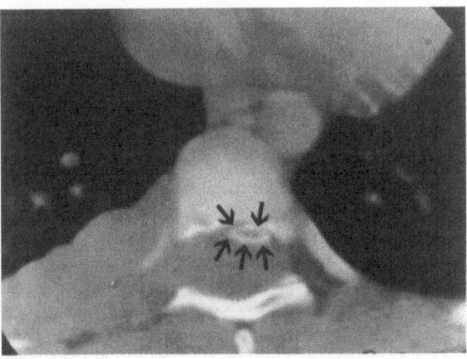

Fig. 6.16. A 3-mm CT section through a thoracic vertebra of the same patient as shown in Fig. 6.15. This image shows the compression of the spinal cord within the theca (*arrowheads*) and the extent of tumour extending into the right thoracic cavity. The patient had no lung metastases, and tumour spread had presumably been through Batson's plexus

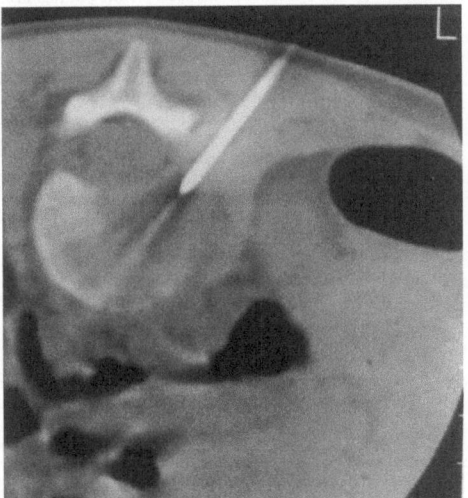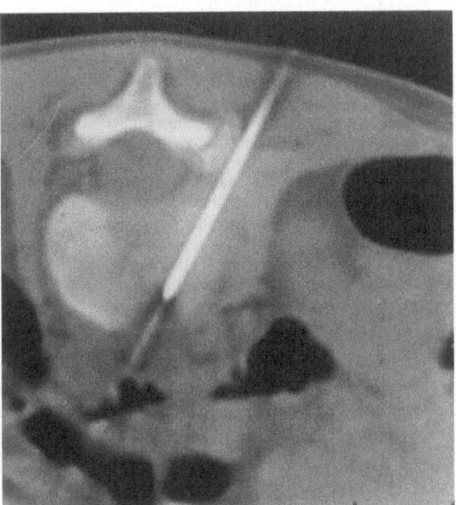

Fig. 6.17a,b. Five-millimeter CT sections through a lumbar vertebra of a boy aged 4 years with a painful lytic lesion approximately 15 mm in diametre in the first lumbar vertebra. The patient is prone. **a** The end-cutting (Franseen) needle on the proximal side of the tumour; **b** the position of the needle at the end of its traverse through the lesion. In this particular patient the lesion was shown to be histiocytosis

References

Aitchison FA, Poon FW, Hadley MD, Gray HW, Forrester AW (1992) Vertebral metastases and an equivocal bone scan: value of magnetic resonance imaging. Nucl Med Commun 13:429-431

Avrihami E, Tadmor R, Dally O, Hadar H (1989) Early MR demonstration of spinal metastases in patients with normal radiographs and CT and radionuclide scans. J Comput Assist Tomogr 13:598-602

Batson OV (1940) The function of the vertebral veins and their role in the spread of metastases. Ann Surg 112:138-149

Batson OV (1957) The vertebral vein system.   Am J Roentgenol 78:195-212

Boesen J, Johnsen A, Helweg-Larsen S, Sorensen PS (1991) Diagnostic value of spinal computer tomography in patients with intraspinal metastases causing complete block on myelography. Acta Radiol 32:1-2

Bohmig R (1930) Die Blutgefäßversorgung der Wirbelbandscheiben. Arch Klin Chir 158:374-424

Boring CC, Squires TS, Tong T (1992) Cancer statistics. Cancer 42:19-38

Bouliere-Najean B, Siles S, Panuel M, Cammilleri S, Faur F, Devred P, Kaphan G (1992) Value of MRI and MIBG-I123 scintigraphy in the diagnosis of spinal bone marrow involvement in neuroblastoma in children. Pediatr Radiol 22:443-446

Breschet G (1819) Essai sur les veines du rachis. Mequignon-Marvis, Paris.

Brugieres P, Gaston A, Heran F, Voisin MC, Mesault C (1990) Percutaneous biopsies of the thoracic spine under CT guidance: transcostovertebral approach. J Comput Assist Tomogr 14:446-448

Brugieres P, Gaston A, Voisin MC, Ricolfi F, Chakir N (1992) CT guided percutaneous biopsy of the cervical spine: a series of 12 cases. Neuroradiology 34:358-360

Cohen M (1992) Imaging of children with cancer. Mosby Year Book, St Louis, pp 99-100

Coman DR, DeLong RP (1951) The role of the vertebral venous system in the metastasis of cancer in the spinal column. Cancer 4:610-618

Crock HV, Yoshizawa H (1976) The blood supply of the lumbar vertebral column. Clin Orthop Rel Res 113:6-21

Crock HV, Yoshizawa H, Kame SK (1973) Observations on the venous drainage of the human vertebral body. J Bone Joint Surg [BR] 55:528-533

Ferguson WR (1950) Some observations on the circulation in foetal and infant spines. J Bone Joint Surg [AM] 32:640-656

Gerrard M, Eden OB, Merrick MV (1987) Imaging and treatment of disseminated neuroblastoma with ^{131}I-metaiodobenzylguanidine. Br J Radiol 60:393-395

Godersky JC, Smoker WR, Knutson R (1987) Use of magnetic resonance imaging in the evaluation of metastatic spinal disease. Neurosurgery 21:676-680

Gosfield E, Alavi A, Kneeland B (1993) Comparison of radionuclide bone scans and magnetic resonance imaging in detecting spinal metastases. J Nucl Med 34:2191-2198

Harris RS, Jones DM (1956) The arterial supply to the adult cervical vertebral bodies. J Bone Joint Surg [BR] 38:922-930

Helweg-Larsen S, Wagner A, Kjaer L, Johnsen A, Boesen J, Palner T, Sorensen PS (1992) Comparison of myelography combined with postmyelographic spinal CT and MRI in suspected metastatic disease of the spinal canal. J Neurooncol 13:231-237

Jacobs A, Delree M, Desprechins B, et al (1990) Consolidating the role of ^{131}I-MIBG scintigraphy in childhood neuroblastoma: five years of clinical experience. Pediatr Radiol 20:157-159

Jamiolkowska K (1979) Arterial vascularisation of the arches of lumbar vertebrae in man. Folia Morphol (Warsz) 38:65-76

Kattapuram SV, Khurana JS, Scott JA, el Khoury GY (1990) Negative scintigraphy with positive magnetic resonance imaging in bone metastases. Skeletal Radiol 19:113-116

Klein SL, Sanford RA, Muhlbauer MS (1991) Pediatric spinal epidural metastases. J Neurosurg 74:70-75

Knutson F (1961) Growth and differentiation of the postnatal vertebra. Acta Radiol 55:401-408

Miller RW (1989) Frequency and environmental epidemiology of childhood cancer. In: Pizzo PA, Poplack DG (eds) Principles and practice of pediatric oncology. Lippincott, Philadelphia, pp 3-18

Mineiro JD (1965) Coluna vertebral humana. MD thesis, Lisbon

Moyes JSC, Babich JW, Carter R, et al (1989) Quantitive study of radio-iodinated MIBG uptake in children with neuroblastoma. J Nucl Med 30:474-479

Ratcliffe JF (1978) Microarteriography of the cadaveric human lumbar spine. Acta Radiol 19 656-668

Ratcliffe JF (1980) The arterial anatomy of the adult human lumbar vertebral body. J Anat 131:57-79

Ratcliffe JF (1980) The arterial anatomy of the developing human dorsal and lumbar vertebral body. J Anat 133:625-638

Ratcliffe JF (1982) An evaluation of the intraosseous arteries in the human vertebral body at different ages. J Anat 134:373-382

Ratcliffe JF (1985) The anatomical basis for the pathogenesis and radiological features of vertebral osteomyelitis and its differentiation from childhood discitis. Acta Radiol 26: 137-143

Ratcliffe JF (1986) Arterial changes in the human vertebral body associated with aging. Spine 11:235-240

Sarpel S, Sarpel G, Yu E, Hyder S, Kaufman B, Hindo W, Ezdinli E (1987) Early diagnosis of spinal-epidural metastases by magnetic resonance imaging. Cancer 59:1112-1116

Sebag GH, Dubois J, Tabet M, Bonato A, Lallemand D (1993) Pediatric spinal bone marrow: assessment of normal age-related change in the MRI appearance. Pediatr Radiol 23: 515-518

Sze G (1991) Magnetic resonance imaging in the evaluation of spinal tumors. Cancer 67:1229-1241

Viessens R (1685) Neurographia universalia. Johannen Certe, Lugduni, p 146

Wagoner G, Prendergrass EP (1932) The intrinsic circulation of the vertebral body. Am J Roentgenol 27:818-829

Wiklund TA, Blomqvist CP, Raty J, et al (1991) Postirradiation sarcoma: analysis of a nationwide cancer registry material Cancer 68:524-531

Wiley AM, Trueta J (1959) The vascular anatomy of the spine and its relationship to pyogenic osteomyelitis. J Bone Joint Surg[Br] 41:796-809

7 Interventional Procedures of Vertebral Tumors

K.W. FRASER, C.F. DOWD, and M.J. DONOVAN POST

CONTENTS

7.1
Introduction

Interventional image-guided procedures of the spine and spinal cord continue to expand as technology provides better tools for less invasive techniques in

K. W. FRASER, MD, St. Francis Medical Center, Department of Radiology, 530 NE Glen Oak Avenue, Peoria, IL 61637, USA
C. F. DOWD, MD, Neurovascular Medical Group, Department of Radiology UCSF Medical Center, Room L352, 505 Parnasus Avenue, San Francisco, CA 94143-0628, USA
M.J. DONOVAN POST, MD, Department of Radiology, University of Miami School of Medicine, P.O. Box 016960 (R-109), Miami, FL 33101, USA

diagnosing and treating vascular lesions. This chapter will provide the reader with details of current techniques using radiologic guidance with respect to biopsy and embolization of vertebral and spinal cord lesions. Tumors of the spine are accessible for biopsy using fluoroscopic and computer tomography (CT) techniques with a variety of approaches. The issues of safety and accuracy will be discussed with an emphasis on avoidance of iatrogenic injury. The recent method of endovascular embolization of vascular lesions of the spine and percutaneous acrylic stabilization of the vertebral column will be presented.

Spinal angiography and embolization of spinal vascular malformations have also continued to be advanced with newer technology. A brief description of basic spinal vascular anatomy and the classification of the various types of vascular malformations of the spine and spinal cord should provide an introduction to the treatment of these lesions. Interventional neuroradiologic advances are providing safer and effective adjunctive, as well as definitive therapy of these complex vascular malformations of the spine.

7.2
Image-Guided Spinal Biopsy

7.2.1
Metastatic Tumor Involvement of the Spine

MALAWER and DELANEY (1989) identified the vertebral bodies as the most common site of metastatic disease, diagnosed in nearly a million US patients. The incidence of metastatic deposits in the spine approaches 70% of those patients succumbing to cancer. TATSUI et al. (1996) retrospectively studied 425 patients with scintigraphic detection of spinal metastases. The detection of spinal metastasis from the time of primary lesion diagnosis was shortest in lung cancer (3.6 + 6.1 months) and longest in breast cancer (29.4 + 33.5 months) 7.5% of patients presented with spinal metastases prior to the diagnoses of the primary lesion. The use of bone scintigraphy is useful in detection of metastatic bone tumors 3-18 months earlier than radiographs (RAMSDELL et al. 1977). The 1-year survival after spinal metastasis was high in prostate cancer (83%) and breast cancer (78%) but low in lung cancer (22%) and gastric cancer (0%; TATSUI et al. 1996). This data is important in selecting the optimal therapeutic methods based on the features of the primary lesions and expected prognosis. Therefore, after biopsy confirmation of the metastatic lesion, several options exist in the treatment of the spinal lesions. Even though bone scintigraphy can detect as little as 5-10% change in ratio in an area of normal bone representing an abnormal focus, MR imaging is more sensitive in identifying metastatic lesions for image guided biopsy. ALGRA et al. (1991) demonstrated higher sensitivity of MR than bone scintigrams for detection of vertebral metastases. In a double blind prospective study of 71 patients, bone scintigraphy identified 499 abnormal vertebrae and with MR imaging 818 abnormal vertebral lesions were identified, depicting an additional abnormal vertebra in 49 patients (70%). Four different types of metastasis were detected on MR, including focal sclerotic, focal lytic, diffuse homogeneous, and diffuse inhomogeneous lesions. MR analysis of metastatic involvement of the spine has rapidly replaced CT scanning for early detection of vertebral marrow replacement by tumor (Fig. 7.1; METHA et al. 1995). Different MR sequences are currently being evaluated for sensitivity, as well as for specificity in determining benign versus malignant replacement of the bone marrow. AN et al. (1995) evaluated serial MR studies of patients with benign or malignant compression fractures of the spine using the interpretations of two neuroradiologists with a sensitivity rate of 88.5% and a specificity rate of 89.5%. The diagnosis accuracy of percutaneous bone biopsy has been reported as high as 72% (DOLLAHITE et al. 1989), 78% (OTTOLENGHI 1955), and 93% (AYALA and ZORNOSH 1983).

Cervical spine vertebral biopsy can present more difficulty in developing a safe approach to specimen acquisition. Percutaneous biopsy of the cervical spine can be performed with either c-arm fluoroscopy (VALLS et al. 1948) or with CT guidance. TAMPIERI et al. (1991) described an anterolateral approach for lesions of C2-C7 with c-arm fluoroscopy in nine patients presenting with neck pain and varying degrees of myelopathy. In eight patients a definitive diagnosis was made histologically, with one patient having a nonspecific inflammatory process. The procedure was performed with local anesthesia with the patient in a supine position. The biopsy needle was directed medial to the anterior margin of the sternocleidomastoid muscle while retracting the muscle laterally to displace the common carotid artery as well. Therefore, the needle path bisects the plane between the airway and the common carotid artery. With the needle 2-3 mm from the vertebra, the stylet is removed and the trocar is advanced. The trocar is rotated in order to cut and then retracted from the specimen using slight negative vacuum effect. Prior to removal the c-arm fluoroscope is rotated to confirm the trajectory of the needle tip, and anteroposterior and lateral films are obtained to document the final position within the lesion.

OTTOLENGHI et al. (1964) described aspiration biopsy of the cervical spine by a posterolateral approach between the posterior margin of the sternocleidomastoid muscle and a vertical line originating from the tip of the mastoid for lesions of C4 to C7. This approach, however, is more difficult when approaching lesions of the anterior aspect of the cervical vertebral body. The uncovertebral joint can cause obstruction of the needle path with the posterolateral approach. Additionally, the vertebral artery in the foramen transversum may also be encountered.

Thoracic vertebral biopsy requires careful anatomic considerations to avoid iatrogenic complications of the pleural space, nerve roots, and spinal canal. Different approaches have been developed using fluoroscopic or CT-guided biopsies of the vertebral body, discs, or paraspinal soft tissues. The choice of CT or c-arm fluoroscopy depends on the skills of the physician, but more often CT is utilized in patients where there is difficulty in identifying the path of proposed navigation of the biopsy needle through the pedicle. (BRUGIERES et al. 1992) JELINEK et al. (1996) described a series of 32 patients undergoing percutaneous transpedicular biopsy of thoracic and lumbar vertebral body lesions; c-arm fluoroscopy was utilized in 25 patients and CT in 7 patients using 14- to 17-G osty-cut (Bard/Angiomed, Germany) biopsy needles. CT was selected in four patients with compression fractures, two with scoliosis, and one with severe osteopenia to provide a more accurate visualization of the needle path. The diagnosis was established in all patients but two patients required a second biopsy owing to suspicious but nondiagnostic cytological findings on the initial biopsy. There were no complications and all patients were discharged after a 2-h observation.

LAREDO and BARD (1986), using single-plane fluoroscopic guidance, performed 41 percutaneous biopsies of thoracic vertebral bodies from T3 to T12 without complication. The heads of the ribs deter-

Fig. 7.1a-c. A 34-year-old female with initial work-up for biopsy proven breast carcinoma. **a** Abnormal uptake in the left T6 transverse process; **b** MR demonstration of abnormal signal in the left T6 transverse process; **c** CT-guided biopsy of the left T6 transverse process was positive for solitary metastatic breast carcinoma. Note lack of findings on CT

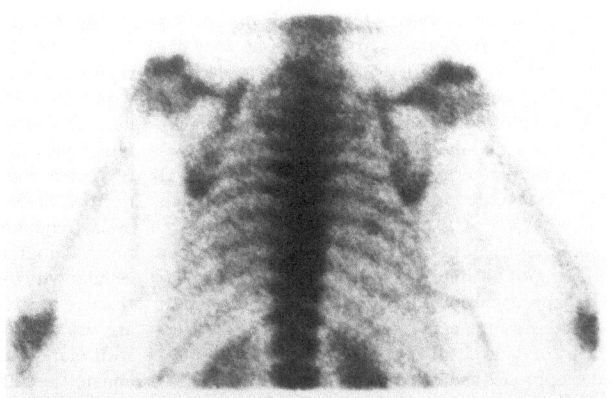

a

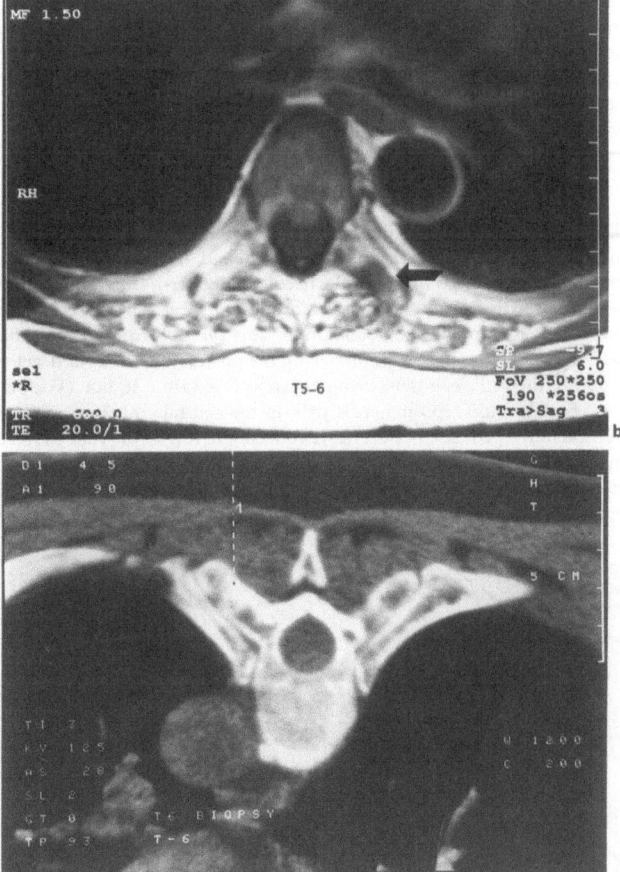

b

c

mine the path of the needle biopsy with the patient in a 35° angle from the sagittal plane, as first described by OTTOTENGHI (1969). This technique avoids the pleural space and spinal canal but is limited to lesions inferior or superior to a perpendicular line drawn along the margins of the pedicles. However, more than 50% of the volume of the vertebral body is accessible from the transpedicular approach (STRINGHAM et al. 1994).

Some spinal lesions of the thoracic or lumbar spine cannot be approached by a standard posterolateral approach. Specifically, if a lesion is located in the posterocentral aspect of the vertebral body, adjacent to or between the pedicles, then a transpedicular approach is utilized. The fluoroscopic radiographic anatomy of the thoracic pedicle has been described by PHILLIPS et al. (1994). The maximum diameter of the waist of the pedicle is visualized 15 (rotated in an axial fashion from a true lateral position. RENFREW et al. (1991) described CT-guided transpedicular vertebral biopsy in six patients. The pedicle is approached in a posterior-oblique fashion with the needle inserted posteriorly into the long axis of the pedicle (Fig. 7.2). Advantages of the CT-guided transpedicular approach cited by RENFREW et al. include (1) shorter needle tract, (2) guidance of the needle toward the pedicle via the acute angle formed by the adjacent transverse process and the mamillary process, (3) the tip of the needle being perpendicular to the cortex allows better torque control at the side of entry into the bone, and (4) the cortical surface of the bone is slightly thinner along the posterior aspect of the pedicle. It must be emphasized that care must be taken to keep the needle path in the central portion of the pedicle since the nerve roots are in intimate contact with the pedicle and a slightly medial path could interrupt the interior cortex with resultant epidural hemorrhage (McLAUGHLIN et al. 1976).

The disadvantages of percutaneous bone biopsy include sampling bias such as obtaining a small nonrepresentative area for histology. Other problems with processing the samples include crush artifact, necrotic debris, and possible nonrepresentative sampling bias. Lesions with sclerotic, blastic or cartilaginous components provide scant cells. Areas of necrosis or cystic lesions, such as aneurysmal bone cysts, frequently yield insufficient material for diagnosis. Benign lesions are often cystic, generally less cellular with less striking features when compared to reactive adjacent or normal bone. Malignant lesions are usually more cellular, less cystic – more solid with marked differences to normal bone. With adequate sampling a high accuracy rate of diagnosis can be expected with malignant lesions and giant cell tumors. However, if the bone lesion appears both benign and cystic, open excisional biopsy for more tissue may be necessary for an accurate diagnosis DOLLAHITE et al. 1989).

7.3
Vascularity of Vertebral Bone Tumors

The differentiation of benign from malignant bone tumors can be difficult. Angiography can provide additional information in the evaluation of tumors. Malignant tumor vascularity has been described as neovascularity, arteries with irregular caliber, abrupt angulations, distorted anatomic behavior, vascular lakes and arteriovenous (AV) shunting within the tumor (VOEGELI and FUCHS 1976). Benign tumors are more apt to have displacement of vessels, absence of venous lakes, and neovascularity. Nonspecific arteriographic findings which can be visualized in benign or malignant tumors (or even in infection) include hypervascularity with enlarged, regularly

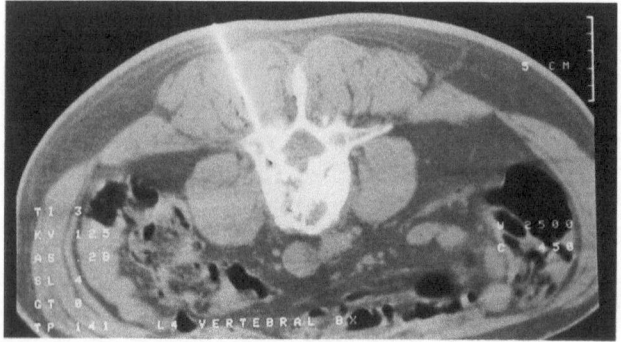

Fig. 7.2. CT-guided transpedicular approach in needle biopsy of metastatic lung carcinoma

shaped arterial pedicles, contrast medium accumulation with parenchymal staining during the capillary phase of angiography, and early regional venous drainage. The lack of tumor vessels or a mass with hypovascularity does not completely exclude malignancy (VIAMONTE et al.1973). The finding of the most vascularized areas within a particular tumor corresponding to the most malignant components has previously been confirmed with micro-angiographic studies (LAGERGREN et al. 1961). Thus, angiography can provide a guide for determining the site of biopsy prior to possible preoperative tumor embolization. Angiographic patterns of primary tumors of the vertebral body are nonspecific except for vertebral hemangiomas. The angiographic appearance of hemangiomas include normal sized arterial pedicles and heterogenous opacification with venous lakes involving portions of the vertebral body with contrast medium pooling late into the venous phase without AV shunting.

7.3.1
Primary Mass Lesions Involving the Vertebral Bodies

The variety of primary bone tumors involving the spinal axis encompasses benign as well as malignant types. Some of the benign tumors may behave in malignant fashion with progressive mass effect causing significant disturbance of neurologic function, or pain.

7.3.2
Vertebral Hemangiomas

Vertebral hemangiomas represent a spectrum of vascular disturbance of the bony matrix visualized radiographically (BALEY and BUEY 1929; PERMAN 1926) or histologically in 11% of the population at autopsy (SCHMORL and JUNGHANNE 1971). Classification of vertebral hemangiomas encompasses clinical, radiologic, angiographic, and histologic characteristics. Clinically, vertebral hemangiomas are classified as noninvasive, active, or intermediate (LAREDO et al. 1990). The pathophysiologic mechanisms by which vertebral hemangiomas can cause myeloradicular compression include expansion of the vertebra with narrowing of the central canal and direct spinal cord compression. Extension of soft tissue tumors into the epidural space or epidural

hematoma can compromise the central spinal canal (KOSARY et al. 1977, MCALLISTER et al. 1975). Fracture compression with mass effect can also encroach on the spinal cord (BELL 1955).

Asymptomatic vertebral hemangiomas (inactive) predominate in the lower thoracic and lumbar spine. With CT evaluation, thickened reinforced vertical trabeculae appear in axial images with a somewhat "polka-dot" appearance (DAHLIN and UNNI 1986). With intravenous contrast medium, the lesions enhance with pooling of contrast medium in the venous lake components. The MR appearance varies with the selected sequence, degree of fatty marrow replacement, and vascularity of the lesion (ROSS et al. 1987, LAREDO et al. 1986).

LAREDO et al. (1986) correlated the significance of fatty marrow replacement in 57 solitary vertebral hemangiomas. Those with the greatest fatty involution were more likely to be asymptomatic and without soft tissue epidural extension. Angiography by selective arterial injection demonstrated sites of dense, homogeneous, extensive hypervascularity with multiple venous lakes filling during the capillary phase and dense opacification of the entire vertebra rather than hemivertebra. There was no identified AV shunting (LAREDO et al. 1990).

Therapeutic interventional modalities for symptomatic vertebral hemangiomas consist of surgery (LANG and PERSERICO 1960; HEMMY et al. 1977; NGUYEN et al. 1987), radiotherapy (EISENSTEIN et al. 1986; FARIA et al. 1985; YANG et al. 1985), and embolization (GRAHAM and YANG 1984; HEKSTER et al. 1972; GROSS et al. 1976; PICARD et al. 1989; SMITH et al. 1993; DOPPMAN and PEVSNER 1983; RACO et al. 1990; NGUYEN et al. 1987; IDE et al. 1996; COTTEN et al. 1996). The treatment of vertebral hemangiomas involves a variety of approaches. Adjunctive preoperative endovascular transarterial embolization has been described with muscle particles (HEKSTER et al. 1972), gelfoam (GROSS et al. 1976; ESPARZA et al. 1978), polyvinyl alcohol (PVA) particles (SMITH et al. 1993), and alcohol (HEISS et al. 1994; DOPPMAN 1995). Embolization techniques for vertebral hemangiomas include transarterial catheter-directed materials (GROSS et al. 1976; HEKSTER et al. 1972; PICARD et al. 1989; SMITH et al. 1993; DOPPMAN and PEVSNER 1983) and direct percutaneous delivery of liquid agents (NICOLA and LINS 1987; HEISS et al. 1994; DOPPMAN 1995): the transarterial approach provides temporary devascularization prior to surgery but is relatively ineffective since hemangiomas have slow flow, with an intervening capillary bed trapping the particles. Additionally, multiple arterial pedicles usually increase the risk of transarterial embolization since collateral iatrogenic nontargeted emboli may reach arterial sources of the spinal cord. Therefore, direct percutaneous ablation of the vertebral hemangioma may provide the safest definitive approach.

Direct percutaneous treatment of vertebral hemangioma was designed to stabilize the inherent lattice structure of the abnormal trabeculae by the use of acrylic cement (NICOLA and LINS 1987; GANGI et al. 1994; COTTEN et al. 1996; IDE et al. 1996). The disadvantages of direct methyl methacrylate injection include the lack of destruction of the vascular cellular elements of the hemangioma and possible aggravation of the soft tissue mass effect on the epidural elements (HEISS et al. 1994).

HEISS et al. (1994) described the relief of spinal cord compression from vertebral hemangioma by intralesional absolute alcohol injection in two patients. The technique of ethanol ablation of vertebral hemangioma requires careful delivery of the agent. Ideally, the transpedicular route is safer than the lateral paraspinous approach, avoiding the potential iatrogenic effects with the pleural and retropleural spaces, or intercostal neurovascular structures. Using CT guidance, cannulation of the pedicle is performed with a smaller needle than required by the method of methyl methacrylate delivery. Evaluation of potential collateral venous effluents is performed with injection of nonionic contrast medium, defining the morphologic features including the volume and rate of delivery of ethanol. Careful, gentle injection technique is required to avoid retrograde filling of the capillaries or arteries. Cannulation of the largest well-vascularized venous lake is performed. The alcohol is injected with metrizamide to opacify the vertebral body. It is important to fill the entire lesion on the initial injection owing to the inherent risk of thrombosis, which can occur near the needletip with slow infusions which will subsequently fail to treat the remaining communicating venous lakes. A 30-min interval is allowed prior to removal of the needle to avoid tracking of the ethanol along the needletrack, potentially causing fascial necrosis. DOPPMAN (1995) described a 3-year follow-up in two patients which demonstrated reossification of the involved vertebral bodies, which can undergo reconstitution in postmenopausal women.

7.3.3
Benign and Malignant Vertebral Tumors

Aneurysmal bone cysts usually present with focal spinal pain in children and young adults (CORY et al. 1989). The aneurysmal bone cysts account for 1.4% of all bone tumors of which 20% are localized to the spine (DYSART et al. 1992). These tumors are benign histologically but can be locally aggressive, resulting in major neurologic deficit or death. The tumor usually originates in the posterior elements with contiguous involvement of the vertebral body. Angiographic analysis demonstrates diffuse inhomogeneous tumor staining with indistinct lakes of contrast medium opacification in cystic areas of the tumor (CHUANG et al. 1981; DISCH et al. 1986; DYSART et al. 1992; LINDBOM et al. 1961; Fig. 7.3).

Other rare vertebral tumors have been described angiographically, including chordoma (FIROOZNIA et al. 1976; PINTO et al. 1975; SUNDARESAN et al. 1979), osteosarcoma (VOEGELI and FUCHS 1976; YAGHMAI 1977), osteoid osteoma (KAMANO and FUKUSHIMA 1976; FUKUSHIMA et al. 1972), hemangiopericytoma (MURASZKO et al. 1982), giant cell tumors (LAURIN 1977; DJINDJIAN et al. 1981) and hemangioblastoma. Those tumors with hypervascularity and "safe" angioarchitecture may be embolized similar to previously described hemangiomas.

Transcatheter arterial embolization of primary vertebral bone tumors has been extensively documented with aneurysmal bone cysts (CHUANG et al. 1981; CORY et al. 1988; DECRISTOFARO et al. 1992; DEROSA et al. 1990; DISCH et al. 1986; KONYA and SZENDROI 1992; KUDO et al. 1984; SUBY-LONG et al. 1988). Many of these authors demonstrated some cases of regression and "cure" following embolization, with reossification of the tumor site. However, others have documented "recurrence" of the tumor 4 years after embolization (KOCI et al. 1995). SOO et al. (1982) demonstrated some bone reossification in four patients after embolization in six patients with giant cell tumors with gelfoam, PVA, and steel coils. Five of the six patients were pain free for a duration of from 3 months to 4 years after embolization.

7.3.4
Embolization of Metastatic Vertebral Tumors

Palliative embolization for vertebral metastases is usually for pain management, as well as to improve

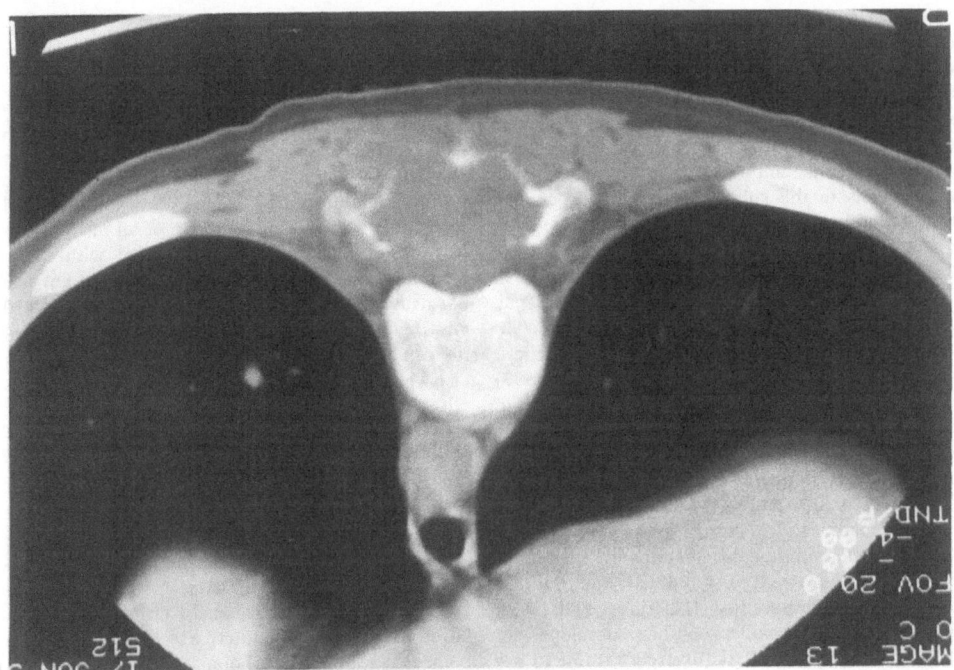

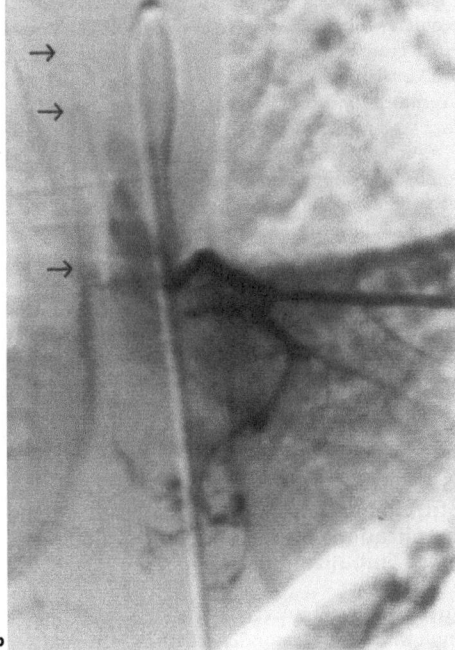

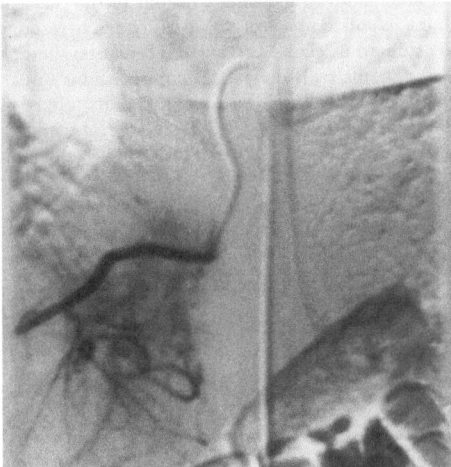

Fig. 7.3. a Non contrast enhanced CT with bony destruction and soft tissue encroachment of the central canal secondary to a thoracic aneurysmal bone cyst. **b** A pre-embolization spinal angiogram demonstrates an arterial pedicle supplying both the tumor and anterior spinal axis (*arrows*). Due to the risk of iatrogenic injury to the cord this pedicle was not embolized. **c** This arterial pedicle only opacified the blood supply to the tumor and was safely embolized with polyvinyl alcohol (PVA)

of the quality of life of the terminally ill patient (COURTHEOUX et al. 1985). Embolization of metastatic lesions to the vertebrae requires careful definition of the angioarchitecture of the tumor, adjacent structures, and, most importantly, by collateral avenues to the spinal arteries (Fig. 7.4). If the arterial anatomy permits, embolization of vascular metastatic lesions to the spine can decrease operation time, blood loss, and occasionally improve the margin of dissection of the tumor (BROADDUS et. al. 1990; GELLAD et al 1990; SUNDARESAN et al. 1990; KING et al. 1991; OLERUD et al. 1993; SOO et al. 1982; SMITH et al. 1995). SUNDARESAN et al. (1990) documented an average 5 units replacement in patients without preoperative embolization. OLERUD et al. (1993) demonstrated an average of two-thirds reduction in blood loss when comparing patients with metastatic renal cell carcinoma undergoing a posterior surgical approach with preoperative embolization with PVA or gelfoam to those patients without embolization.

Other methods of treatment of primary or metastatic lesions should be considered with a team approach. A new method of stereotactic radiosurgery has been recently described (HAMILTON et al. 1995). HAMILTON and his colleagues have developed an extracranial stereotactic radiosurgery frame to deliver a precise beam of radiation with a modified linear accelerator to metastatic lesions of the cervical, thoracic, and lumbar vertebrae which fail to respond to standard external fractionated radiation therapy. Five patients with metastatic spinal lesions underwent skeletal fixation with small clamps affixed to the spinous processes one to two vertebral segments above and below the targeted lesion. The calculated localization error was approximately 1.00 mm, with an isocentricity error of 1.0 mm for an overall radiation treatment error of 1.4-2.0 mm. This spinal stereotactic frame thus approaches the treatment accuracy of cranial radiosurgery (LUXTON et al. 1993).

7.4
Intrathecal Spinal Tumors

Intrathecal spinal tumors can be divided into intramedullary and extramedullary intradural lesions. Although, endovascular embolization of these lesions is rarely needed, an angiographic description and the role of embolization should be considered. The tumors of the spinal cord and dura possess a complex vascular supply usually from the anterior or posterolateral spinal arteries. These arteries are usually slightly enlarged but not as much as seen with

vascular lesions such as arteriovenous malformations (AVMs). Additionally, the drainage veins are usually prominent but without the rapid AV shunting visualized with AVMs. Of the intrathecal tumors, hemangioblastomas, meningiomas, paragangliomas, and neuromas have been the most frequently described.

Hemangioblastomas are an uncommon spinal cord tumor accounting for 2-4% of all intramedullary tumors. The tumor can present with intramedullary or subarachnoid hemorrhage at any age but usually occurs in young adults (average age 30 years). The tumor is usually intramedullary (80%) but can be extramedullary as well (20%). DJINDJIAN et al. (1981) detailed his experience with 135 patients with 163 intradural hemangioblastomas. As a rule, small intramedullary hemangioblastomas are supplied by only the anterior spinal artery. Moderate-size hemangioblastomas can be supplied by either the anterior or posterior spinal arteries, while large tumors were supplied by both. Angiographically, the anterior and/or posterolateral spinal arteries are enlarged, but not as greatly as seen with AVMs. Enlarged draining veins are usually visible. Slow circulation time is also a distinctive feature, with 12-35 s before the venous phase being identified, as opposed to AVMs.

Hemangioblastomas are usually solitary intramedullary tumors. However, in one-third of patients spinal cord hemangioblastoma may be associated with Von-Hippel Lindau disease. These patients may have more than one hemangioblastoma, as well as other visceral tumors.

Tumors of the cauda equina such as ependymoma, neurofibroma, or meningioma usually are not supplied by the lumbar arteries. The anterior and posterior lumbrosacral radicular arteries can be identified with the formation of an anastomotic network surrounding the conus medullaris as the posterolateral spinal arteries from L2 to L4. When evaluating these tumors angiographically, the artery of Adamkiewicz should be identified with regard to its location and possible existence as a vascular supply to the tumor.

7.5
Contraindications and Avoidance Iatrogenic Complications of Vertebral Body and Spinal Tumor Embolizations

Vertebral body biopsy carries a small risk of complication which is operator dependent. Selection of the

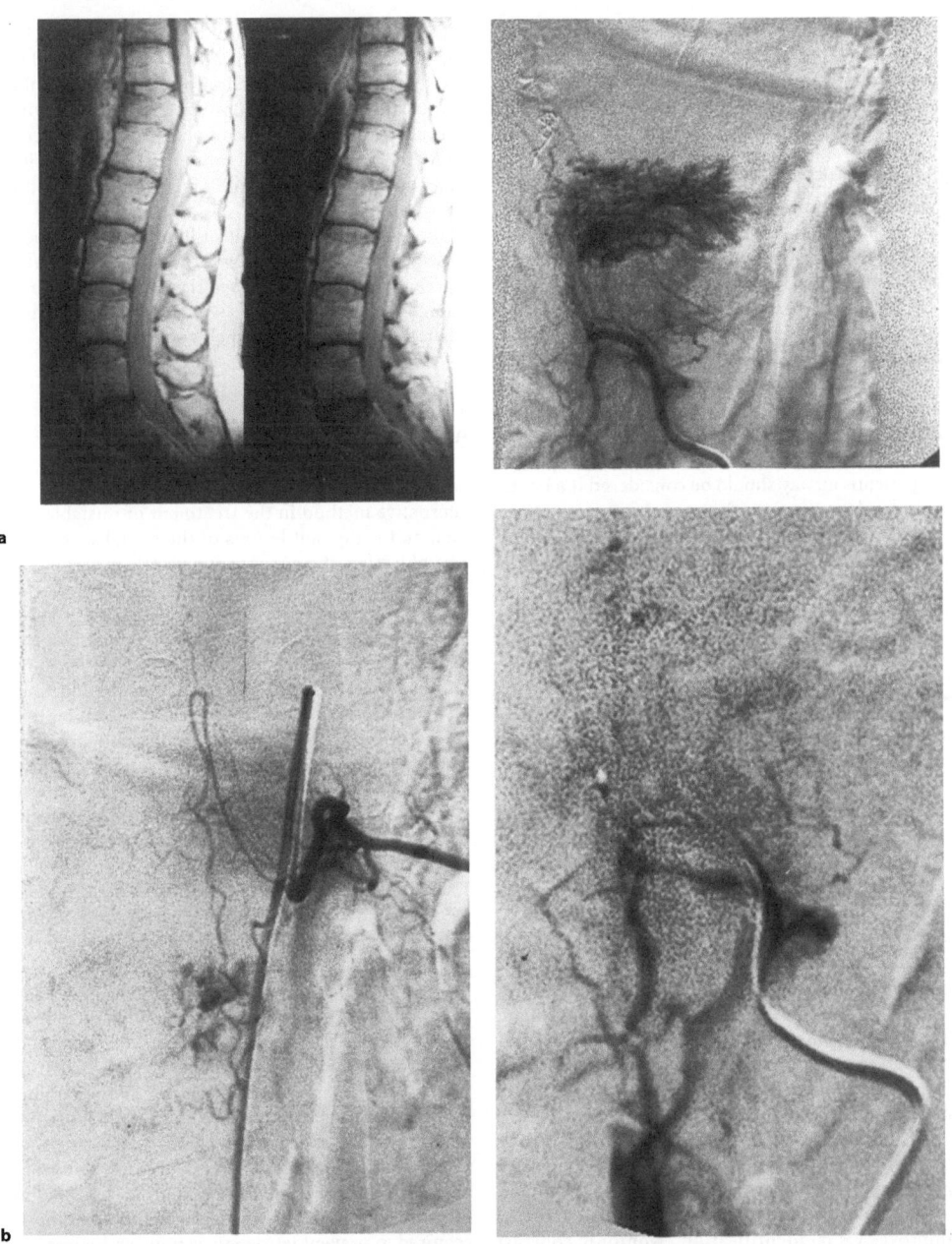

Fig. 7.4. a A sagittal MR image of T12 vertebral renal cell metastases with the central canal encroachment. b An anteroposterior (AP) supine angiogram with the arterial pedicle supplying both the anterior spinal artery and the tumor vascular system. This pedicle was not embolized. c An AP spinal angiogram with tumor neovascularity to the T12 vertebral body with metastatic renal cell carcinoma. Note coil embolization of the arterial pedicle at T11 to prevent collateral iatrogenic embolization to the anterior spinal axis. d Following post PVA embolization to metastatic renal cell carcinoma to T12 (AP)

optimal imaging modality is important. C-arm or biplane fluoroscopy provides dynamic real-time visual monitoring of the biopsy needle's path into the lesion. This can be less optimal with underlying demineralized bone with osteolysis or with osteoporosis. CT-guided biopsy provides a concise two-dimensional imaging of the needle's path with respect to various anatomic structures. The disadvantage with CT is the increased time and expense, as well as nondynamic real-time monitoring of the needle's movement. The possible vascular injury of brachiocephalic vessels with cervical vertebral biopsy usually can be reduced by use of contrast medium-enhanced CT mapping with respect to the vertebral or carotid arteries and their branches. If the carotid artery is punctured on an anterolateral approach to the cervical spine, gentle pressure is applied and held for 10-15 min. Careful monitoring of the patient's airway should be considered if a hematoma develops.

With spinal tumors and vertebral tumor embolizations, the risk of nontargeted occlusion must be carefully weighed against the benefits of devascularizing the tumor. To reduce potential adjacent normal tissue necrosis, a distal coil or gelfoam pledget is placed in the nontargeted branches prior to the embolization of the primary arterial pedicle supplying the tumor. Occasionally, temporary balloon occlusion is utilized during the embolization process to protect against distal iatrogenic embolization.

The selection of embolic agent is based upon the vascular characteristics of the lesion, the goal of therapy, and the personal experience of the interventionalist with the agents associated potential risks. The tumor or vascular lesion can be more deeply penetrated with smaller particles (< 150 u) and liquid embolic agents. However, these agents may also harbor the greatest risk of tissue necrosis and possibly thrombosis of the vasa nervosum of spinal nerves, causing neurological impairment. Therefore, agents greater than 150 u are recommended to provide adequate distal penetration with less risk to the capillary bed of adjacent soft tissues and spinal nerves.

The agents should also be well visualized during fluoroscopic delivery, preferably with a digital blank road map. The addition of tantalum powder to liquid adhesives such as normobutyl-cyanoacrylate (NBCA) improves visual identification. Nonionic contrast medium used in particulate embolization should be diluted to prevent clumping of the material in the microcatheter, decreasing the risk of catheter occlusion. If the microcatheter, does become occluded

with particulate, gentle probing with a microwire should be performed. If the operator tries instead to use forceful syringe injection pressure to clear the microcatheter, proximal rupture of the catheter with iatrogenic nontargeted embolization will occur. Sometimes the occlusion cannot be cleared easily, necessitating removal and replacement of the microcatheter.

Embolization of thoracic or lumbar arterial pedicles should be limited to two consecutive ipsilateral arteries. There is an increased risk of injury to spinal intercostal nerves, as well as of soft tissue ischemia when three contiguous pedicles are embolized.

7.6
Acrylic Vertebroplasty

Percutaneous acrylic vertebroplasty is becoming an alternative method in the treatment of unstable benign and malignant lesions of the spinal vertebrae. The objective of percutaneous vertebroplasty is to stabilize or prevent the collapse of unhealthy vertebral bodies. Currently, acrylic vertebroplasty is reserved for patients with pain without neurological deficit. Previously, patients with unstable vertebral bodies were treated with open reduction and stabilization with either bone grafts, metallic prostheses, or even operative methyl methacrylate reconstruction. The use of a combination of CT and fluoroscopy for the injection of methyl methacrylate to stabilize pathologic vertebral bodies has recently been described (GANGI et al. 1994; IDE et al. 1996; GALIBERT et al. 1987; COTTEN et al. 1996; KAEMMERLEN et al. 1989a, 1989b; DERAMOND et al. 1990). GANGI et al. (1994) described ten patients undergoing CT and fluoroscopic percutaneous vertebroplasty for severe osteoporosis, hemangiomas, and metastases. There were no complications and all ten patients were relieved of their back pain with follow-up of 4-17 months.

The technique of percutaneous acrylic vertebroplasty requires the evaluation of the anatomic boundaries of the central spinal canal, the adjacent neuroforamen, and the lateral recess in order to avoid encroachment on these structures. Additionally, upon injection of the pre-setting semi-liquid form of methyl methacrylate, real-time imaging is required to prevent iatrogenic venous embolization. The patient is placed in the prone position while titrating neuroleptanalgesic with local anesthesia during the placement of a large-bore cannula (10- to 12-g trocar needle). The patient should undergo close monitoring not only for sedation purposes, but for hypotension which can be related to the injection of the methyl methacrylate. The thoracic level is approached via a transpedicular or intercostovertebral pathway (Fig. 7.5a). The lumbar level can be approached by the transpedicular or posterolateral route. After placing the cannula in the optimal portion of the vertebral body (the mid-anterior third), fluoroscopy is then utilized with the gentle injection of 10-15 ml of nonionic contrast medium to identify the vertebral venous plexus (Fig. 7.5b). The components of the draining vertebral body plexus include the basivertebral vein, the anterior internal vertebral veins, the infra- and suprapediculate radicular veins, the ascending lumbar veins, and the lumbar segmental veins which ultimately drain into the inferior vena cava (HANLEY et al. 1994). After ascertaining the volume of contrast medium needed to replace the vascular elements of the vertebral body without reflux into the capillary or overinjection into the venous effluents, the methyl methacrylate is mixed with contrast medium (metrizamide, barium, tantalum, and/or tungsten). The acrylate cement rapidly polymerizes and must be injected within 2-3 min. The initial consistency of the acrylate is thin, but rapidly becomes pasty. The pasty consistency is important to prevent distal venous migration upon injection (GANGI et al. 1994). Additional small volumes are injected with Luer-Lok syringes mounted with a pressure regulator to facilitate the injection of the viscous methyl methacrylate. The injection is discontinued when epidural or paravertebral opacification is visualized with fluoroscopy to prevent spinal cord compression or venous embolization. When the cast of methyl methacrylate is inadequate, a contralateral injection should be considered to stabilize the vertebral body. It is important to remove the needle after the stylet has been replaced before the cement adheres the trocar into place. Within 6-7 min after mixing, the methyl methacrylate begins to solidify (Fig. 7.5c). Patients are monitored overnight, with discharge from the hospital after 1-2 days. Patients monitor their temperatures twice a week for 8 weeks to detect fever which may be a sign of infection. Post embolization plain films are obtained to provide a baseline study of the methyl methacrylate cast. After embolization the patients' pain should be relieved. However, some patients may still require surgical decompression of any soft tissue component or posterior decompression laminectomy (GANGI et al. 1994; COTTEN et al. 1996).

7.7
Spinal Angiography

Spinal angiography was introduced by DJINDJIAN et al. in 1962. Digital subtraction spinal angiography is replacing spinal subtraction angiography, introduced by DOPPMAN and DI CHIRO in 1965 (YEATES et al. 1985). Assessment of the angioarchitecture of the spine and the cord requires techniques with high-resolution filming, as well as timing of the contrast medium's passage from the arterial to the venous phases.

Most centers using digital subtraction spinal angiography utilize suspended apnea in patients who are under general endotracheal anesthesia. Since it is crucial to have minimal motion during the injection of contrast medium and long filming times (25-30 sec), apnea is induced during each arterial pedicle injection. To assess adequate injection of each artery, a vertebral blush should be visualized. The vertebral column derives its arterial supply from four main sources (CROCK and YOSHIZAWA 1977; CHIRAS et al. 1979). The craniocervical junction receives its blood supply from the muscular branches of the occipital artery, posterior branch of the ascending pharyngeal artery, and the anterior meningeal branch of the vertebral artery. The posterior ipsilateral half of each vertebral body is supplied by the anterior spinal canal artery branches from the vertebral artery in the cervical region, the intercostal arteries in the thoracic region, lumbar arteries in the lumbar region, and the iliolumbar arteries in the lumbosacral region. The posterior supply to the vertebral body is from the dorsospinal arterial branch of the radicular artery, and posterior spinal canal arteries supply the posterior elements including the lamina and posterior spinous process (CHOI and BERENSTEIN 1988). Since each vertebra sustains its primary arterial supply with vertebral, ascending cervical, intercostal, lumbar or hypogastric artery, an adequate arterial injection of each pedicle is measured by the ipsilateral hemi-vertebral blush. If the pedicle has been injected with enough contrast medium volume, a hemi-vertebral blush is visualized during the mid to late venous phase of the injection. Commonly, there is additional visualization of collateral opacification of adjacent craniad or caudad arterial pedicles on the ipsilateral side and occasionally of the contralateral arterial pedicles.

The arterial supply to the spinal cord is diverse and complicated. There are 31 pairs of vessels (62 arteries) entering the spinal canal through the intervertebral foramina. Most of these 31 radicular

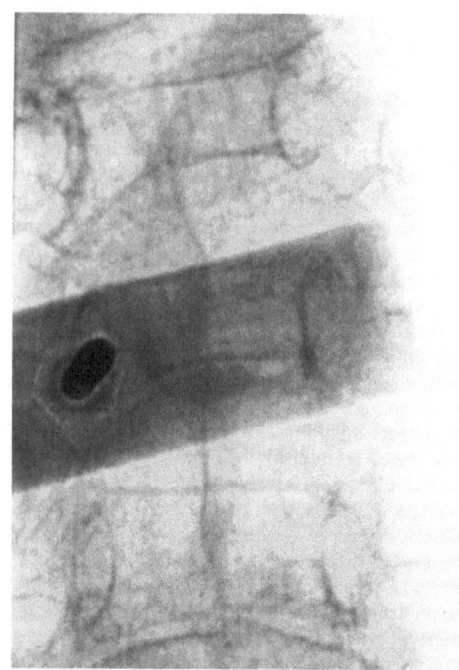

a

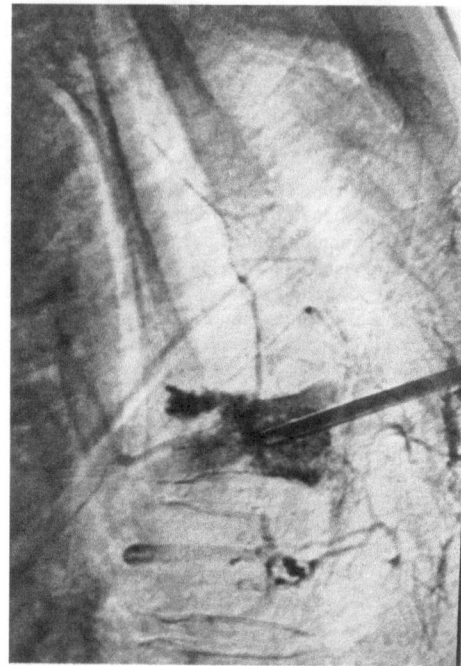

b

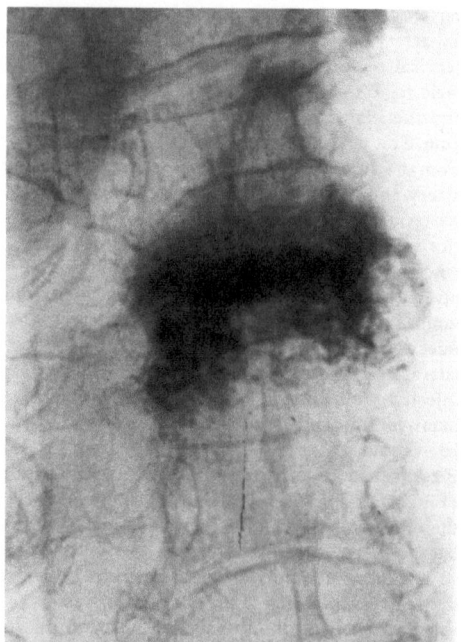

c

Fig. 7.5. a Fluoroscopically directed transpedicular cannulation of a thoracic vertebra in an elderly patient with pain from an osteoporotic insufficiency fracture (courtesy of Dr. Mary E. Jensen, University of Virginia). b Fluoroscopically monitoring of contrast evaluation with a transpedicular cannula. Note the epidural draining veins (courtesy of Dr. Mary E. Jensen, University of Virginia). c Following acrylic vertebroplasty with stabilization of the vertebral body: the patient was pain free, returning to ambulation within 24 h (courtesy of Dr. Mary E. Jensen, University of Virginia)

arteries have branches supplying the nerve roots, dura and pia mater, but rarely with medullary branches supplying the spinal cord. Fewer than eight radiculomedullary branches supply the entire spinal cord. However, angiographic identification of the arterial anatomy of the spinal cord is paramount in avoiding iatrogenic injury during endovascular therapies directed at vascular lesions of the spinal column and the cord. The spinal cord is nourished in its anterolateral two-thirds by the anterior spinal artery. The anterior spinal artery by definition originates from the terminal portions of one or both vertebral arteries prior to the junction with the basilar artery. The concept of two equal-size arterial branches from the distal vertebral arteries merging into a single large anterior spinal artery is usually the exception (THRON 1988). The anterior spinal artery proceeds in a caudad longitudinal fashion in the ventral median sulcus. Several studies have documented a continuous anterior spinal artery throughout the length of the spinal cord (DOMMISSE 1974; BASSETT et al. 1996), while others suggest a discontinuous course (LAZORTHES et al. 1971).

The spinal cord is angiographically defined by three arterial regions distinguished by the number of radicular spinal arterial branches and the predominance of collateral circulation. Simplistically, the spinal cord can be divided into the cervicothoracic, mid-thoracic, and thoracolumbar regions. Anatomically, the midthoracic spinal cord region has the least abundant arterial supply. The anterior spinal artery in the midthoracic region is usually supplied by a single radiculomedullary collateral vessel from the intercostal or right bronchial artery. From the anterior spinal artery, the central arteries penetrate into the gray and white matter of the cord. The size and number of these central arteries are reduced in the midthoracic region of the cord in comparison to the cervicothoracic and thoracolumbar areas. For the midthoracic region, a 20-cm length of cervical or cervicothoracic segment, possesses 80-100 central penetrating arterial branches (BASSETT et al. 1996). Additionally, the perimedullary anastomosis between the anterior spinal artery and the two posterior spinal arteries is virtually nonexistent in the midthoracic region.

The lower spinal cord and conus derives its arterial supply from the anterior and posterolateral spinal arteries from an arcade around the caudal aspect of the cord. The inferior aspect of the cord and conus is also variably supplied by infra-aortic collateral arteries (PARKE et al. 1994). The abdominal aorta usually bifurcates anterior to the fourth lumbar verte-

bra. Therefore the last segmental arteries are constituted as the fourth lumbar arteries. The median sacral artery usually arises from the posterior surface of the abdominal aortic bifurcation, supplying the promontory of the sacrum and the coccyx. The posterior division of the internal iliac artery supplies the sacral segments, the fourth and fifth vertebral bodies, and their respective neural elements. The branches of the posterior division of the internal iliac hypogastric artery include the superior gluteal, the iliolumbar, and the lateral sacral artery (MOORE 1980). Therefore, the important arterial supply to the spinal region caudal to L4 is derived from the iliolumbar, median sacral, and lateral sacral arteries. This anatomy is important to consider during the angiographic analysis of dural arteriovenous fistula (AVF) and for preoperative evaluation for surgery of the lower spine (PARKE et al 1994).

The venous anatomy and drainage pathways occupy a central role in the clinical presentation secondary to the hemodynamic consequences of the valveless intrathecal venous system (FRIED et al. 1971; GILLILAN 1970). The spine and intrathecal cord in general drain toward the heart. Therefore, the lumbrosacral and lower thoracic cord drain in a craniad direction. Retrograde venous reflux from the epidural (Batsonís) plexus is normally prevented at the level of dural penetration of the medullary veins. The dural segment of the medullary vein between its intra- and extradural location functions as a physiologic valve owing to the differential venous pressures. The spinal cord is drained by centrifugal radial veins coursing outward to the coronal venous plexus on the surface of the cord. These veins converge to drain into the anterior or posterior medullary veins which exit the thecal sac at the root sleeve. The medullary veins ultimately drain blood from the spinal veins into the epidural plexus.

LAUNAY et al. (1979) described spinal veins as draining the spinal cord and lying on its surface. These include the median, anterior or posterior, lateral anterior or posterior veins. The anterior spinal vein is small, lying in the midline with a straight course. The posterior spinal veins are larger with more of a serpentine course, near midline. The lateral spinal veins, anteriorly or posteriorly, are usually too small to be visualized on angiography. The anterior spinal vein at the cervical level is usually visualized at 9-10 s with disappearance of contrast by 20-21 s. The posterior venous plexus circulation time is slower, with appearance at 12 s and slightly longer time of disappearance.

In the lumbar region there is a difference of circulation time in reference to the spinal cord and vertebral column. The spinal and epidural veins remain opacified while the epidural and external vertebral veins (azygos, intercostal, and ascending lumbar) can no longer be visualized. Of course, the hemodynamic state of the patient will also influence the timing of the venous opacification by the size of the artery injected, volume and rate of contrast medium injected, anesthesia agent, and the relative circulating hydration state of the patient.

7.8
General Principles of Spinal Neurovascular Embolization

The general technique of spinal embolization usually involves coaxial catheter systems with a guiding catheter positioned in the origin of the arterial pedicle. A microcatheter is placed through a rotating hemostatic valve connected to the hub of the guiding catheter which allows infusion of heparinized saline (1000 units heparin in 1000 ml normal saline) around the microcatheter to prevent thrombus within the dead space at the coaxial interface. A three-way stopcock on the sidearm of the valve allows contrast medium injection for serial angiograms or road mapping.

7.8.1
Agents Used for Embolization

The choice of embolic agents for endovascular spinal therapy is dependent upon the intended goal of treatment. The therapeutic strategy should be patientspecific depending upon the symptoms, current neurological status, and prognosis. Embolization is rarely a curative procedure but can be enlisted as an adjunctive measure prior to surgery or as a palliative procedure to improve the quality of life. The goal of embolization with regard to tumors is to devascularize the lesion without injury to the cord or nerve roots. This can provide improved surgical visibility, shorten operative time and reduce blood loss for resectable tumors. Palliative procedures are performed to promote necrosis with shrinkage of the tumor with resultant relief of pain and improved neurological function. The embolic agents for endovascular spinal therapy are currently limited. The use of polyvinyl alcohol (PVA) is ineffective for long-term closure of arterial pedicles associated with

dural AVFs (TOUHO et al. 1995; NICHOLS et al. 1992; HALL et al. 1981). NICHOLS et al. (1992) described the Mayo Clinic experience of using PVA particles (100-500 (m size) to embolize 14 patients with spinal dural arteriovenous fistula (SDAVF). Postembolization angiography demonstrated complete occlusion of the feeding arterial pedicles, with initial clinical improvement in all cases. After the initial improvement, 11 patients developed subsequent deterioration within a mean of 7 months. Of the 11 patients with clinical deterioration, 9 demonstrated recanalization or recurrence of their SDAVF on angiography. This has led to the recommendation of using a more permanent agent. Isobutyl 2-cyanoacrylate (IBCA) and, currently, normobutyl-cyanoacrylate (NBCA) have been proposed as the permanent agents of choice (BROTHERS et al. 1989). The safe use of these liquid adhesives requires extensive practice and experience owing to the rapid polymerization time induced with microcatheter delivery. The timing of polymerization requires adjustment of the ratio of the glue to the iophendylate (BERENSTEIN and LASJAUNIAS 1992). To be effective, NBCA must navigate from the arterial component of the nidus or fistula and polymerize in the most proximal portion of the draining vein(s). This must be carefully controlled so as to avoid distal migration of the acrylic cast into the efferent segment of the draining coronal or medullary vein(s). Distal migration of the glue cast can result in occlusion or impedance of normal venous drainage of the cord with aggravation of the venous hypertension or even hemorrhage. Sudden occlusion of a large draining vein in a lesion such as a type IV-C spinal AVM, can result in Foix-Alajouanine syndrome with possible cord infarction: if the NBCA cast polymerizes proximal to the nidus or fistula, the lesion will continue to recruit collateral arterial pedicles.

7.9
Classification of Spinal Arteriovenous Malformations

Classifications and descriptions of spinal vascular malformations are as numerous as they are confusing (RICHE et al. 1985; ANSON and SPETZLER 1992). RODESCH (1996) has simplified the approach to understanding the anatomic distinction between intramedullary, perimedullary, and extramedullary spinal arteriovenous malformations (AVM) by comparing their location with respect to neural tissue as subpial (RODESCH et al. 1994). The concept of subpial or "extra-axial" anatomic location of vascular malformations has been previously described in cerebral AVM as defined by pathologic and surgical specimens (HASSLER et al. 1989). In this chapter, classification will follow the Barrow Institute (ANSON and SPETZLER 1992). The Barrow classification of spinal vascular malformations is based on the arterial and venous anatomy, as well as hemodynamic flow patterns (Table 7.1). The spinal cord AVMs are divided into four categories: types I to IV with subtypes of type I and type IV. Type I spinal AVM is the spinal dural arteriovenous fistula (SDAVF), which is further subdivided by the number of arterial feeders (Fig. 7.6). Type I-A is with a single artery and type I-B possesses multiple arterial feeders. Most SDAVFs are located posteriorly with respect to the cord, with a single rostrally directly dilated venous drainage. However, 15% may have tortuous anterior drainage. Associated arteriolar venous aneurysms have not been described with SDAVFs. Type II spinal AVM represents a true intramedullary AVM with compact nidus previously labeled as a ìglomusî malformation (Fig. 7.7). The type II spinal AVM may be supplied by branches of the anterior spinal artery, posterior spinal artery, or both. Hemodynamic studies suggest these lesions have high pressure with low flow. Angiographically, the AVM fills rapidly with early venous opacification. There is an equal male to female ratio but symptoms usually occur much earlier than in patients with type I spinal AVMs. Type III spinal AVMs were previously known as "juvenile" AVMs (Fig. 7.8). They are com-

plex intramedullary lesions with some extramedullary extension. Typically, these are supplied from multiple vertebral levels with multiple arterial pedicles. These are quite rare in comparison to type I and type II spinal AVMs, present most often in adolescents or young adults, and have an extremely poor prognosis.

Type IV spinal AVMs are also known as perimedullary AVMs, originally described by DJINDJIAN et al. (1977a) and classified as type IV AVMs (HEROS et a.l 1986; BARROW et al. 1994; Fig. 7.9). Perimedullary AVMs (AVFs) comprise 14-20% of spinal cord arteriovenous malformations (BERENSTEIN and LASJAUNIAS 1992; ROSENBLUM et al. 1987). Type IV AVMs are intradural and entirely extramedullary. The AVM nidus resides outside the spinal cord and pia, with arterial supply from the anterior spinal artery. Rarely, the type IV AVM can receive arterial pedicles from the posterior spinal artery since its most common location is at the level of the conus medullaris. The type IV AVMs present most frequently in the 3rd to 6th decades of life with progres-

Table 7.1 The Barrow classification of spinal vascular malformations

Type	Subtype
Type I (dural arterio-venous fistula)	I-A (Single arterial feeder) I-B (Multiple feeders)
Type II (glomus)	
Type III (juvenile)	
Type IV (perimedullary)	IV-A (Small) IV-B (Medium) IV-C (Giant)

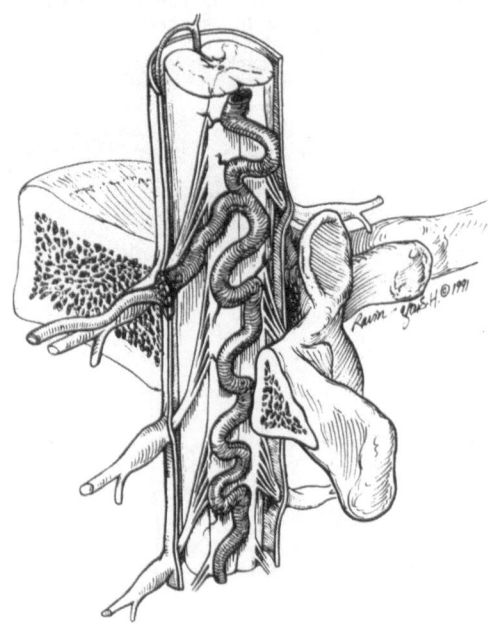

Fig. 7.6. Type I spinal arteriovenous malformation (AVM): A single arterial feeder forms at the dural root sleeve, then drains into an enlarged coiled intradural arterialized vein (with permission of the Barrow Neurological Institute)

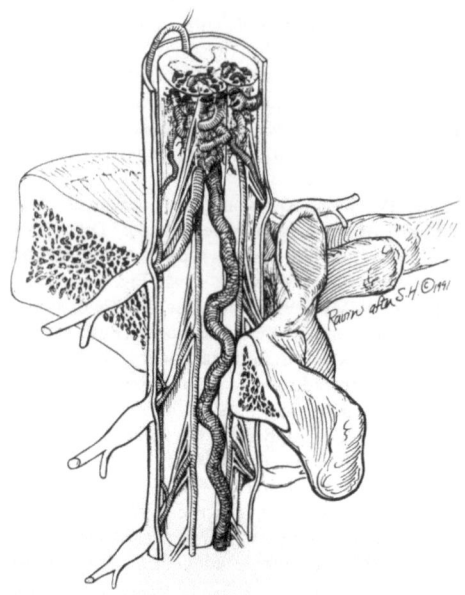

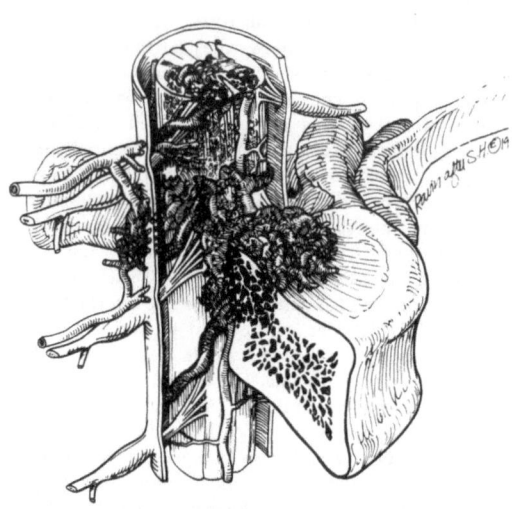

Fig. 7.7. Type II spinal AVM: A compact intramedullary nidus is supplied by branches of both the anterior and posterior spinal arteries and drains into a dilated coronal venous plexus: (with permission of the Barrow Neurological Institute)

Fig. 7.8. Type III spinal AVM: Multiple feeders supply these large and diffuse lesions that often extend into surrounding dura and bone (with permission of the Barrow Neurological Institute)

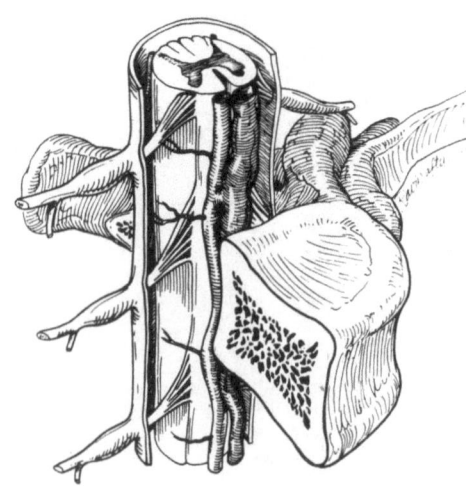

Fig. 7.9. Type IV spinal AVM: A direct arteriovenous fistula is present between the anterior spinal artery and an extra-medullary draining vein (with permission of the Barrow Neurological Institute)

sive neurologic deficit or hemorrhage (Mourier et al. 1993a).

Merland and Reizine (1987) classified type IV spinal AVMs into three subtypes (Fig. 7.10). Type IV-A AVMs have a single arterial pedicle frequently from the artery of Adamkiewicz. This is a low-flow shunt with moderate venous enlargement. Type IV-B spinal AVMs are intermediate in size with one or more arterial pedicles. Typically, a major arterial pedicle is from the anterior spinal artery. AV shunting and transient time is increased with dilated draining veins. Type IV-C spinal AVM are giant multiple arterial AVFs. The anterior spinal artery usually supplies the AVM with marked AV shunting into dilated tortuous draining veins. These giant AVFs have highflow rate and may truly represent "stealphenomenon" as part of their pathophysiology.

There are two reported syndromes of hereditary cutaneous hemangiomas associated with vascular malformations of the spine and spinal cord: KLIPPEL-TRÈNAUNAY-WEBER syndrome and Rendu-Osler-Weber syndrome / hereditary hemorrhagic telangiectasia. Klippel-Trénaunay-Weber syndrome is a congenital phakomatosis with cutaneous angiomas, unilateral superficial varices, and extremity giantism. This syndrome may have peripheral AVMs or AVFs of the hypertrophic limb or possess intramedullary spinal cord AVMs. Only 16 cases have been reported (NAKSTAD et al. 1993; DJINDJIAN et al. 1977b). DJINDJIAN et al. (1977b) describe five cases of this syndrome with intramedullary spinal AVM out of 150 cases of spinal AVMs in their series.

Spinal vascular malformations with a cutaneous hemangioma in the same dermatome is a distinct but rare entity usually classified as the Cobb syndrome. It is expressed as the triad of skin, bone, and spinal cord involvement and represents cutaneous vertebral medullary angiomatosis. The metameric lesion is usually of capillary or arterial type with frequent high-flow arteriovenous fistulization. The location of the cutaneous lesion may be suggestive of the involved spinal cord myelomere but does not necessarily correlate with the segmental dermatome (DOPPMAN et al. 1969). Patients with metameric AVMs should be clinically evaluated to direct therapy toward the symptomatic lesion, i.e., toward the area of spinal cord involvement or the cutaneous lesion.

Fig. 7.10. The three subtypes of type IV AVM are classified on the basis of the size of the arterial feeder and draining vein and the degree of increased flow through the shunt

7.10
Endovascular Treatment of Spinal Vascular Malformations

7.10.1
Type I Spinal AVM (Spinal Dural AVF)

Spinal dural arteriovenous fistulas (SDAVFs) or type I spinal AVM usually present in middle-aged men (85%; mean age 55 years) with slowly progressive sensorimotor myelopathy with progressive sphincter dysfunction. (CRISCUOLO et al. 1989; RODESCH et al. 1992; DEEN et al. 1994; HURST et al. 1995; SYMON et al. 1984; ROSENBLUM et al. 1987). These rarely, if ever, hemorrhage. The most common location is the midthoracic to thoracolumbar level supplied by radicular branches of the intercostal, lumbar, or hypogastric arteries (SYMON et al. 1984; ROSENBLUM et al. 1987; MERLAND et al. 1980; LARSEN et al. 1995; BURGUET et al. 1985; STEIN et al. 1972). Usually the SDAVF has one site of involvement near the dural reflection of the proximal nerve root sleeve by a branch of a radicular artery supplying the dura (ROSENBLUM et al. 1987). At the same level, the ipsilateral and contra+lateral arterial pedicles above and below the level of the fistula should be injected to identify crossing tributaries to the fistula. However, several reports have documented patients with two separate level SDAVFs (BARNWELL et al. 1991; PIEROT et al. 1993). Patients with SDAVFs may dem-

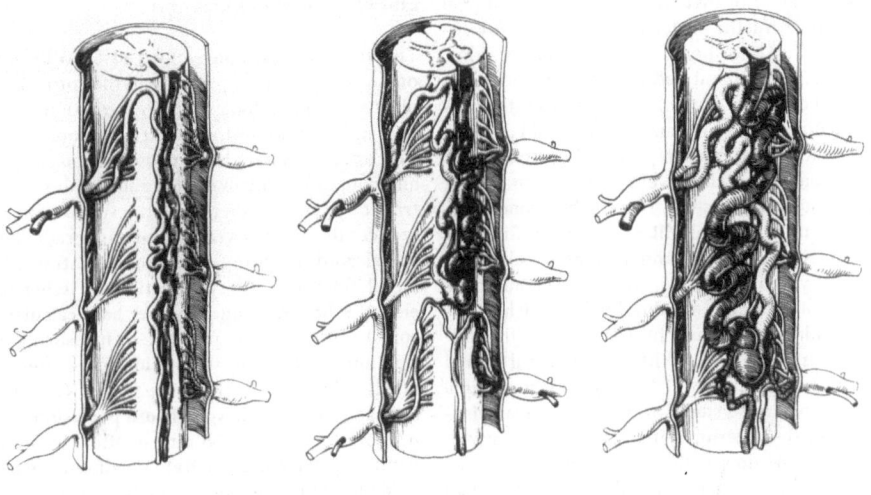

IV-A   IV-B   IV-C

onstrate T2 spin-echo intramedullary hyperintensity of the cord (usually the conus), focal cord enlargement or enlarged serpentine draining veins (CHEN et al. 1995; MASARYK et al. 1987; ISU et al. 1989; GILBERTSON et al. 1994; LARSSON et al. 1991). Gilbertson et al. demonstrated flow voids of dilated coronal veins in up to 45% of the MR evaluations of patients with SDAVF. However, the MR findings may frequently be normal. Therefore, most investigators recommend supine spinal myelography as the radiologic screening exam of choice (LARSEN et al. 1995; MEDER et al. 1984; N'DIAYE et al. 1984). Myelography will frequently demonstrate a serpentine, enlarged dorsal coronal vein draining along the posterior aspect of the cord (N'DIAYE et al. 1984, GILBERTSON et al. 1994). Selective spinal angiography is performed to identify the level of the dural AVF and the artery of Adamkiewicz. The use of MR angiography has recently been introduced for the diagnosis and localization of SDAVF in patients with suspicious MR and appropriate clinical findings (BOWEN et al. 1995; GELBERT et al. 1992; MASCALCHI et al. 1995a; MOURIER et al. 1993b; PROVENZALE et al. 1994). BOWEN et al. (1996) demonstrated the use of postcontrast-enhanced 3-D time-of-flight MR angiography of the thoracolumbar spine to evaluate normal spinal vascularity confirmed by contrast catheter angiography. They found MR angiography detects primarily the largest veins at the cord surface which extend into the epidural venous system. On the ventral aspect of the spinal cord, the visualized intradural veins are the anterior median vein draining into the anterior medullary veins. On the dorsal aspect of the cord, the posterior median vein is visualized draining into the posterior medullary veins. Therefore, the dominant midline vessel on the posterior aspect of the cord on MR angiograms is the posterior median vein, which may possess mild tortuosity over several vertebral segments but drains into the posterior medullary veins with their rather straight angio architecture. Bowen thus concluded, in view of these normal MR angiography findings, that excessive tortuosity and increased caliber or number of vessels on the dorsal surface should raise suspicion of enlarged intradural veins which in the proper clinical setting may be associated with a spinal AVM or dural AVF. With conventional digital subtraction angiography (DSA), the anterior spinal artery demonstrated slow flow with prolonged visualization of the anterior spinal vein (WILLINSKY et al. 1990a). Slow flow with enlarged dorsal coronal veins is usually seen in a rostral direction. Almost all the type I spinal AVMs (SDAVFs) will have rostrally

directed venous outflow which is exacerbated by greater hydrostatic pressure in the upright position. This may explain the clinical findings of worsening of symptoms with prolonged standing. Spetzler has measured the venous pressure in the draining vein and demonstrated in ten type I spinal AVMs increased venous pressure with artificially induced systemic hypertension (ANSON and SPETZLER 1993). This can be correlated with worsening of symptoms during exercise (HASSLER et al. 1989; ROSENBLUM et al. 1987) In contrast to type I AVM, type II and III spinal cord AVMs usually have bi directional rostral-caudal directed venous drainage, but clinical symptoms usually do not change with exercise or altered position (ROSENBLUM et al. 1987; ANSON and SPETZLER 1993). Additionally, other radiculomedullary communications can occur at the cervical (WILLINSKI et al. 1990b) and thoracolumbar levels (CLAVIER et al. 1986; AGGARWAL et al. 1992; DREYER et al. 1994). These collateral anastomoses are important prior to consideration of possible embolization treatment. Therefore, a complete DSA spinal angiogram is performed under general anesthesia with suspended apnea on injection of every intercostal and lumbar artery in addition to both thyrocervical, costocervical, vertebral, and internal iliac arteries. Both lateral and oblique filming projections are sometimes necessary to identify the anatomy of the vascular malformation with specific anatomic reference if surgical treatment is anticipated.

7.10.2
Endovascular Embolization

The accepted pathophysiology of SDAVFs is based on increased venous pressure in the coronal venous plexus and medullary veins (AMINOFF and LOGUE 1974a; STECKER et al. 1966). The venous hypertension of the coronal plexus causes venous stagnation and congestion involving the radial veins of the intrinsic system. Furthermore, the venous congestion reduces the arterial-venous pressure gradient of the spinal cord, resulting in decreased intramedullary blood flow with the production of ischemic myelopathy. Bederson and Spetzler have calculated the spinal cord perfusion pressure by measuring the intraluminal venous pressure prior to and after closure of the dural AVF in ten patients (ANSON and SPETZLER 1993). The spinal cord perfusion pressure improved from 39 to 58 mmHg after closure of the fistula. Spetzler demonstrated a diminished spinal cord blood flow and autoregulation below 50 mmHg of perfusion pressure gradient. This can be correlated with loss of somatosensory evoked potentials below a gradient perfusion pressure of 40 mmHg (LASCHINGER et al. 1987).

Of 90 reported cases of SDAVF, 85 were of mid-thoracic to thoracolumbar location (MERLAND et al. 1980; ROSENBLUM et al. 1987; SYMON et al. 1984); 4 cases were sacral and 1 cervical in location. A special type of SDAVF is one with its arterial supply entirely from the infra-aortic arterial branches (BURGUET et al. 1985; HEINDEL et al. 1975; KIM et al. 1991; LARSEN et al. 1995; PARTINGTON et al. 1992; STEIN et al. 1972; SUGIYAMA et al. 1982; TAKAHASHI et al. 1977). LARSEN et al. (1995) described four male patients with type I SDAVFs supplied exclusively by arterial branches of the posterior division of the internal iliac artery. The lateral sacral artery was the supply in three of the four patients, who were all successively treated by transcatheter embolization with NBCA. The other patient underwent surgical ablation with neurologic recovery. As previously described by the authors, embolization with a permanent liquid adhesive (NBCA) was equally as effective as surgery. However, because this SDAVF was located far removed from the spinal cord, embolization with NBCA was particularly safe. This type of location and arterial supply to the SDAVF were found in 12.5% of their 32 previously reported patients. The significance of this finding is of interest since only eight previous cases have been described in the literature. Therefore, the UCSF group suggest this subtype of SDAVF may be underdiagnosed in patients with underlying progressive myelopathic disorders which may carry a misdiagnosis of transverse myelitis, multiple sclerosis, spinal cord tumor, degenerative disc disease, or spinal cord AVM.

Another particularly rare presentation of spinal dural AVF occurs in the cervical region and may or may not have an intracranial source of spinal venous congestion (BRET et al. 1994; GAENSLER et al. 1990; GLASER et al. 1993; GOBIN et al. 1992; PARTINGTON et al. 1992; SYMON et al. 1994; VERSARI et al. 1993; WILLINSKI et al. 1990b; WROBEL et al. 1988). WILLINSKI et al. (1990b) described four patients with dural AVFs of the upper spinal axis, two at the level of the foramen magnum and two of the lower cervical spine. Wrobel et al. (1988) reported three cases of patients with intracranial dural AVFs who presented with myelopathy secondary to retrograde venous drainage into spinal medullary veins. Therefore, study of the vertebral, thyrocervical, costocervical, external carotid, and possibly the internal carotid arteries may be necessary when cervical myelopathy exists without an identified etiology.

Treatment options for SDAVFs should be carefully weighed up with risk-benefit considerations. Low thoracic, thoracio-lumbar, and sacral SDAVFs without arterial pedicle communication to the artery of Adamkiewicz may be carefully embolized with a permanent liquid adhesive such as NBCA (BERENSTEIN et al. 1984; LARSEN et al. 1995) Inadvertent distal migration of the NBCA glue cast may cause venous occlusion distal to the nidus and result in venous congestion, stagnation, and thrombosis of normal spinal cord venous drainage with possible infarction.

Embolization of type II or III AVMs is usually limited to palliative treatment owing to the morbidity of these intramedullary lesions (GOBIN et al. 1993: HALBACH et al. 1987; SPETZLER et al. 1989). The angioarchitecture of these lesions needs to be assessed for flow-related arterial aneurysms, nidus aneurysms, or venous aneurysms which represent the major risk with spinal hemorrhage. Additionally, these lesions may have significant mass effect with outflow venous varices with cord compression. BIONDI et al. (1990, 1992) existing embolized 14 patients an average of five times for palliative treatment with existing intramedullary AVMs associated with anterior spinal artery aneurysms. Embolization was usually performed with PVA particulate to decrease the flow in these lesions with respective improvement of neurologic function. BIONDI et al. (1992) did note two subsequent findings with postembolization and recurrent recanalization of these intramedullary AVMs. The group with "flow-related" anterior spinal artery aneurysms had reduction or resolution of their aneurysms without subsequent recanalization of the AVM nidus. In a second group of patients, specifically those with metameric angiomatosis, the evolution or resolution of aneurysms of the anterior spinal artery was not influenced by the particulate treatment of the intramedullary AVMs. Therefore, BIONDI et al. concluded there were two types of spinal artery aneurysm associated with intramedullary AVMs.

Embolization of type IV perimedullary AVMs is often complex and difficult (Fig. 7.11). Adjunctive, staged embolization of various arterial pedicles is usually performed in conjunction with surgery because of the association with the anterior spinal artery. The prognosis of patients with this type of AVM is directly related to early diagnosis and therapeutic action rather than the type of fistula or therapeutic method selected (GUEGUEN et al. 1987; AMINOFF and LOGUE 1974a, b). Perimedullary AVMs without treatment progress to disabling partial medullary

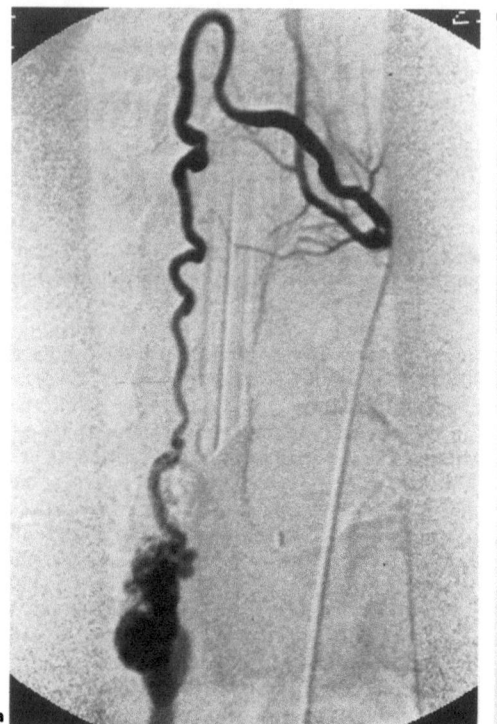

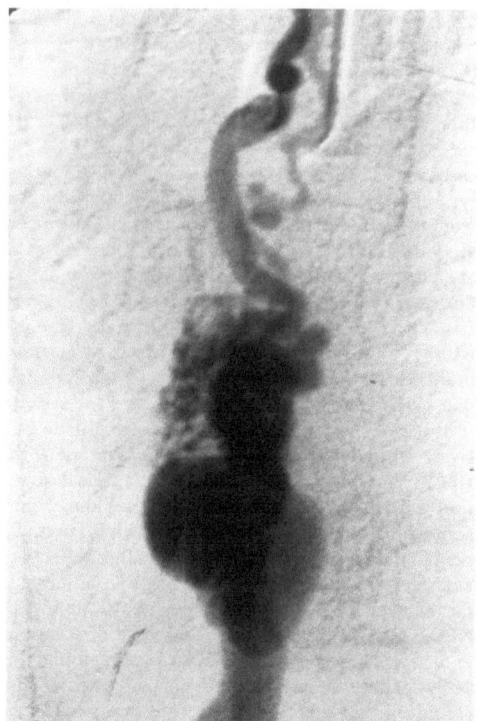

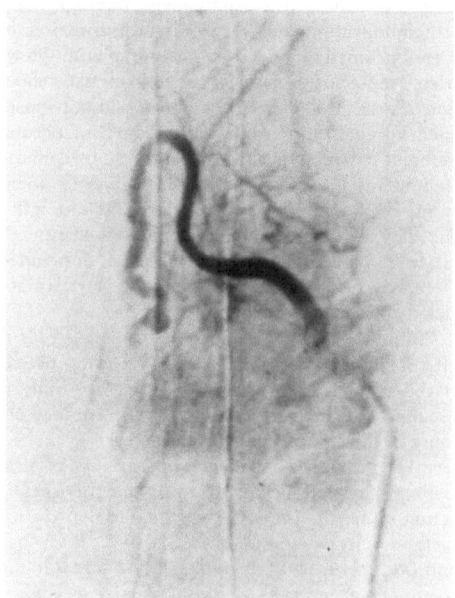

Fig. 7.11. a An AP spinal angiogram showing the anterior spinal artery supply to a type IVB AVM of the thoracic spinal cord. Note venous varices or aneurysms of the nidus. **b** An AP spinal angiogram of a type IVB AVM with intranidus aneurysms and venous varices. **c** A spinal AP angiogram postembolization with Normobutyl-cyanacrylate with slow but antegrade flow in the anterior spinal artery (ASA). Note proximal ASA flow-related aneurysm continuing to fill at the distal aspect of the contrast column

syndrome and ultimately to complete spinal transection in 7-9 years. The partial medullary syndrome may have three different clinical sequelae: (1) radicular pain syndrome with sensorimotor signs, (2) spastic paraparesis with symmetric or (3) asymmetric sensory losses. The sensory changes are associated with pain and temperature, with touch less affected. Joint position is rarely if ever involved as these sensory changes relate to the anterior spinal artery syndrome. Uni- or bilateral lower extremity radicular sensorimotor defect may be clinically apparent. Further progression results ultimately in complete spinal transection with spastic paraplegia with a sensory level and sphincter dysfunction. Type IV perimedullary AVMs usually require embolization in combination with surgery to achieve occlusion (DJINDJIAN et al. 1977a; MOURIER et al. 1993a, HALBACH et al. 1993, TOUHO et al. 1995).

7.11
Complications and Contraindications to Spinal Vascular Embolization

Complications of modern diagnostic spinal angiography are rare (FORBES et al. 1988; KENDALL 1986). Forbes et al. reported a prospective study of 134 consecutive spinal angiograms with an 8.2% complication rate. The neurologic complication rate was 2.2%, with full recovery of deficits in all patients. The authors compared spinal angiography to cerebral angiography with similar rates of complications. The methods to decrease the risk of complications include avoidance of repetitive injections in the same artery over a short period of time, control of the amount and rate of injection, use of nonionic contrast medium, and avoidance of obstruction of continuous flow with small vessel lumen by the catheter.

Complications of spinal angiography and embolization usually are secondary to spinal cord ischemia (BERENSTEIN and LASJAUNIAS 1987, 1992; KERBER 1980). Meticulous technique is required not to iatrogenically introduce air, blood clot, or atheromatous debris (older patients). Furthermore, with the use of coaxial catheter technique with selective distal embolizations, wedging of the guiding catheter for prolonged periods may induce ischemia or thrombosis of the arterial pedicle.

To avoid iatrogenic complications to the spinal cord or nerve roots, contraindications to spinal vascular embolization must be considered (HARE et al. 1983; RICHE et al. 1983; SATTAN 1988). Probably the paramount contraindication to embolization is the proximity of the proposed arterial pedicle embolization to the anterior or posterior spinal artery. DREYER et al. (1994) reported five patients with type I spinal AVMs with opacification of the lesion and the anterior spinal artery by selective injection of the intercostal or lumbar artery. These patients all underwent surgical ablation with intraoperative spinal angiography. The intraoperative spinal angiography was performed initially to identify the site of the dural AVF, shortening the operative time. The patient then underwent a completion angiogram at the level of the surgery and for both arterial pedicles above and below the site to ensure no dural AVF remained.

7.11.1 Intraoperative Physiologic Monitoring During Spinal Embolization

Embolization of spinal vascular lesions requires sophisticated physiologic monitoring to avoid iatrogenic injury to the patient. A variety of provocative testing methods exists to evaluate potential injury to the normal arterial pedicles which supply the spinal cord. Electrophysiologic monitoring of the spinal cord can utilize somatosensory evoked potentials (SSEPs; BASSETT et al. 1996; BERENSTEIN et al. 1984; STECHISON et al. 1995; YOUNG and BERNESTEIN 1985) or transcranial electrical motor evoked potentials (ANDERSON et al. 1994; YANG et al. 1994; JELLINEK et al. 1991).

SSEP monitoring is a measure of dorsal column sensory function which is the vascular territory of the posterior spinal arteries. Amplitude changes of more than 50% for the P40 signal have been documented during temporary occlusion of segmental arteries (APEL et al. 1991). Most investigators accept the criteria of 10% increase in wave latency and 50% decrease in wave amplitude as significant potential for provocative intraoperative event of the spinal cord while in a state of reversible dysfunction (BROWN and NASH 1991, KEITH et al. 1990). BERENSTEIN et al. (1984) described the use of SSEP monitoring in 42 angiographic examinations during 33 therapeutic embolizations in 41 patients. During contrast medium injections with opacification of the anterior spinal artery, there were immediate changes in the amplitudes of the waveforms in all but two patients without residual neurologic deficit. After angiography withdrawal of the catheter tip engaged in the artery resulted in recovery of the baseline waveform within 2-4 min, except in a patient with a cervical AVM, which required 24 min after discontinuation of the procedure. Embolizations were performed in 12 patients with spinal canal tumors. Despite the reports of SSEP monitoring "posterior" spinal artery integrity, Berenstein demonstrated sensitivity of this technique for compromised anterior spinal artery function. Use of SSEP is not without risk for loss of detection of anterior column or motor function of the cord (DAUBE et al. 1989). Focal motor deficits have been documented when monitoring posterior column function with normal SSEPs (BEN-DAVID et al. 1987; KATSUTA et al. 1993; KRISHNA et al. 1991; LESSER et al. 1986; MUSTAIN and KENDIG 1991; GINSBURG et al. 1985). Other reports have suggested transcranial magnetic evoked potential should be utilized or even supplemented with SSEPs during monitoring of the spinal cord during invasive procedures (ANDERSON et al. 1994; EDMONDS et al. 1988; JELLINEK et al.1991; YANG et al. 1994).

Some reports have suggested an increased sensitivity to anterior spinal artery dysfunction can be improved with the addition of pharmacologic provocative testing of the proposed arterial pedicle to be closed with SSEP monitoring (KHAYATA et al. 1995; CHOI 1995). DOPPMAN et al. (1986) have investigated the spinal WADA test to monitor motor and reflex changes in monkeys, using various doses of pentobarbital and lidocaine injected selectively into the artery of Adamkiewicz, as well as the right bronchial artery. Pentobarbital produced acute paraplegia while lidocaine produced transient paraplegia followed by hyperreflexia and muscular fasciculations for from 5 to 60 min which was completely reversible in all the animals. However, the study did not determine the most appropriate drug or concentration of drug for use in human subjects. Thus, the current provocative use of lidocaine or barbiturate injections into the spinal arteries in human patients should be made with careful consideration and caution. KHAYATA et al. (1992) have suggested 20 mg of lidocaine or 30-40 mg of amoborbital (Amytal) for testing each arterial pedicle prior to embolization.

7.12 Conclusions

The continued advancement of "minimally" invasive image-guided techniques in the diagnosis and treatment of spinal tumors and vascular lesions will provide a greater role of the interventional neuroradiologist in patient care. The technologies we select will be further adapted to the cost-containment and managed-care environment. Patient outcomes will be weighed up and should be evaluated with respect to the patient's quality of life before and after

interventional techniques are applied in the course of their treatment. The close cooperative collaboration with our colleagues in other disciplines, including radiology, neurosurgery, neurology, orthopedics, and nursing, should be expanded to provide the best care possible for the patient. The careful application of current methods requires clinical judgment which is as critical as the interventional skills of the physician. The wise and prudent practice of medicine should always be in the forefront of our actions. It is incumbent upon our specialty to temper our enthusiasm of treatment with the consideration of future technology and innovative therapies.

References

Aggarwal S, Willinsky R, Montanera W, Terbrugge K, Wallace MC (1992) Superselective angiography of a spinal dural arteriovenous fistula having a common segmental origin with the artery of Adamkiewicz. Neuroradiology 34:352-354

Algra PR, Bloem JL, Tissing PR, Falke TH, Arndt JW, Verboom LJ (1991) Detection of vertebral metastases: comparison between MR imaging and bone scintigraphy. Radiographics 11:219-232

Aminoff MJ, Logue V (1974a) Clinical features of spinal vascular malformation. Brain 97:197-210

Aminoff MJ, Logue V (1974b) The prognosis of patients with spinal vascular malformations. Brain 97:211-218

An HS, Andreshak TG, Nguyen C, Williams A, Daniels D (1995) Can we distinguish between benign versus malignant compression fractures of the spine by magnetic resonance imaging? Spine 20:1776-1782

Anderson LC, Hemler DE, Luethke JM, Latchaw RE (1994) Transcranial magnetic evoked potentials used to monitor the spinal cord during neuroradiologic angiography of the spine. Spine 19:613-616

Anson JA, Spetzler RF (1992) Classification of spinal arteriovenous malformations and implications for treatment. Barrow Neurol Inst Q 8:2-8

Anson JA, Spetzler RF (1993) Spinal dural arteriovenous malformations. In: Awad IA, and Barrow DL (eds) Dural arteriovenous malformations. American Association of Neurological Surgeons Publications Committee, Park Ridge, Ill, pp 175-192

Apel DM, Marrero G, King J, Tolo VT, Bassett GS (1991) Avoiding paraplegia during anterior spinal surgery. Spine 16:365-370

Ayala AG, Zornosa J (1983) Primary bone tumors: percutaneous needle biopsy. Radiologic - Pathologic study of ZZZ biopsies. Radiology 149:675-679

Baley P, Buey PC (1929) Cavernous hemangioma of the vertebra. JAMA 92:1748-1751

Barnwell SL, Halbach VV, Dowd CF, Higashida RT, Hieshima GB, Wilson CB (1991) Multiple dural arteriovenous fistulas of the cranium and spine. AJNR Am J Neuroradiol 12:441-445

Barrow DL, Colohan ART, Dawson R (1994) Intradural perimedullary arteriovenous fistulas C Type IV spinal cord arteriovenous malformations. J Neurosurg 81:221-229

Bassett G, Johnson C, Stanley P (1996) Comparison of preoperative selective spinal angiography and somato-sensory-evoked potential monitoring with temporary occlusion of segmental vessels during anterior spinal surgery. Spine 21:1996-2000

Bell RL (1955) Hemangiomas of a dorsal vertebrae with collapse and compression myelopathy. J Neurosurg 12:570-576

Ben-David B, Hauer G, Taylor P (1987) Anterior spinal fusion complicated by paraplegia. A case report of a false negative somatosensory-evoked potential. Spine 12:536-539

Berenstein A, Lasjaunias P (1992) Spine and spinal cord vascular lesions. In: Berenstein A, Lasjaunias P (eds) Endovascular treatment of spine and spinal cord lesions. Surgical neuroangiography, Vol. 5 Springer, Berlin Heidelberg pp 1-109

Berenstein A, Young W, Ransohoff J, Benjamin V, Merkin H (1984) Somatosensory evoked potentials during spinal angiography and therapeutic transvascular embolization. J Neurosurg 60:777-785

Biagini R, Decristofaro R, Ruggieri P, Boriani S (1990) Giant-cell tumor of the spine. J Bone Joint Surg: 1102-1107

Biondi A, Merland JJ, Reizine D, et al (1990) Embolization with particles in thoracic intramedullary arteriovenous malformations: long-term angiographic and clinical results. Radiology 177:651-658

Biondi A, Merland JJ, Hodes JE, Aymard A, Reizine D (1992) Aneurysms of spinal arteries associated with intramedullary arteriovenous malformations. II. Results of AVM endovascular treatment and hemodynamic considerations. AJNR Am J Neuroradiol 13:923-931

Bowen BC, Fraser KW, Kochen JP, Pattany PM, Green BA, Quencer RM (1995) Spinal dural arteriovenous fistulas: evaluation with magnetic resonance angiography. AJNR Am J Neuroradiol 16:2029-2043

Bowen BC, Deprima S, Pattany PM, Marcillo A, Madsen P, Quencer RM (1996) MR angiography of normal intradural vessels of the thoracolumbar spine. AJNR Am J Neuroradiol 17:483-494

Breslau J, Eskrige JM (1995) Pre-operative embolization of spinal tumors. JVasc Interv Radiol 6:871-875

Bret P, Salzmann M, Bascoulergue Y, Guyotat J (1994) Dural arteriovenous fistula of the posterior fossa draining into the spinal medullary veins – an unusual cause of myelopathy. Case report. Neurosurgery 35:965-969

Broaddus WC, Grady MS, Delashaw JB, Ferguson RDG, Jane JA (1990) Pre-operative superselective arteriolar embolization: a new approach to enhance respectability of spinal tumors. Neurosurgery 27:755-759

Brothers M, Kaufmann J, Fox A, Deveikis J (1989) N-Butyl-2-cyanoacrylate-substitute for IBCA in interventional neuroradiology. AJNR Am J Neuroradiol 10:777-

Brown RH, Nash CL (1991) Intraoperative spinal cord monitoring. In: Frymoyer JW (ed) The adult spine: principles and practice. Raven, New York, pp 549-562

Brugieres P, Gaston A, Voisin MC, Ricolfi F, Chakir N (1992) CT-guided percutaneous biopsy of the cervical spine: A series of 12 cases. Neuroradiology 34:358-360

Burguet JL, Dietermann JL, Wackenheim A, Kehr P, Buchheit F (1985) Sacral meningeal arteriovenous fistula fed by branches of the hypogastric arteries and drained through medullary veins. Neuroradiology 27:232-237

Cahan LD, Higashida Rt, Halbach VV, Hieshima GB (1987) Variants of radiculomeningeal vascular malformations of the spine. Neurosurgery 66:333-337

Chen CJ, Ro L-S, Cheng W-C, Chen S-T (1995) MRI/myelo-graphic localization of fistulous tract in spinal dural arte-riovenous malformations prior to arteriography. J Comput Assist Tomogr 19:893-896

Chiras J, Movan G, Merland JJ (1979) The angiographic appearance of the normal intercostal and lumbar arteries. Analysis of the anatomic correlation of the lateral branches. J Neuroradiol 6:169-196

Choi I (1995) Embolization of intracranial and spinal tumors. In: Maciunas RJ (ed) Endovascular neurological intervention. American Association of Neurological Surgeons Publications Committee, Springfield, Il., pp 263-278

Choi I, Berenstein A (1988) Surgical neuroangiography of the spine and spinal cord. Radiol Clin North Am 26:1131-1141

Chuang VP, Os CS, Wallace S, Benjamin RS (1981) Arterial occlusion: management of giant cell tumor and aneurysmal bone cyst. AJR Am J Roentgenol 136:1127-1130

Clavier E, Tadie M, Thiebot J, Presles O, Benozio M (1986) Common origin of the arterial blood flow for an arteriovenous medullar fistula and the anterior spinal artery: a case report. Neurosurgery 18:660-663

Cory DA, Fritsch SA, Cohen MD, et al (1989) Aneurysmal bone cysts: imaging findings and embolotherapy. AJR Am J Roentgenol 153:369-373

Cotten A, Deramond H, Cortet B, et al (1996) Preoperative percutaneous injection of methyl methacrylate and N-butyl cyanoacrylate in vertebral hemangiomas. AJNR Am J Neuroradiol 17:137-142

Courtheoux P, Alachkar F, Casasco A, et al (1985) Chemoembolization of lumbar spine metastases: A preliminary study. J Neuroradiol 12:151-162

Criscuolo GR, Oldfield EH, Doppman JL (1989) Reversible acute and subacute myelopathy in patients with dural arteriovenous fistulas: Folx-Alajouanine syndrome reconsidered. J Neurosurg 70:354-359

Crock HV, Yoshizawa H (1977) Origins of arteries supplying the vertebral column. In: Crock HV, Yoshizawa H (eds) The blood supply of the vertebral column and spinal cord in man. Springer, Berlin Heidelberg New York, pp 1-21

Dahlin DC, Unni KK (1986) Benign vascular tumors In: Dahlin DC, Unni KK (eds) Bone tumors, 4th ed. Charles Thomas, Springfield, pp 167-180

Daube Jr (1989) Intraoperative monitoring by evoked potentials for spinal cord surgery: the pros. Electroencephalogr Clin Neurophysiol 73:374-377

DeCristofaro R, Biagini R, Boriami S, et al (1992) Selective arterial embolization in the treatment of aneurysmal bone cyst and angioma of bone. Skeletal Radiol 21:523-527

Deen HG, Nelson KD, Gonzales GR (1994) Spinal dural arteriovenous fistula causing progressive myelopathy: clinical and imaging considerations. Mayo Clin Proc 69:83-84.

Deramond H, Galibert H, Debussche-Depriester C (1990) Percutaneous vertebroplasty with methyl-methachrylate: technique, method, and results (abstract) Radiology 117 : 352

DeRosa GP, Graziano GP, Scott J (1990) Arterial embolization of aneurysmal bone cyst of the spine. J Bone Joint Surg Am 72:777-780

Disch SP, Grabb RL, Gaso MH, Strecker WB, Marbarger JP (1986) Aneurysmal bone cyst of the cervicothoracic spine: computed tomographic evaluation of the value of preoperative embolization. Case report. Neurosurgery 19: 290-293

Djindjian M, Djindjian R, Rey A, Hurth M, Houdart R (1977a) Intradural extramedullary spinal arterio-venous malformations fed by the anterior spinal artery. Surg Neurol 8:85-93

Djindjian M, Djindjian R, Hurth M, Rey A, Houdart R (1977b) Spinal cord arteriovenous malformations and the Klippel-Trénaunay-Weber syndrome. Surg Neurol 8:229-237

Djindjian R, Dumesnil M, Faure C, Lefebre J, Leveque P (1962) Etude angiographique dfun angiome intra-rachidiaen. Rev Neurol (Paris) 106:278-285

Djindjian R, Merland JJ, Djindjian M, Stoeter P (1981) Angiography of spinal column and spinal cord tumors. Thieme-Stratton, New York, pp 1-237

Dollahite HA, Tatum L, Moinuddin SM, Carnesale PG (1989) Aspiration biopsy of primary neoplasms of bone. J Bone Joint Surg 71-A:1166-1169

Dommisse GF (1974) The blood supply of the spinal cord. J Bone Joint Surg [Br] 56:225-235

Doppman JL (1995) Percutaneous treatment of symptomatic vertebral hemangiomas by direct injection of alcohol. Course in interventional neuroradiology syllabus, ASNR, Chicago, 21-22 April 1995, pp 49-54

Doppman JL, di Chiro G (1965) Subtraction-angiography of spinal cord vascular malformations. Report of a case. J Neurosurg 23:40-43

Doppman JL, Pevsner P (1983) Embolization of arteriovenous malformations by direct percutaneous puncture. AJR AM J Roentgenol 140:773-778

Doppman JL, Wirth FP, Dichiro G, et al (1969) Value of cutaneous angioma in the arteriographic localization of spinal cord arteriovenous malformations. N Engl J Med 281: 1440-1444

Doppman JL, Girton M, Oldfield EH (1986) Spinal WADA test. Radiology 161:319-321

Dreyer FW, Higashida RT, Dowd CF, Deprima SJ, Fraser KW, Hieshima GB (1994) Intraoperative spinal angiography for arteriovenous malformations (abstract). Radiology. 193:157

Dysart SH, Swengel RM, Van Dam BE (1992) Aneurysmal bone cyst of a thoracic vertebra: treatment by selective arterial embolization and excision. Spine 17:846-848

Edmonds HL, Paloheimo MPJ, Backman MH, Johnson JR, Holt RT, Shields CB (1988) Transcranial magnetic motor evoked potentials (tc MMEP) for functional monitoring of motor pathways during scoliosis surgery. Spine 14:683-686

Eisenstein S, Spiro F, Browde S, Allen CM, Grobler L (1986) The treatment of a symptomatic vertebral hemangioma by radiotherapy. Spine 11:640-642

Esparza J, Castro S, Portillo JM, Roger R (1978) Vertebral hemangiomas: spinal angiography and preoperative embolization. Surg Neurol 10:171-173

Faria SL, Schulpp WR, Chiminazzo H Jr (1985) Radiotherapy in the treatment of vertebral hemangiomas. Int J Radiat Oncol Biol Phys 11:387-390

Firooznia H, Pinto RS, Lin JP, Baruch HH, Zawsner J (1976) Chordoma: radiologic evaluation of twenty cases. AJR 127:797-805

Forbes G, Nichols DA, Jack CR, et al (1988) Complications of spinal cord arteriography: prospective assessment of risk for diagnostic procedures. Radiology 169:479-484

Fried LC, Doppman JL, Dichiro G (1971) Venous Phase in spinal cord angiography. Acta Radiol 11:393-401

Fukushima T, Kamano S, Sakurai I, Chigasaki H (1972) A case of osteoid osteoma affecting the T8 neural arch: with special reference to selective spinal angiography. No To Shinkei 24:213-219

Gaensler EHL, Jackson DE, Halbach VV (1990) Arteriovenous fistulas of the cervicomedullary junction as a cause of myelopathy: radiographic findings in two cases. AJNR Am J Neuroradiol 11:518-521

Galibert P, Deramond H, Rosat P, Legars D (1987) Note preliminaire sur le traitement des angiomes vertebraux par vertebroplatie acrylique percutanée. Neurochirurgie 33:166-168

Gangi A, Kastler BA, Dietermann JL (1994) Percutaneous vertebroplasty guided by a combination of CT and fluoroscopy. AJNR Am J Neuroradiol 15:83-86

Gelbert F, Guichard JP, Mourierkletal (1992) Phase-contrast MR angiography of vascular malformations of the spinal cord at O.5.T. J Magn Reson Imaging 2:631-636

Gellad FE, Sadato N, Namaguchi Y, Levine AM (1990) Vascular metastatic lesions of the spine: pre-operative embolization. Radiology 176:683-686

Gilbertson JR, Miller GM, Goldman MS, Marsh WR (1994) Spinal dural arteriovenous fistulas: MR and myelographic findings. AJNR Am J Neuroradiol 16:2049-2057

Gillilan LA (1970) Veins of the spinal cord: anatomic details: Suggested clinical applications. Neurology 20: 860-868

Ginsburg HH, Shetter AG, Raudzens PA (1985) Postoperative paraplegia with preserved intraoperative somatosensory evoked potentials. J Neurosurg 63:296-300

Glasser R, Masson R, Mickle JP, Peters KR (1993) Embolization of a dural arteriovenous fistula of the ventral cervical spinal canal in a nine year-old boy. Neurosurgery 33:1089-1094

Gobin YP, Rogopoulos A, Aymard A et al (1992) Endovascular treatment of intracranial dural arteriovenous fistulas with spinal perimedullary venous drainage. J Neurosurg 77: 718-723

Gobin YP, Houdart E, Casasco A, Merland JJ (1993) Endovascular therapy for arteriovenous malformations and fistulas in the spinal cord. Semin Interv Radiol 10: 227-241

Graham JJ, Yang YC (1984) Vertebral hemangioma with compression fracture and paraparesis treated with pre-operative embolization and vertebral resection. Spine 9:97-101

Gross CE, Hodge CJ, Binet EF, Kricheff II (1976) Relief of spinal block during embolization of a vertebral body hemangioma. J Neurosurg 45:327-330

Gueguen B, Merland JJ, Riche MC, Rey A (1987) Vascular malformations of the spinal cord: intrathecal perimedullary arteriovenous fistulas fed by medullary arteries. Neurology 37:969-979

Halbach VV, Higashida RT, Dowd CF, Fraser KW, Edwards MS, Barnwell SL (1993) Treatment of giant intradural (perimedullary) arteriovenous fistulas. Neurosurgery 33: 972-980

Halbach VV, Higashida RT, Hieshima GB (1987) Treatment of vertebral arteriovenous fistulas. AJNR Am J Neuroradiol 8:1121-1128

Hall WA, Oldfield EH, Doppman JL (1981) Recanalization of spinal arteriovenous malformations following embolization. J Neurosurg 70:714-720

Hamilton AJ, Lula BA, Fosmire H, Stea B, Cassady JR (1995) Preliminary clinical experience with linear accelerator-based spinal stereotactic radiosurgery. Neurosurgery 36: 311-319

Hanley EN, Howard BH, Brigham CD, Chapman TM, Guilford WB, Coumas JM (1994) Lumbar epidural varix as a cause of radiculopathy. Spine 19:2122-2126

Hare W, Lond F, Holland C (1983) Paresis following internal iliac artery embolization. Radiology 146:47-51

Hassler W, Thron A, Grote E (1989) Hemodynamics of spinal arteriovenous fistulas. An intraoperative study. J Neurosurg 70:360-370

Heindel CC, Dugger GS, Guito FC (1975) Spinal arteriovenous malformation with hypogastric blood supply. Case report. J Neurosurg 64:134-139

Heiss JD, Doppmann JL, Oldfield EH (1994) Brief report: relief of spinal cord compression from vertebral hemangioma by intralesional injection of absolute ethanol. N Engl J Med 331:508-511

Hekster REM, Luyendijk W, Tan TI (1972) Spinal cord compression caused by vertebral hemangioma relieved by percutaneous catheter embolization. Neuroradiology 3:160-164

Hemmy DC, McGee DM, Armbrust FH, Larson SJ (1977) Resection of a vertebral hemangioma after preoperative embolization: case report. J Neurosurg 47:282-285

Heros RC, Debrun GM, Ojemann RG, et al (1986) Direct spinal arteriovenous fistula: a new type of spinal AVM. Case report. J Neurosurg 64:134-139

Hurst RW, Kenyon LC, Lavi E, Raps EC, Marcotte P (1995) Spinal dural arteriovenous fistula: the pathology of venous hypertension myelopathy. Neurology 45:1309-1313

Ide C, Gangi A, Rimmelin A, et al (1996) Vertebral hemangiomas with spinal cord compression: the place of preoperative percutaneous vertebroplasty with methyl methacrylate. Neuroradiology 38:585-589

Isu T, Iwasaki Y, Akino M, Koyanagi I, Abe H (1989) Magnetic resonance imaging in cases of spinal dural arteriovenous malformation. Neurosurgery 24:919-923

Jellinek JS, Kransdorf MJ, Gray R, Aboulafia AJ, Malawer MM (1996) Percutaneous transpedicular biopsy of vertebral body lesions. Spine 21:2035-2040

Jellinek D, Jewkes D, Symon L (1991) Noninvasive intraoperative monitoring of motor evoked potentials under propofol anesthesia: effects of spinal surgery on the amplitude and latency of motor evoked potentials. Neurosurgery 29: 551-557

Kaemmerlen P, Thiesse P, Bouvard H, et al (1989a) Percutaneous vertebroplasty in the treatment of metastases: technique and results. J Radiol 70:557-562

Kaemmerlen P, Thiesse P, Bouvard H, Biron P, Mornex F, Jonas P (1989b) Vertebroplastie percutanée dans le traitement des métastases. J Radiol 70:557-562

Kamano S, Fukushima T (1976) Angiographic demonstration of vertebral osteoid osteoma. Surg Neurol 6:167-168

Katsuta T, Morioka T, Hasuo K, Miyahara S, Fukui M, Masuda K (1993) Discrepancy between provocative test and clinical results following endovascular obliteration of spinal arteriovenous malformation. Surg Neurol 40:142-145

Keith RW, Stamboogh JL, Awender SH (1990) Somatosensory cortical evoked potentials: a review of 100 cases of intraoperative spinal surgery monitoring. J Spinal Disord 3:220-226

Kendall B (1986) Spinal angiography with iohexol. Neuroradiology 28: 72-73

Kerber CW (1980) Flow-controlled therapeutic embolization: a physiologic and safe technique. AJR Am J Roentgenol 134:557-561

Khayata M, Aymard A, Guichard JP et al (1992) Interventional neuroradiology. Curr Opin Radiol 4:71-78

Khayata MH, McKenzie J, Vishteh AG, Dean B, Spetzler RF (1995) Endovascular approach to spinal vascular lesions. In: Maciunas RJ (ed) Endovascular neurological intervention. American Association of Neurological Surgeons Publication Committee, Springfield, pp 247-261

Kim D, Choi I, Berenstein A (1991) A sacral dural arteriovenous fistula presenting with an intermittent myelopathy aggravated by menstruation. Case report. J Neurosurg 75:947-949

King GJ, Kostuik JP, McBroom RJ, Richardson W (1991) Surgical management of metastatic renal carcinoma of the spine. Spine 16:265-271

Koci TM, Mehringer CM, Yamagata N, Chiang F (1995) Aneurysmal bone cyst of the thoracic spine: evolution after particulate embolization. Am J Neuroradiol 16:857-860

Konya A, Szendroi M (1992) Aneurysmal bone cysts treated by superselective embolization. Skeletal Radiol 21:167-172

Kosary IA, Braham J, Shaked I, Shaked R (1977) Spinal epidural hematoma due to hemangioma of vertebra. Surg Neurol 7:61-62

Krishna M, Taylor JF, Brown MC, Farrell J, Morley TR, Edgar MA, Young D (1991) Failure of somatosensory-evoked-potential monitoring in sensorimotor neuropathy. Spine 16:479

Kudo S, Chuang VP, Wallace S, Bechtel W, Mir S (1984) Middle sacral arteriography: diagnostic and therapeutic implications. Radiology 151:65

Lagergren C, Lindbom A, Soderberg G (1961) The blood vessels of osteogenic sarcomas. Acta Radiologica 55:161-176

Lang EF Jr, Perserico L (1960) Neurologic and surgical aspect of vertebral hemangiomas. Surg Clin North Am 40:817-823

Laredo JD, Bard M (1986) Thoracic spine: percutaneous trephine biopsy. Radiology 160:485-489

Laredo JD, Reizine D, Bard M, Merland JJ (1986) Vertebral hemangiomas: radiologic evaluation. Radiology 161:183-189

Laredo JD, Assouline E, Gelbert F, Wybier M, Merland JJ, Tubiana JM (1990) Vertebral hemangiomas: fat content as a sign of aggressiveness. Radiology 177:467-472

Larsen DW, Halbach VV, Teitelbaum GP, McDougall CG, Higashida RT, Dowd CF, Heishima GB (1995) Spinal dural arteriovenous fistulas supplied by branches of the internal iliac arteries. Surg Neurol 43:35-41

Larsson E-M, Desai P, Hardin CW, Story J, Jinicins JR (1991) Venous infarction of the spinal cord resulting from dural arteriovenous fistula: MR imaging findings. AJNR Am J Neuroradiol 12:739-743

Laschinger JC, Cunningham JN Jr, Baumann FG, et al (1987) Monitoring of somatosensory evoked potentials during surgical procedures on the thoracoabdominal aorta. II. Use of somatosensory evoked potentials to assess adequacy of distal aortic bypass and perfusion after thoracic aortic bypass and perfusion after thoracic aortic cross-clamping. J Thorac Cardiovasc Surg 94:266-270

Lasjaunias P, Berenstein A (1987) Functional vascular anatomy of the brain, spinal cord and spine. In: Lasjaunias P, Berenstein A (EdsS) Surgical neuroangiography, Springer, Berlin, Heidelberg New York, pp 15-87

Launay M, Chiras J, Bories J (1979) Angiography of the spinal cord: venous phase normal features. Pathological application. J Neuroradiology 6:287-315

Laurin S (1977) Angiography in giant cell tumors. Radiology 17:118-123

Lazorthes G, Couaze A, Zadeh JO, Santini JJ, Lazorthes Y, Burdin P (1971) Arterial vascularization of the spinal cord. J Neurosurg 35:253-262

Lesser RP, Raudzens P, Luders H, et al (1986) Postoperative neurological deficits may occur despite unchanged intraoperative somatosensory evoked potentials. Ann Neurol 19:22-25

Lindbom A, Soderberg G, Spjut, et al (1961) Angiography of aneurysmal bone cyst. Acta Radiol 55:12-16

Luxton G, Petrovich Z, Josef G, Nedzi LA, Apuzzo MLJ (1993) Stereotactic radiosurgery: principles and comparison of treatment methods. Neurosurgery 32:241-259

Malawer MM, Delaney TF (1989) Treatment of metastatic cancer to bone. In: Devita VT, Hellman DS, Rosenberg SA (eds) Cancer: principles and practice of oncology, 3rd ed. Lippincott, Philadelphia, pp 2298-2317

Masaryk TJ, Ross JS, Modic MT, Ruff RL, Selman WR, Ratcheson RA (1987) Radiculomeningeal vascular malformations of the spine: MR imaging Radiology 164:845-849

Mascalchi M, Bianchi MC, Quilici N, et al. (1995a) MR angiography of spinal vascular malformations. AJNR Am J Neuroradiol 16:289-297

Mascalchi M, Bianchi MC, Quilici N, Mangiafico S, Ferrito G, Padolecchia R, Bartolozzi C (1995b) MR angiography of spinal vascular malformations. AJNR Am J Neuroradiol 16:289-297

McAllister VL, Kendall BE, Bull JWD (1975) Symptomatic vertebral hemangiomas. Brain 98:71-80.

McLaughlin RE, Miller WR, Miller CW (1976) Quadriparesis after needle aspiration of the cervical spine. Report of a case. J Bone Joint Surg [Am] 58:1167-1168

Meder JF, Chiras J, Barth MO, NíDaiye M, Bories J (1984) Myelographic features of the normal external spinal veins. J Neuroradiol 11:315-325

Mehta RC, Marks MP, Hincks RS, Glover GH, Enzmann DR (1995) MR evaluation of vertebral metastases; T1-weighted, short-inversion-time inversion recovery, fast spin-echo, and inversion-recovery fast spin-echo sequences. AJNR Am J Neuroradiol 16:281-288

Merland JJ, Reizine D (1987) Treatment of arteriovenous spinal-cord malformations. Semin Intervent Radiol 4:281-290

Merland JJ, Riche MC, Chiras J (1980) Les fistules arterioveneuses intra-canalaires, extra-medullaires à drainage veineux medullaire. J Neuroradiol 7:271-320

Moore KL (1980) The perineum and pelvis. In: Moore KL (ed) Clinically oriented anatomy. Williams and Wilkins, Baltimore

Mourier KL, Gobin YP, George B, et al (1993a) Intradural perimedullary arteriovenous fistulae: results of surgical and endovascular treatment in a series of 35 cases. Neurosurgery 32:885-891

Mourier KL, Gelbert F, Reizine D, et al (1993b) Phase contrast magnetic resonance of the spinal cord arterio-venous malformations. Acta Neurochir (Wien) 123:57-63

Muraszko KM, Antrunes JL, Hilal SK, Michelsen WJ (1982) Hemangiopericytomas of the spine. Neurosurgery 10:473-479

Mustain WD, Kendig RJ (1991) Dissociation of neurogenic motor and somatosensory evoked potentials. A case report. Spine 16:851-853

Nakstad PH, Hald JK, Bakke SJ (1993) Multiple spinal arteriovenous fistulas in Klippel-Trénaunay-Weber syndrome treated with platinum fibre coils. Neuroradiology 35:163-165

N'Diaye M, Chisas J, Meder JF, Barth MO, Koussa A, Bories J (1984) Water-soluble myelography for the study of dural arteriovenous fistulae of the spine draining in the spinal venous system. J Neuroradiol 11:327-339

Nguyen JP, Djindjian M, Gaston A, et al (1987) Vertebral hemangiomas presenting with neurologic symptoms. Surg Neurol 27:391-397

Nichols DA, Rufenacht DA, Jack CR Jr, Forbes GS (1992) Embolization of spinal dural arteriovenous fistula with polyvinyl alcohol particles: experience in 14 patients. AJNR Neurorad 13:933-940

Nicola N, Lins E (1987) Vertebral hemangioma: retrograde embolization-stabilization with methyl methacrylate. Surg Neurol 27:481-486

Olerud C, Jonsson H, Löfberg A, Lörelius L, Sjöstrom L (1993) Embolization of spinal metastases reduces preoperative blood loss. Acta Orthop Scand 64:9-12

Ottolenghi CE (1955) Diagnosis of orthopaedic lesions by aspiration biopsy. Results of 1,061 punctures. J Bone Joint Surg Am 37:443-464

Ottolenghi CE (1969) Aspiration biopsy of the spine. J Bone Joint Surg Am 51:1531-1544

Ottolenghi CE, Schajowicz F, Deshant FA (1964) Aspiration biopsy of the cervical spine. Technique and results in thirty-four cases. J Bone Joint Surg Am 46:715-733

Parke WW, Whalen JL, VanDemark RE, Kambin P (1994) The infra-aortic arteries of the spine; their variability and clinical significance. Spine 19:1-5

Partington MD, Rufenacht DA, March WR, Piepgras DG (1992) Cranial and sacral dural arteriovenous fistulae as a cause of myelopathy. J Neurosurg 76:615-622

Perman F (1926) An hemangioma in spinal column. Acta Chir Scand 61: 91-105

Phillips JH, Kling TF, Cohen MD (1994) The radiographic anatomy of the thoracic pedicle. Spine 19:446-449

Picard L, Bracard S, Roland J, Moreno A, Per A (1989) Embolisation des hemangiomes vertebraux: technique-indications-resultats. Neurochirurgie 35:289-293, 305-308

Pierot L, Vlachopoulos T, Attal N, Martin N, Bert S, Chiras J. (1993) Double spinal dural arteriovenous fistulas: report of two cases. AJNR Am J Neuroradiol 14:1109-1112

Pinto RS, Lin JP, Firooznia H, LeFleur RS (1975) The osseous and angiographic features of vertebral chordomas. Neuroradiology 9:231-241

Provenzale JM, Tien RD, Felsberg GJ, Hacien-Bey L (1994) Spinal dural arteriovenous fistula: demonstration using phase contrast MRA. J Comput Assist Tomogr 18:811-814

Raco A, Cipippetta P, Artico M, Salvati M, Guidetti G, Gugliemi G (1990) Vertebral hemangiomas with cord compression: the role of embolization in 5 cases. Surg Neurol 34:164-168

Ramsdell JW, Peters RM, Taylor AJ (1977) Multiorgan scans for staging lung cancer. Correlation with clinical evaluation. J Thorac Cardiovasc Surg 73:653-658

Renfrew DL, Whitten CG, Wiese JA, El-Khoury GY, Harris KG (1991) CT-guided percutaneous transpedicular biopsy of the spine. Radiology 180:574-576

Riche MC, Melki JP, Merland JJ (1983) Embolization of spinal cord vascular malformations via the anterior spinal artery. AJNR Am J Neuroradiol 4:378-381

Riche MC, Reizine D, Melki JP, et al (1985) Classification of spinal cord vascular malformations. Radiat Med 3:17-24

Rodesch G, Berenstein A, Lasjaunias P (1992) Vasculature and vascular lesions of the spine and spinal cord. In: Manelfe C (ed) Imaging of the spine and spinal cord. Raven, New York, pp 565-598

Rodesch G, Lasjaunias P, Berenstein A (1994) Embolization of arteriovenous malformations of the spinal cord. In:

Rodesch G, Alvarez H, Chaskis C, Peters J, Lasjaunias P (1996) Clinical manifestations in paraspinal arteriovenous malformations. Spinal cord symptoms, pathophysiology, and treatment objectives. Int J Neuroradiol 2:430-436

Rosenblum B, Oldfield EH, Doppman JL, Di Chiro G (1987) Spinal arteriovenous malformations: a comparison of dural arteriovenous fistulas and intradural AVMs in 81 patients. J Neurosurg 67:795-802

Ross JS, Masaryk TJ, Modic MT, Carter JR, Mapstone T, Dengel FH (1987) Vertebral hemangiomas : MR imaging. Radiology 165:165-169

Satran R (1988) Spinal cord infarction. Stroke 19:529-532

Schmorl G, Junghanne H (1971) The human spine in health and disease, 2nd edn. Grune and Stratton, New York

Smith TP, Gray L, Weinstein JN, Richardson WJ, Payne CS (1995) Pre-operative transarterial embolization of spinal column neoplasms. J Vasc Interv Radiol 6:863-869

Smith TP, Koci T, Mehringer CM et al (1993) Transarterial embolization of vertebral hemangioma. J Vasc Interv Radiol 4:681-685

Soo GS, Wallace S, Chuang UP, Carrasco CH, Phillies G (1982) Lumbar artery embolization in cancer patients. Radiology 145:655-659

Spetzler RF, Zabramski JM, Flom RA (1989) Management of juvenile spinal AVMs by embolization and operative excision. J Neurosurg 70:628-632

Stechison MT, Panagis SG, Reinhart SS (1995) Somatosensory evoked potential monitoring during spinal surgery. Acta Neurochir (Wien) 135:56-61

Stecker MM, Marcotte P, Hurst R, Patterson T (1996) Spinal dural arteriovenous malformations: intraoperative evoked potential evidence for pathophysiology. A case report. Spine 21:512-515

Stein SC, Ommaya AK, Doppmann JL, Di Chiro G (1972) Arteriovenous malformation of the cauda equina with arterial supply from branches of the internal iliac arteries. Case report. J Neurosurgery 36:639-651

Stringham DR, Hadjipavlou A, Dzioba R, Lander P (1994) Percutaneous transpedicular biopsy of the spine. Spine 19: 1985-1991

Suby-Long T, Bos GD, Rosch J (1988) Biopsy proven eradication of an aneurysmal bone cyst treated by superselective embolization: a case report. Cardiovasc Intervent Radiol 11:292-295

Sugiyama Y, Kondo H, Tanabe Y, Sakai N, Yamada H, Ilkeda K (1982) Arteriovenous malformation of the spinal cord and cauda equina fed by branches of the internal iliac artery and associated with vertebral hemangiomas. Surg Neurol 18:97-101

Sundaresan N, Choi IS, Hughes JEO, Sachdev VP, Berenstein A (1990) Treatment of spinal metastases from kidney cancer by presurgical embolization and resection. J Neurosurg 73:548-554

Sundaresan N, Galicich JH, Chu FCH, Huvos AG (1979) Spinal chordomas. J Neurosurg 50:312-319

Symon L, Kuyama H, Kendall B (1984) Dural arteriovenous malformations of the spine. J Neurosurg 60:238-247

Takahashi H, Jooshita I, Saito I, Sano S, Akagi Y (1977) Spinal arteriovenous malformation fed by branches of the internal iliac artery. No Shinkei Geka 5:285-289

Tampieri D, Weill A, Melanson D, Ethier R (1991) Percutaneous aspiration biopsy in cervical spine lytic lesions. Indications and technique. Neuroradiology 33:43-47

Tatsui H, Onomura T, Morishita S, Oketa M, Inoue T (1996) Survival rates of patients with metastatic spinal cancer after scintigraphic detection of abnormal radiographic accumulation. Spine 21:2143-2148

Thron AK (1988) Vascular anatomy of the spinal cord. Neuroradiological investigations and clinical syndromes. Springer, Vienna New York, pp 1-105

Touho H, Monobe T, Ohnishi H, Karasawa J (1995) Treatment of type II perimedullary arteriovenous fistulas by intraoperative transvenous embolization: case report. Surg Neurol 43:491-496

Valls J, Ottolenghi CE, Shajowicz F (1948) Aspiration biopsy in the diagnosis of lesions of vertebral bodies. JAMA 136:375-382

Versari PP, DíAliberti G, Talamonti G, Branca V, Boccardi E, Collice M (1993) Progressive myelopathy caused by intracranial dural arteriovenous fistula: report of two cases and review of the literature. Neurosurgery 33:914-919

Voegeli E, Fuchs W (1976) Arteriography in bone tumors. Br J Radiol 49:407-415

Willinski R, Lasjaunias P, TerBrugge KN, Hurth M (1990a) Angiography in the investigation for spinal dural arteriovenous fistula. A protocol with application of the venous phase. Neuroradiology 32: 114-116

Willinski R, TerBrugge K, Lasjaunuas P, Montaneraw (1990b) The variable presentations of craniocervical and cervical dural malformations. Surg Neurol 34:118-123

Willinski R, TerBrugge KN, Montanera W, Wallace MC, Gentili F (1993) Spinal epidural arteriovenous fistulas: arterial and venous approaches to embolization. AJNR Am J Neuroradiol 14:812-817

Wrobel CJ, Oldfield EH, Di Chirog, Tarlov EC, Baker RA, Doppman JL (1988) Myelopathy due to intracranial dural arteriovenous fistulas draining intrathecally into spinal medullary veins. Report of three cases. J Neurosurg 69:934-939

Yaghmai I (1977) Angiographic features of osteosarcoma. Am J Roentgenol Radiat Ther Nucl Med 129:1073-1081

Yang Z-Y, Zhang L-J, Chen A-X, Hu H-Y (1985) Hemangioma of the vertebral column: a report on twenty-three patients with special reference to functional recovery after radiation therapy. Acta Radiol Oncol 24:129-132

Yang LH, Lin SM, Lee WY, Liu CC (1994) Intraoperative transcranial electrical motor evoked potential monitoring during spinal surgery under intravenous ketamine or etomidate anesthesia. Acta Neurochir (Wien) 127: 191-198

Young W, Berenstein A (1985) Somatosensory evoked potential monitoring of intraoperative procedures. In: Schramm J, Jones SJ (eds) Spinal Cord Monitoring. Springer, Berlin Heidelberg New York, pp 197-203

Yeates A, Drayer B, Heinz ER, Osborne D (1985) Intra-arterial digital subtraction angiography of the spinal cord. Radiology 155: 387-390

8 Current Concepts of Surgical Therapy of Vertebral Tumours

M.W. Fidler

CONTENTS

More specifically, whether surgery is to be curative or palliative will depend on the staging of the tumour (ENNEKING 1986) and whether or not a "radical" resection is technically feasible. Unfortunately, the meaning of "radical" is subject to various interpretations. "Radical" is frequently used to mean extra-lesional excision with a tumour-free margin but, if one follows the classification of ENNEKING (1986), "radical" resection (i.e. en bloc resection of the whole compartment or the whole vertebra) with preservation of the spinal cord or cauda equina is impossible. The more specific terms "marginal" or "wide" may be more appropriate (marginal excision: en bloc extracapsular within the reactive zone; wide excision: en bloc, through normal tissue beyond the reactive zone). Malignant tumours are often treated by combining surgery with chemotherapy, radiotherapy and hormone therapy.

8.1
Introduction

The majority of vertebral tumours requiring surgical treatment are metastases. Of the 200 consecutive personally treated tumours on which this chapter is based, 22 (11%) were benign, 1 (0.5%) was intermediate, 23 (11.5%) were primary malignant tumours and 154 (77%) were metastases (149 "palliative" operations and 5 "curative" resections). This last percentage corresponds with the 5:1 ratio of metastases to primary tumours quoted by ROSENBERG and SCHILLER (1990).

As with any tumour, the surgical treatment of a vertebral tumour is basically governed by whether it is benign or malignant, primary or secondary.

M.W. FIDLER, MS FRCS FRCS Ed, Orthopaedic Department, Onze Lieve Vrouwe Gasthuis, 1e Oosterparkstraat 179, 1091 HA Amsterdam, The Netherlands
Netherlands Cancer Institute, Amsterdam, The Netherlands

8.2
General Presentation of Vertebral Tumours

Vertebral tumours usually present with local pain, radiating pain, a painful pathological fracture or the development of neurological symptoms and signs singly or in combination. Asymptomatic vertebral metastases, previously, were usually discovered on routine radiological survey but this has now given place to a screening bone scan in patients with known malignant disease.

8.3
Imaging

The imaging techniques are described in detail in Chap. 2 and only the surgically relevant aspects are summarized here.

8.3.1
Radiographs

Plain anteroposterior and lateral radiographs are still the basis of investigations but it must be remembered that some 50% of the bone must be destroyed before a lesion is visible (EDELSTYN et al. 1967). Osteolytic lesions in the sacrum, in particular, are easily overlooked. Routine chest radiographs are essential.

8.3.2
Bone Scan

As well as localizing the lesion, the bone scan identifies lesions in neighbouring vertebrae and in remote areas. This last is particularly important if bone grafting is to be part of the surgical procedure. It is important to know that cold as well as hot spots can occur. A rotating display of reconstructed single photon emission computer tomography (SPECT) images is ideal for localizing areas of intense activity such as produced by an osteoid osteoma.

8.3.3
CT Scanning

This is the best method for depicting changes due to tumour in the cortical bone.

8.3.4
MRI

MRI has now replaced CT myelography in tumour surgery. It simplifies the construction of a mental three-dimensional picture of the lesion, giving accurate localization of the zone of any neural compression and any soft tissue extension of the tumour. The extent of infiltration of the tumour through the cancellous bone is open to discussion. On the one hand, the "MRI abnormal bone" is partly due to a local inflammatory reaction, and on the other hand, even an MRI probably misses minute fingers of advancing tumour. At present it would probably be wise to remove all bone which appears abnormal on MRI if one is planning a resection of all macroscopic tumour in combination with post-operative radiotherapy. A curative "wide" resection should have a wider margin.

When planning the surgical treatment of vertebral metastases, MRI is the best method of detecting other metastases in neighbouring vertebrae (ALGRA 1992).

MRI can help in differentiating between tumour and an osteoporotic fracture (RUPP et al. 1995). Normal marrow almost certainly excludes tumour, whilst pedicle involvement and an associated soft tissue mass are fairly specific for tumour. A repeat MRI scan after 2–3 months will show diminished contrast enhancement in benign lesions and an increase in malignant lesions (AN et al. 1995).

8.4
Pre-operative Investigations

8.4.1
Blood Examination

Blood examination is routine. Depression of bone marrow activity due to any recent chemotherapy or radiotherapy can be assessed. Metastatic bone tumour, in particular, may cause hypercalcaemia.

8.4.2
Selective Angiography and Embolization

These are indicated in relation to the malignant lesions and the hypervascular benign lesions, such as aneurysmal bone cysts, osteoblastomas and haemangiomas. Angiography reveals the feeder arteries and any vascular abnormalities near the tumour. If hypervascular, the feeder arteries and the tumour bed are embolized with Ivalon (polyvinyl alcohol); any segmental artery which also gives rise to an important medullary artery (DOMMISSE 1980), such as the artery of Adamkiewicz, is, of course, not embolized. Angiography and embolization are carried out within 4 or 5 days of the definitive operation. If performed earlier, there is a definite risk of collaterals opening up or of recanalization occurring.

Embolization prior to a biopsy should be within 24 h of operation, preferably only a few hours before, in order to minimize necrosis of the specimen and improve the chance of an accurate histological diagnosis.

Embolization used to be restricted to the thoracic and lumbar spine and the sacrum, but nowadays, with modern techniques and special catheters, many cervical spine tumours can also be embolized. Embolization is especially helpful if the feeder arteries on the side of the spine contralateral to the operative approach can be occluded prior to any intralesional resection. Ipsilateral feeders can be directly ligated during the operation. During radical resections, all feeders will eventually be ligated and divided prior to removal of the tumour, but embolization probably diminishes the blood flow through the tumour into the epidural venous plexus with consequent decrease in blood loss when these veins have to be dealt with.

8.4.3
Biopsy

If there is any doubt about the nature of the lesion, biopsy is essential. Until recently, for vertebral body lesions which could not be curatively resected a percutaneous postero-lateral approach to the thoracic and lumbar spine was used, with a wide-bore Harlow Wood biopsy set under bi-planar image intensification. Nowadays, CT guidance is more usual. A core diameter of at least 3.5 mm is recommended for optimal histological assessment (WARD et al. 1996). At present an open biopsy is performed for anterior cervical spine tumours, though this will also be superseded by a CT-guided percutaneous technique (BABU et al. 1994).

If a resectable primary vertebral body lesion is suspected, open transpedicular biopsy (FIDLER and NIERS 1990; ROY-CAMILLE et al. 1990) is preferred. This method restricts contamination to an area which can be excised at the time of the radical operation. Furthermore, the posterior cortical defect can be blocked with bone wax to prevent the formation of a contaminated haematoma. Although oncologically not perfect, this open technique seems better than the postero-lateral percutaneous one, which transgresses and contaminates several compartments.

Posterior tumours at all levels are, if possible, initially biopsied with a Tru-Cut needle (Travenol) under CT guidance. If this would be dangerous or if it fails, resort is made to open operation.

A combination of cytology and fine-core biopsy (JELINEK et al. 1996) or cytology alone (KREICBERGS et al. 1996) using a percutaneous technique under radiological control can be successful in achieving a diagnosis in some 80% of cases in specialized centres. It is possible that one of these techniques will become the primary choice, recourse being had to wide-bore biopsies or open biopsies only in cases of doubt.

Finally, it must be stressed that spine tumours should only be biopsied in special centres by surgeons or their colleagues experienced in the total management of these difficult problems. This recommendation was made by WEINSTEIN and McLAIN

in 1987 and still holds true today. An inappropriate biopsy can compromise a possible radical resection.

8.5
Individual Tumours: Treatment Guidelines

8.5.1
Benign Tumours

8.5.1.1
Osteoid Osteoma

This small and painful tumour is usually seen in patients between 10 and 20 years of age and occurs more commonly in males (PETTINE and KLASSEN 1986). Ten per cent of osteoid osteomas occur in the spine (JACKSON et al. 1977).

An osteoid osteoma consists of a central nidus of osteoid tissue surrounded by a zone of reactive hyperostosis. These features are responsible for the typical radiological appearance. The osteoma gives rise to an intense hot spot on a bone scan and especially on a rotating display of reconstructed SPECT images.

An osteoid osteoma usually occurs in the posterior elements where it can be precisely localized by CT (Fig. 8.1) following the bone scan. It can be approached directly, and only the nidus has to be removed. Very rarely, the hot spot cannot be identified on the CT image and, in this case, a block of bone, calculated to contain the microscopic hot spot, will have to be removed (FIDLER and HOEFNAGEL 1984). Intra-operative bone scanning may help in localizing the lesion or checking that a lesion has been completely excised (OSEBOLD et al. 1993), but this technique should rarely be required. If a facet joint has to be sacrificed, a local fusion is necessary to maintain spinal stability. Pain is usually relieved immediately following operation.

A vertebral osteoid osteoma is one of the more common causes of a painful scoliosis, convex to the opposite side, in children. Following excision, the scoliosis resolves if the lesion presents around the time of or after skeletal maturity, but, in adolescence, a prolonged delay in treatment may result in a progressive structural scoliosis (RANSFORD et al. 1984). PETTINE and KLASSEN (1986) suggest that 15 months is the critical duration of symptoms with respect to whether a scoliosis will regress or progress following excision of the tumour.

Osteoid osteomas in the limbs have been successfully treated with long-term (2 years or more) nonsteroidal anti-inflammatory drugs (NSAID; KNEISL

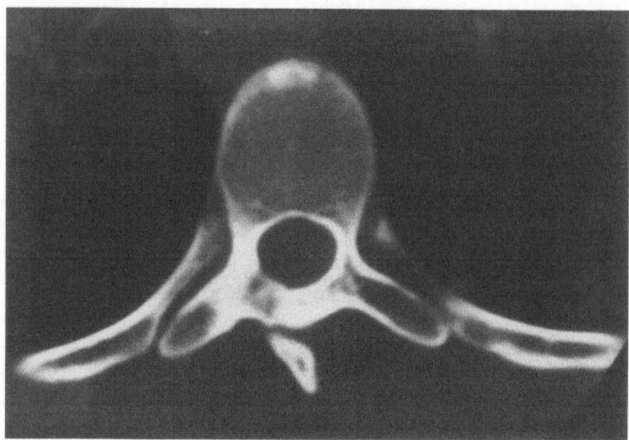

Fig. 8.1. A CT image showing an osteoid osteoma in the left lamina. The central nidus is surrounded by sclerosis

and SIMON 1992). On this basis, when a spinal lesion presents at the time of skeletal maturity or later and when there is probably no danger of a structural scoliosis developing, perhaps medical rather than surgical treatment should be contemplated.

8.5.1.2
Osteoblastoma

Osteoblastomas are less common and tend to develop in patients who are slightly older than those developing osteoid osteomas (PETTINE and KLASSEN 1986). They occur more commonly in males and 35% are situated in the spine (JACKSON et al. 1977).

An osteoblastoma is similar to but larger than an osteoid osteoma. The differentiating diameter is 2 cm. Like osteoid osteoma, it also has a predilection for the posterior elements of the spine and can cause scoliosis. Whereas osteoid osteoma remains localized, osteoblastoma is usually destructive and expansile, though part of the tumour frequently becomes sclerotic and appears to be burnt out (Fig. 8.2). Conservative treatment has never been shown to be effective.

An osteoblastoma can be highly vascular, and preoperative angiography is advisable. If embolization is not possible, any large feeder arteries should be ligated at the commencement of the operation. The recurrence rate following intralesional surgery is in the order of 15% (SCHAJOWICZ 1994, p. 62) and, rarely, malignant transformation to an osteosarcoma has been observed, though in some cases this fol-

lowed post-operative radiotherapy (SCHAJOWICZ 1994, pp. 57–58). While, owing to this unpredictable behaviour, a wide en bloc excision is the recommended treatment, such an excision may increase morbidity so much that the risks of intralesional surgery are preferable. In such a case, an extralesional dissection is carried out as far as possible; this further devascularizes the tumour, which is then removed piecemeal. The walls of the cavity are either resected or curetted, burred and biopsied. Sclerotic bone can probably be left in situ if its removal would be dangerous.

8.5.1.3
Aneurysmal Bone Cyst

This lesion most commonly occurs in patients between 5 and 20 years of age and is found somewhat more often in the neural arch with 60% compared with 40% in the vertebral body (HAY et al. 1978). It is an expansile osteolytic lesion which is frequently highly vascular. It can be extremely aggressive, sometimes involving more than one vertebra. Angiography usually reveals definite feeder arteries, which should be embolized. This is followed by biopsy to confirm the diagnosis. The combination of embolization and biopsy may be sufficient to cause regression and ossification of the lesion so that no further treatment is necessary (MISASI et al. 1982; MURPHY et al. 1982; FIDLER and NIERS 1990; Fig. 8.3). In the absence of impending mechanical failure or a neurological deficit, this should be the first line of treatment. Otherwise, or if this simple treatment

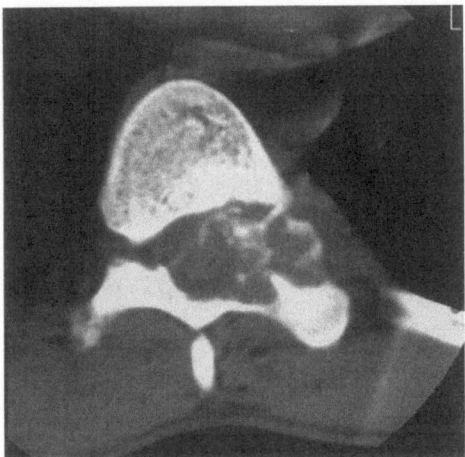

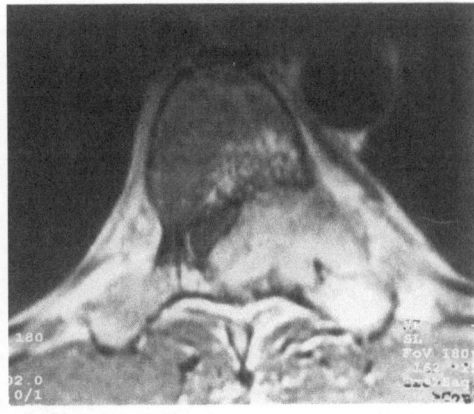

a

Fig. 8.2. CT (**a**) and MRI (**b**) scans of an osteoblastoma arising from the left side of T9. The spinal cord is compressed

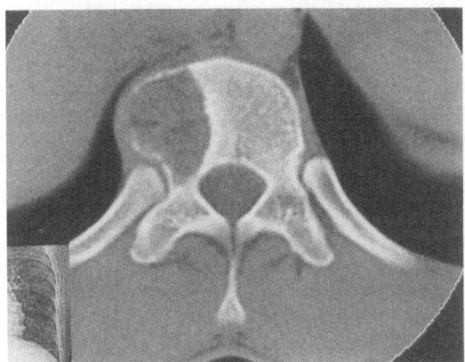

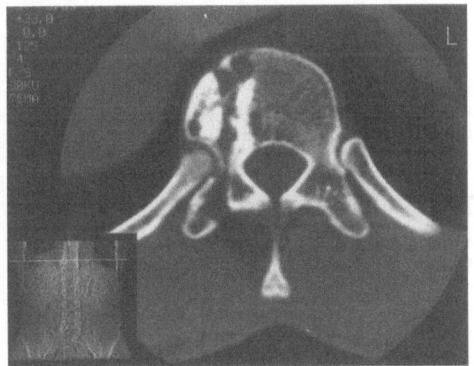

a

b

Fig. 8.3. CT images of an aneurysmal bone cyst: a prior to treatment and b 2 years following embolization and open transpendicular biopsy. Most of the lesion has become sclerotic. The track of the biopsy is still visible

fails, operation is necessary. The lesion should be devascularized as far as possible with an extralesional approach and then removed intralesionally. The walls of the cavity should be vigorously curretted/burred or, where possible, resected. The operation can sometimes be facilitated by using a cavitational ultrasonic surgical aspirator (CUSA or Cavitron); (VANDERTOP et al. 1994). Reconstruction is by means of autograft, if necessary supplemented with internal fixation. With such a technique, even cysts in surgically challenging situations can be safely treated (BONGIOANNI et al. 1996). HAY et al. (1978) reported a recurrence rate of 25% following curettage. The recurrences responded to total excision or partial excision with curettage. Complete

extralesional resection would be curative but the results of vigorous intralesional surgery including the possibility of a second chance justify this more conservative initial approach.

8.5.1.4
Haemangioma

This is a benign lesion affecting the vertebral body and the neural arch (Fig. 8.4). It occurs at all ages and more commonly in females. It can be associated with cutaneous haemangiomas (ASUMU et al. 1996). The primary treatment for pain should probably be embolization (PICARD et al. 1989); radiotherapy has

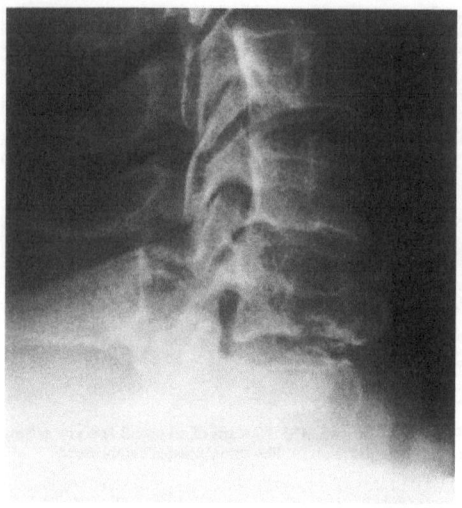

a

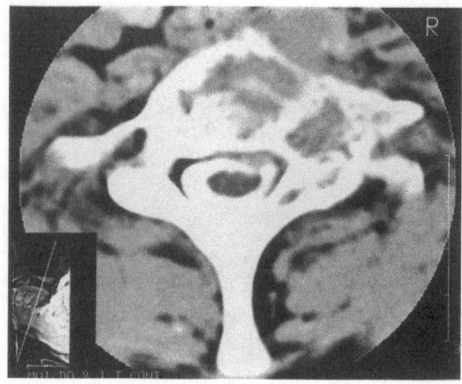

b

Fig. 8.4. A lateral radiograph (a) and a CT image (b) of a haemangioma involving the vertebral body and arch of C7. There is minor indentation of the dura antero-laterally

also proved effective (Fox and ONOFRIO 1993) but one is always wary about the long-term effects of radiotherapy. Surgery is only indicated for unresponsive, intractable pain, mechanical failure or neural compression. Following angiography and, if possible, embolization, the lesion is devascularized as far as possible by an extralesional dissection from the appropriate direction prior to an intralesional excision. As with other benign lesions, if the mechanical integrity of the spine is compromised, autografting is essential for long-term reconstruction. Internal fixation provides temporary support whilst the grafts incorporate.

There is an intervening group between the benign haemangiomas and the malignant angiosarcomas. This group includes the angioblastomas, which should be treated surgically. An intralesional resection appears to be sufficient, followed by stabilization with the inclusion of bone grafts (BEEN et al. 1994).

8.5.1.5
Eosinophilic Granuloma (Solitary Version)

This is mainly a disease of children and adolescents/ young adults (CAMPANACCI 1990, p. 770). It is usually self-limiting and confined to the vertebral body, where it typically causes a "vertebra plana", though in the cervical spine, possibly due to earlier presentation, an osteolytic lesion without collapse is com-

mon (DICKINSON and FARHAT 1991). Apart from biopsy to exclude other diagnoses, surgical treatment is almost never required though injections of cortisone into the lesion have been recommended (CAMPANACCI 1990, p. 788). Bedrest until the acute, painful phase is over, followed by support in an appropriate brace is usually sufficient. Even in advanced cases, cord compression rarely occurs. If it does, and particularly if it is progressive, low-dose radiotherapy (1200 rads; GREEN et al. 1980) or surgery (DICKINSON and FARHAT 1991) is indicated.

8.5.1.6
Neurofibroma and Schwannoma (Neurilemmoma, Neurinoma)

Solitary neurofibromas usually occur in patients between 20 and 40 years of age and schwannomas, between 20 and 50 (CAMPANACCI 1990, pp. 1013–1022). Whether these tumours are really separate entities or not is open to discussion (SMITH and SCHMIDEK 1990), but there is now a tendency to consider them as separate (SANGUINETTI et al. 1993). There does seem to be a surgical distinction. The neurofibroma is intimately connected with the nerve, fibres of which pass through it, whereas the schwannoma is often fairly distinct; the nerve usually has to be sacrified when removing a neurofibroma, but part can often be left intact after a schwannoma is dissected free. The schwannoma frequently arises from the sensory roots of spinal nerves or from the nerves of the periosteum or those accompanying small blood vessels in the bone, whereas the neurofibroma is more a tumour of cutaneous and deep peripheral nerves and usually occurs in connection with von Recklinghausen's disease (SMITH and SCHMIDEK 1990; CAMPANACCI 1990, pp. 1013–1022). These tumours can often be quite large by the time the patient is referred for specialist treatment (Fig. 8.5). Malignant transformation of a schwannoma is very rare but occurs in 2–30% of neurofibromas, especially when associated with von Recklinghausen's disease (CAMPANACCI 1990, pp. 1013–1022.

TREATMENT:

Extra-lesional excision is curative. However, these are benign lesions and if such an excision would entail undue risk or morbidity then an intralesional excision is permissable. The nerve of origin is sacrificed except in the case of a schwannoma arising from an important nerve when the tumour may be dissected free. Where part of the tumour is inside the spinal canal, this is exposed first. (Parts of the tumour inside and outside the spinal canal connected by a narrow segment in the intervertebral foramen constitute a "dumb-bell" tumour which produces the typical widening of the intervertebral foramen.) The dissection is then carried laterally, removing bone as

necessary, until the tumour can be removed. Large tumours require a two-stage intralesional operation; first the posterior part is removed and then an antero-lateral approach is used to remove the remainder of the tumour. If MRI indicates the possibility of an intradural extension, this should be explored and, if present, resected. If the spine is rendered unstable, reconstruction with posterior instrumentation, postero-lateral and anterior autografting is added (Fig. 8.6). Following intralesional surgery, a cure can be expected in 90% of cases (SMITH and SCHMIDEK 1990). A recurrence can be re-operated. There is no place for chemotherapy or radiotherapy.

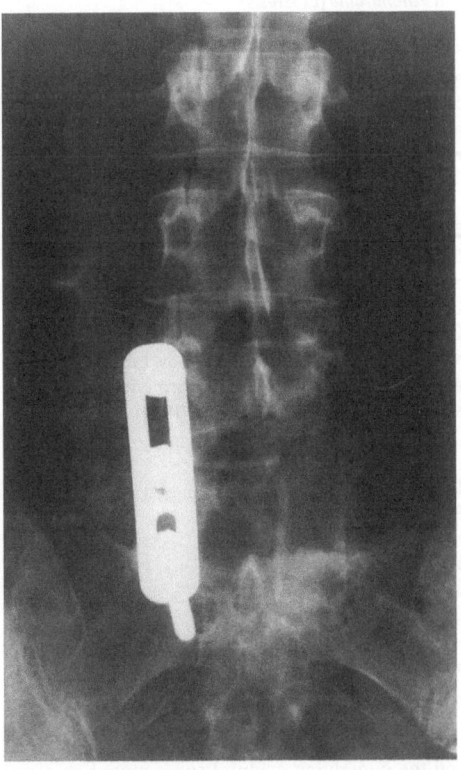

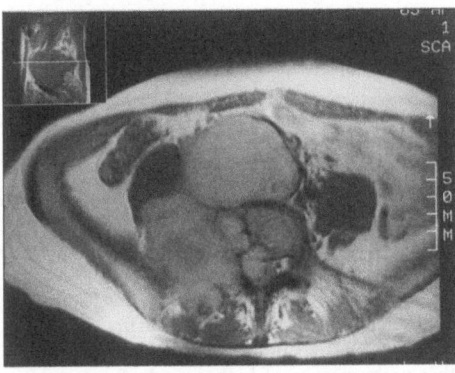

Fig. 8.5. An MRI scan showing a large schwannoma involving the right side of L5. The cauda equina is compressed

Fig. 8.6. An antero-posterior (A–P) radiograph following removal of the schwannoma shown in Fig. 8.5. The defect in the right side of L5 has been bridged with a bone graft from L4 to the sacrum. The instrumentation on the right side was removed at the end of the operation because of the danger of it causing a pressure sore in this thin patient

8.5.1.7
Neurofibromatosis

Occasionally, there is considerable paravertebral involvement with, at some levels, an intraspinal component (dumb-bell tumour) causing cord or cauda equina compression symptoms. Although radical resection is impossible, this type of tumour is treated by a posterior operation to remove the intraspinal component and relieve the neural compression. Via an anterior approach, the paraspinal component is then grossly removed in the hope that there will be less residual tissue which could undergo malignant degeneration.

8.5.1.8
Osteochondroma (Exostosis)

Spinal osteochondromas are uncommon, accounting for some 4% of solitary spinal tumours. Rarely, they cause neurological symptoms due to pressure on neural structures. Complete excision, including the cartilage cap, is curative (ARASIL et al. 1996).

8.5.1.9
Osteoma

Osteomas in the spine are very rare. They can occur from adolescence onward. They usually present with a dull aching pain and there may be symptoms of nerve root compression. Treatment is by total excisional biopsy (PEYSER et al. 1996).

8.5.2
Primary Malignant Tumours

8.5.2.1
Introduction

Any hope of cure requires extralesional and preferably wide resection, if necessary, combined with chemotherapy and radiotherapy. Where such resection means total or almost total vertebrectomy, there are two prerequisites. First, part of the vertebral arch and the underlying epidural space must be normal so that the bony ring around the dura can be broached through healthy tissue to allow the diseased vertebral segment to be rolled away from the dural tube (see Fig. 8.14). Secondly, it must be possible to divide any involved nerve root at its junction

with the dura without overhanging tumour leading to possible contamination of the operation site. The exception is when the lesion occurs in the sacrum, which can be resected at any level though with sacrifice of the appropriate nerve roots. All cases require careful preoperative staging. When curative resection of a malignant primary tumour is technically impossible, the quality of a patient's life may be improved by an intralesional excision, neural decompression and stabilization, as for the treatment of vertebral metastases.

8.5.2.2
Giant Cell Tumour

The giant cell tumour exhibits a wide range of pathological activity, from the very benign to the frankly malignant. Because of its often unpredictable behaviour, it has been included here rather than in the section on benign tumours.

Giant cell tumour (Fig. 8.7) can be considered as a "malignant lesion with a high rate of local recurrence and a low potential for distant metastases" (BENNETT et al. 1993). Giant cell tumours of the spine occur at all ages from the age of 2 years (DAHLIN 1977) onwards, with a peak incidence in young adults; 70% occur in females and 2–10%, in the spine (SIM et al. 1990). Multifocal lesions (PEIMER et al. 1980) are rare and usually involve the appendicular skeleton, though a bifocal lesion in the spine has been treated by the author (Kos et al. 1997). The majority of giant cell tumours of the spine occur in the vertebral body with or without extension into the neural arch. Only 3 of the 24 tumours reported by SANJAY et al. (1993) occurred solely in the neural arch.

Giant cell tumours have been divided histologically into three grades (JAFFE 1958; JAFFE et al. 1940), with grade III being sarcomatous. Although histological grading of the nonsarcomas may give an overall idea as to the behaviour of a tumour, it provides no hard and fast rule about the behaviour of an individual tumour, neither regarding the risk of recurrence after intralesional excision nor its propensity to metastasize (JAFFE 1958). Furthermore, a biopsy specimen may indicate grade I tumour whereas other parts may be of higher grade. Because of its unpredictable behaviour JAFFE, in 1953, had already called the tumour a "rather treacherous lesion". In 1970, GOLDENBERG et al. concluded that constant prediction of the eventual outcome of treatment was not possible on the basis of the histological grading

Fig. 8.7. An MRI view of a giant cell tumour involving the body and the right pedicle of T12

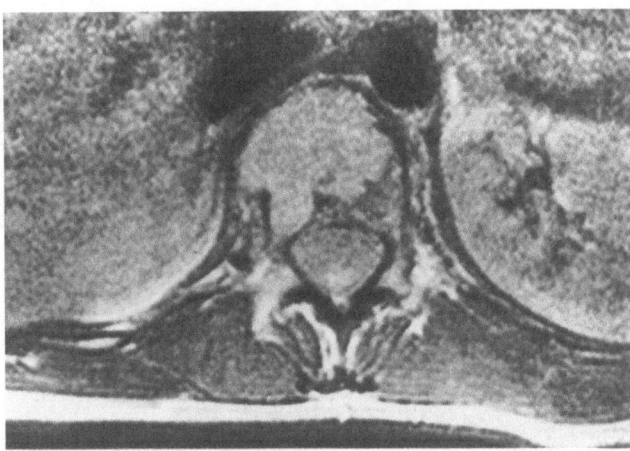

and this was reiterated in 1990 by Campanacci et al. and in 1994 by SCHAJOWICZ (1994, pp. 288–289), who wrote "grading is without practical value".

Any local recurrence following intralesional excision usually occurs within 2 years (GOLDENBERG et al. 1970), though a recurrence in the tibia after 30 years has been recorded (SCULLY et al. 1994).

Metastases are usually restricted to the lung (JAFFE 1958; BERTONI et al. 1988; ROCK et al. 1984; VANEL et al. 1983). They occur in 2% of cases and can occur up to 10 years following removal of the primary tumour (Rock et al. 1984). Pulmonary metastases should be resected whenever technically possible. Metastases to other bones have been reported by WRAY et al. (1990), who also reviewed the preceding literature. Even widespread metastases can occur (JAFFE 1958).

Because of their location, spinal giant cell tumours are often treated by intralesional surgery even though this is associated with a high recurrence rate: 10 of 21 vertebral body tumours described by SANJAY et al. (1993) and 5 of 6 described by SCHRIJVER (1982) in a review of the cases collected by the Dutch bone tumour committee, recurred. Techniques used in limbs to reduce the recurrence rate following intralesional curettage, such as cryotherapy, phenolization and cementation are unattractive in the spine. Recurrences following intralesional surgery of giant cell tumours in the limbs are amenable to re-operation, even amputation is possible. An operation for a recurrent vertebral body tumour is less effective. It is usually far more difficult than the primary operation, with an associated increased risk to neighbouring important

structures, in particular neural structures and the great vessels. For these reasons and because of the unpredictability of individual tumours, the treatment of choice for a vertebral giant cell tumour is an "en bloc" extracapsular resection (FIDLER 1996). This is the most certain method of ensuring the complete excision recommended by SANJAY et al. (1993).

If an en bloc extra-lesional resection would entail life-threatening risk or cause a serious neurological lesion, then the second choice is a complete intralesional excision with any doubtful margin subjected to frozen section analysis and, if positive, immediate resection. If an intralesional excision would clearly be incomplete (Fig. 8.8), then radiotherapy should be considered as described below.

En bloc extralesional resection of a giant cell tumour in the thoracic and lumbar spine often involves sacrifice of one or more segmental nerves, often bilaterally. Except for T1 and perhaps L5 this is, relatively, of little consequence. At the level of the sacrum, bilateral sacrifice of the S2–4 nerves paralyses the sphincters. Unilateral preservation of these nerves maintains the sphincter function and makes a tremendous difference to the patient's subsequent quality of life. The problem is what to do with a large tumour which involves these roots bilaterally (Fig. 8.9). High amputation or even resection of the sacrum with proximal ligation of the dural sac is technically possible (STENER and GUNTERBERG 1978; SUNG et al. 1987; WUISMAN et al. 1989; SHIKATA et al. 1988), but the nerves to the sphincters are destroyed. This should be recommended as the primary treatment for a sarcoma, but probably not for

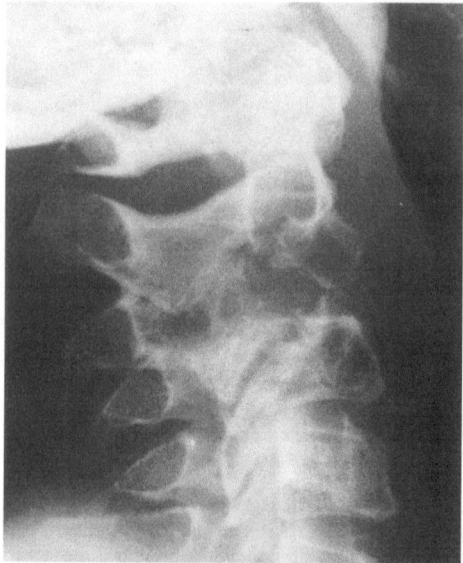

a

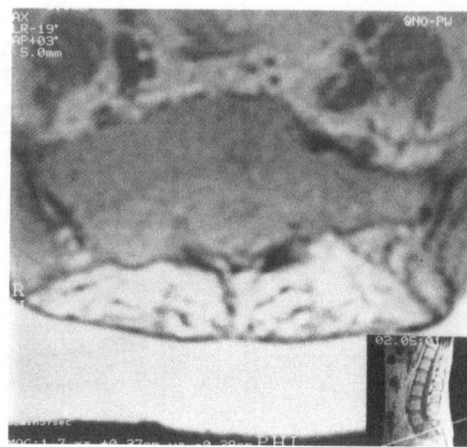

Fig. 8.9. An MRI view of a giant cell tumour which has replaced virtually all of the vertebrae S1 and S2

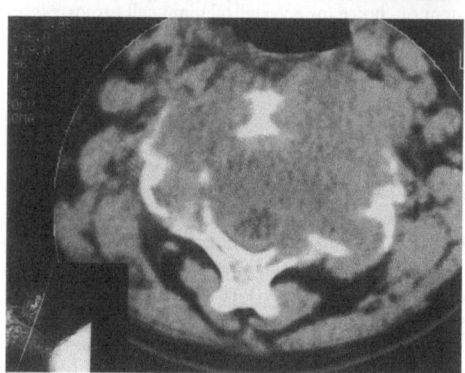

b

Fig. 8.8. A lateral radiograph (a) and CT image (b) of an inoperable giant cell tumour of C2. (By courtesy of Dr. M. Coppes)

the grade I and II tumours. Despite the unpredictability of "non-sarcomatous" giant cell tumours on the basis of their histological grading, it seems reasonable to subject these sacral tumours to a meticulous intralesional excision, with preservation of the nerve roots followed by reconstruction of the vertebrae L4 and L5 to the pelvis (Fig. 8.10). Such excisions are time consuming, involving several operations and multiple frozen sections before the margin is clear. If such an intralesional excision fails, then radiotherapy or a block resection of the recurrence is still possible.

Radiotherapy, at least until recently, has had a poor reputation. It has been successful in only one third of cases and 10% of patients subsequently developed radiation sarcoma (GOLDENBERG et al. 1970; SAVINI et al. 1983; ROCK et al. 1984). However, the recent experience of BENNETT et al. (1993) is less pessimistic. Only one of seven spinal lesions, including the sacrum, recurred following radiotherapy and, in this case, it could still be successfully resected. One patient developed pulmonary metastases. At 2–18 years following radiotherapy there were no post-radiation sarcomas. This is probably due to the use of modern radiation techniques, but the authors point out that "further follow-up is needed to address this issue fully".

When performing an operation, there is no place for "having a go" and relying on post-operative radiotherapy as an excuse for poor pre-operative planning followed by incomplete and impatient surgery. However, if one genuinely does run into trouble then needless risks should not be taken. Radiotherapy may still cure the lesion or, in combination with embolization, reduce it to an operable size (BIAGINI et al. 1990).

In summary, it would seem that, for vertebral giant cell tumours, extralesional en bloc resection is the procedure of choice, with complete and often painstaking intralesional excision as the second choice. Where it is obvious that a total excision will be technically impossible or highly likely to be dangerous or cause unacceptable post-operative morbidity, then modern radiotherapy, as described above, seems preferable. If this fails, then the possibility of surgery should again be assessed. In particular, wide resection of a sacral tumour should still be possible.

8.5.2.3
Osteosarcoma

Osteosarcoma occurs typically between 10 and 30 years of age and is somewhat more common in males (Fig. 8.11). As with lesions in the limbs, a wide (or marginal) resection should be combined with pre-operative and post-operative chemotherapy. At present, the surgical treatment of these lesions is in an early stage of development and no hard and fast rules are available. However, the early results with regard to the local resection of a primary tumour or "solitary" metastasis are encouraging (FIDLER 1994; KRAJBICH and ELDRIGE 1991). Because of the limited resection margin in the spine, even following an extralesional en bloc resection post-operative radiotherapy is advisable. Radiotherapy is also advisable following intralesional surgery (SUNDARESAN et al. 1988) or if surgery proves impossible (SHIVES et al. 1986). Any pulmonary metastases should be excised if possible.

8.5.2.4
Chondrosarcoma

This is primarily a tumour of adulthood, especially between 30 and 70 years of age, and is somewhat more common in males. Extralesional and preferably wide resection is necessary. Chondrosarcomas are unresponsive to chemotherapy. The role of radiotherapy is controversial (SHIVES et al. 1989). If extralesional resection is not possible (Fig. 8.12), then intralesional excision should be complete – with the remaining margins checked by multiple biopsies. The whole field is then irradiated to try and eliminate any residual microscopic tumour tissue. At present, this use of supplementary radiotherapy must be considered experimental. Another possibly promising line of treatment is the use of proton beam therapy (HUG et al. 1995).

8.5.2.5
Chordoma

Chordoma (Fig. 8.13) is a tumour of middle and old age. Occurrence before 25 years of age is exceptional (CAMPANACCI 1990, pp. 639–640). It is more common in males. Extralesional and preferably wide re-

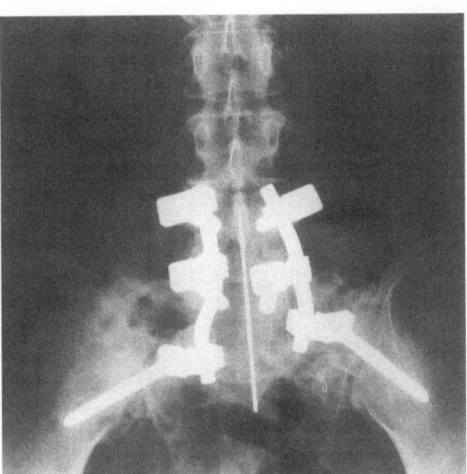

Fig. 8.10. An A–P radiograph showing the reconstruction of L4 and L5 to the iliac wings following intra-lesional excision of the giant cell tumour shown in Fig. 8.9. Multiple frozen section biopsies were necessary before the margins were free of tumour

section is the only established curative treatment (SUNDARESAN 1986; BORIANI et al. 1996a). Failing this, combined proton and photon radiation therapy may lead to considerable palliation and tumour regression (HUG et al. 1995).

8.5.2.6
Ewing's Sarcoma

Primary Ewing sarcoma occurs infrequently in the spine though metastasis to the spine is a common preterminal event. The vast majority of these tumours occurs between 5 and 25 years of age, with a male:female ratio of 2:1. So far, treatment has centred on radiation and chemotherapy, sometimes in association with decompressive laminectomy (GRUBB et al. 1994). The author has no personal experience of a curative resection but, on the basis of lesions in the limbs, would opt for wide (or marginal) resection in combination with pre- and post-operative radiotherapy/chemotherapy, according to the most recent guidelines suggested by the European Intergroup Cooperative Ewing's Sarcoma Study. One incurable lesion following chemotherapy and radiotherapy was treated by intralesional decompression and stabilization, but this provided only temporary neurological improvement and pain relief.

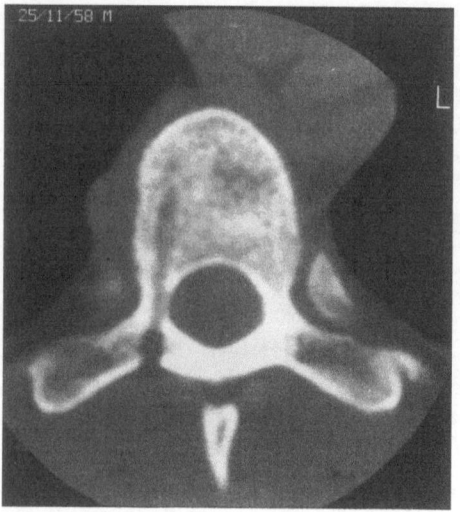

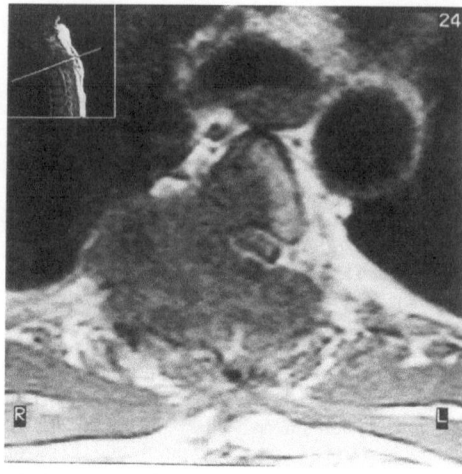

Fig. 8.11. A CT scan of an osteosarcoma in the right side of the body of T7. The open biopsy track is visible. Note the soft tissue extension

Fig. 8.12. Chondrosarcoma of T4, almost encircling and compressing the spinal cord. Only an intralesional excision was possible

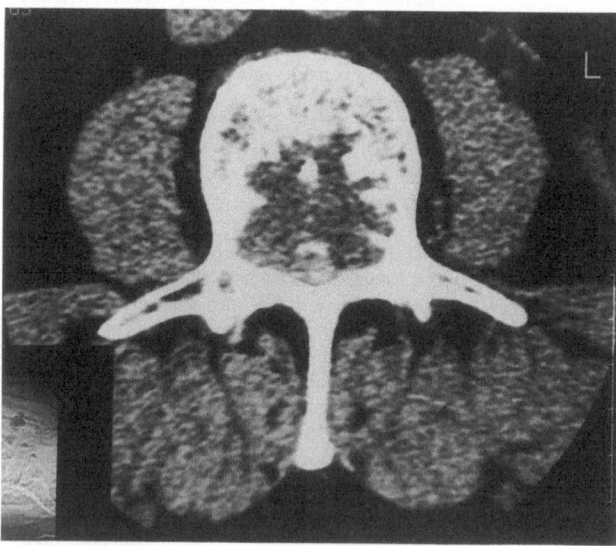

Fig. 8.13. A CT scan of a chordoma of L3

8.5.2.7
Angiosarcoma

Angiosarcoma is rare. If localized, it may be resectable by the technique presently described. If curative resection is not possible, then intractable pain or neurological compression should be treated by the technique described for metastases.

8.6
Surgical Techniques

8.6.1
Curative Resection

8.6.1.1
Thoracic and Lumbar Spines

En bloc resection of a vertebral body tumour by a purely posterior approach has been described by STENER and JOHNSEN (1971), STENER (1971, 1989), ROY-CAMILLE et al. (1981) and TOMITA et al. (1994). The vascular anatomy essential for this procedure has been recently highlighted by KAWAHARA et al. (1996). The author's combined posterior and anterior technique for the en bloc resection of a thoracic or lumbar vertebral body tumour with or without partial involvement of the neural arch is summarized below. A full account of this technique along with the appropriate references is given elsewhere (FIDLER 1994). En bloc resection in association with a surgical staging system has recently been reported by BORIANI et al. (1996b).

Assuming that the tumour resection is curative, the patient will have a normal life expectation. Thus, any reconstruction must rely on the incorporation of bone grafts for long-term stability. Internal fixation is necessary while the bone heals.

8.6.1.1.1
Pre-operative Planning

The basic idea is to remove a segment of healthy neural arch so that, after mobilization, the tumour can be rolled out in an antero-lateral direction away from the dural tube (see also Sect. 8.5.2.1).

The spine is approached posteriorly, as well as from both sides. It is easier to mobilize the aorta and divide segmental vessels from the left side and so, if possible, the left side is chosen for the more major approach and removal of the tumour. If the tumour is predominantly right-sided, or if a large left-sided tumour prevents mobilization of the aorta from this side, the operation is modified accordingly.

Schematic diagrams (Fig. 8.14) based on the radiographs and scans are drawn, and the sites of division of the vertebral arch and the vertebral column are marked. Any bone or soft tissue which MRI shows to be involved is included in the resection.

8.6.1.1.2
The Operation

In stage 1, the patient is positioned prone so as to allow biplanar image intensification. Via a midline incision, the spine is exposed out to the tips of the transverse processes. Any biopsy or previous operation scar is excised and the edges examined by frozen section. A healthy part of the neural arch is removed, the dural tube is mobilized, involved nerve roots are ligated and divided and the postero-lateral parts of the spinal osteotomies or disc divisions are carried out. On one side, usually the right, through the midline incision or through an accessory oblique incision (Fig. 8.15), a relatively minor operation suffices to free the side of the vertebral body and to extend the osteo-

Fig. 8.14a-c. The planned resection of a predominantly left-sided tumour: the laminae are initially removed along *dashed lines "1"*; the uninvolved transverse process and posterior part of the pedicle are removed up to *dashed line "2"*. B is the site of a previous open transpedicular biopsy, D is the involved vertebra. (Reproduced by kind permission of the editor of the *Journal of Bone and Joint Surgery*; 76B, 1994)

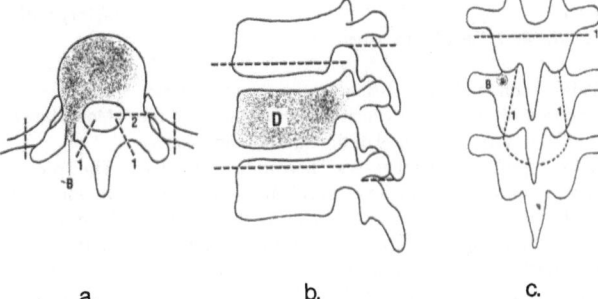

a.   b.   c.

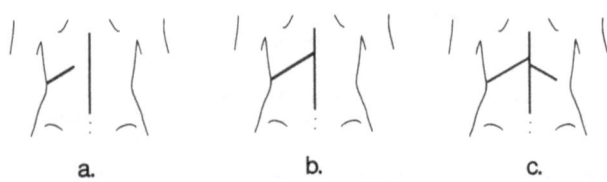

a.   b.   c.

Fig. 8.15a-c. Skin incisions for radical removal of a spinal tumour. **a** Suitable for a thin patient; the view of the tumour during the second stage is impaired by the musculo-cutaneous bridge, but wound closure is easy. **b** The usual incision. **c** Applicable when extra exposure is required. (Reproduced by kind permission of the editor of the *Journal of Bone and Joint Surgery*; 76B, 1994)

tomies or disc divisions. The holes for the pedicle screws are made and tapped. On the side of the minor postero-lateral operation (usually the right) the screws are inserted and the Steffee plate is applied. On the other side, the screw holes are marked with short pieces of catheter for easy identification during the second stage, or screws with short machine threads are inserted (long threads would impede skin closure). The posterior wound is closed.

For stage 2 of the operation, performed either immediately or following an overnight stay in the intensive care unit, the patient is placed in the lateral position. The posterior wound is re-opened. Through a postero-lateral thoracotomy or a lumbotomy, the dissection and osteotomies or disc divisions are completed and the specimen is rolled away from the dura in an antero-lateral direction and removed. Slight loosening of the Steffee nuts facilitates this process.

For reconstruction, the second Steffee plate is applied. Shallow transverse grooves are made in the neighbouring healthy vertebral bodies and a three-cortex iliac crest graft, preferably with its blood supply, is clamped in place as the Steffee system is tightened. The graft vascular anastomosis then completed. Additional cancellous bone graft is added anteriorly as well as postero-laterally on both sides and the wound is closed (Fig. 8.16). The metal is usually removed after the bone grafts have fully consolidated.

8.6.1.2
Curative Resection of the Sacrum

This is achieved by a two-stage anterior and posterior resection of the sacrum which involves ligation of the dural sac at the upper level of the tumour and sacrifice of the appropriate sacral nerves. Thereafter, the lumbar spine is allowed to settle down between the two wings of the ilium, with the formation of a stable fibrous union (SUNG et al. 1987), or the lumbo-pelvic junction is reconstructed with the aid of various metal implants and bone grafts (SHIKATA et al. 1988).

For more caudal tumours, a high amputation of the sacrum rather than a total resection may be possible (STENER and GUNTERBERG 1978; WUISMAN et al. 1989). Preservation of even a half of the S1 vertebra maintains sufficient pelvic girdle strength to permit early post-operative standing (STENER and GUNTERBERG 1978).

The technique for the curative intralesional removal of a low-grade giant cell tumour with preservation of the sacral nerves and reconstruction has already been mentioned (Sect. 8.5.2.2).

8.6.1.3
Cervical Spine

Curative resection of tumours in the cervical spine has personally so far been limited to the intralesional resection of aggressive benign tumours such as aneurysmal bone cysts and haemangiomas. Although the spine can be approached anteriorly and posteriorly, there is much less room for manoeuvre than in the thoracic or lumbar regions, and furthermore the vertebral arteries can cause additional problems. The vessel can be temporarily occluded, mobilized, reconstructed or bypassed (SEN et al. 1995; GEORGE 1995). One vertebral artery can be sacrificed provided that there is a good contralateral flow and a good flow through the circle of Willis. The effect of ligation of a vertebral artery can be estimated pre-operatively by temporarily occluding the artery with a balloon catheter.

8.6.2
Metastases

The spine, especially the lumbar and lower thoracic regions, is the most common site for skeletal metastases (GALASKO 1986; ALGRA 1992, p. 121). The vertebral body is affected seven times more often than the posterior elements (Fig. 8.17). Treatment of spinal metastases (Fig. 8.18) is directed at relieving

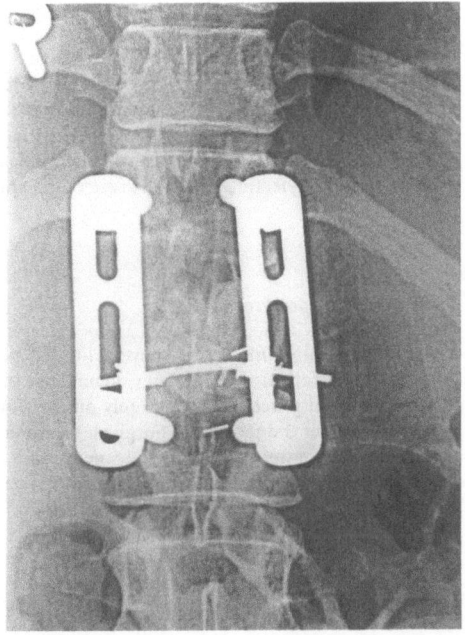
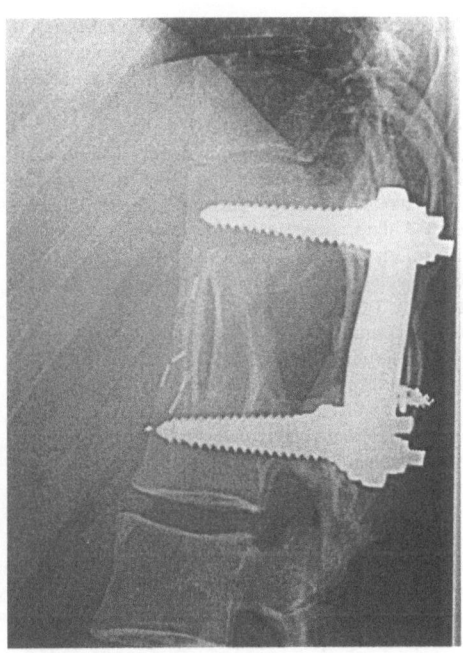

a   b

Fig. 8.16. A–P (a) and lateral (b) radiographs following resection of the giant cell tumour shown in Fig. 8.7. The transverse K wire stabilizes the replaced (uninvolved) laminae of T12 (the patient has 11 ribs)

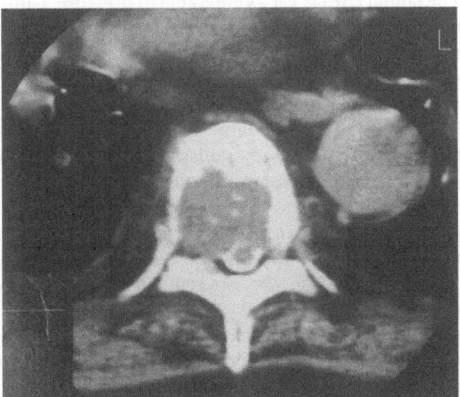

Fig. 8.17. A CT image showing a metastasis in the vertebral body

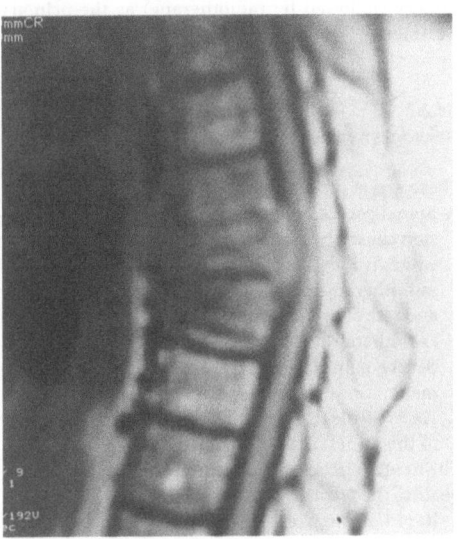

Fig. 8.18. An MRI view showing partial collapse of the vertebral body due to metastasis, with retropulsion of tumour tissue and involved bone causing anterior compression of the spinal cord

pain, restoring or preserving neurological function and stabilizing the spine so that the patients can return home as comfortable and as soon as possible.

The role of corticosteroids in the management of cord compression is discussed in Chap.   . In general, patients presenting with cord compression receive an intravenous (i.v.) bolus of 10–16 mg dexamethasone followed by 4 mg four times daily orally for 3–7 days, after which the dose is tapered off (BOOGERD and VAN DER SANDE 1993), though high doses such as an i.v. bolus of 30 mg dexamethasone daily for 3 days followed by tapering off have also been recommended (T. SIEGAL and T. SIEGAL, personal communication). The stomach is protected with ranitidine (Zantac), 150 mg twice daily.

Some metastases, notably lymphoma, seminoma and myeloma, are particularly radiosensitive or sensitive to chemotherapy. Unless there is a severe neurological or mechanical lesion, non-operative treatment should be the primary treatment for these sensitive tumours.

Moderately radiosensitive tumours, such as those arising from the breast or prostate, usually receive radiotherapy. If this fails, the patients are then referred for surgery, with the inevitable loss of valuable time. If one could predict the effectiveness of radiotherapy in the individual case, then one could choose, without delay, between radiotherapy and surgery (followed by radiotherapy) as the primary treatment.

8.6.2.1
Indications for Operation

These are, at present:
1. Spinal cord, cauda equina or nerve root compression caused by a bone or disc fragment; by tumour which is radioresistant; after a maximum dose of radiotherapy has been given; or where the severity and rate of progression of a cord lesion is such that radiotherapy cannot be expected to be successful.
2. Severe pain despite adequate conservative treatment.
3. An unstable fracture which threatens the integrity of the spinal cord or cauda equina.
The neighbouring vertebrae must be capable of supporting the reconstruction.

Rapid, uncontrollable progression of the disease is a contra-indication to surgery. Solitary metastases related to a treatable osteosarcoma or lesion in the thyroid and kidney should be curatively resected whenever technically possible.

8.6.2.1.1
PROPHYLACTIC SURGERY

At present there is no reliable indication of which metastasis will fracture and, even more importantly, which fracture will produce severe persistent pain or neurological damage. There is thus no indication, at present, for prophylactic palliative surgery for a spinal metastasis.

8.6.2.2
The Aim of the Surgical Procedure

Patients with spinal metastases have a limited life expectancy (TATSUI et al. 1996). They do not have the time for surgical procedures which rely on the slow incorporation of bone grafts. Surgical treatment should restore or maintain adequate neurological function, relieve pain and ensure immediate and permanent spinal stability.

8.6.2.3
Basic Principles

8.6.2.3.1
DECOMPRESSION

The spinal cord is very vulnerable to pressure. Laminectomy for anterior spinal cord compression requires dural and cord retraction and almost always results in neurological deterioration (BLACK 1979; MEIJER 1977); it should be avoided. It also further jeopardizes spinal stability, especially in the presence of vertebral body collapse (FINDLAY 1987). Anterior decompression for anterior cord or cauda equina compression has now become firmly established when conservative treatment is not possible (SIEGAL and SIEGAL 1985; FIDLER 1986a; HARRINGTON 1986; MANABE et al. 1989; SUNDARESAN et al. 1991; COOPER et al. 1993). Anterior decompression is achieved by vertebral body resection, the aim being to remove all visible tumour and involved bone rather than simply to achieve neural decompression. Thereafter anterior stabilization is both biomechanically correct and convenient. Posterior or postero-lateral decompression is, personally, reserved for those uncommon cases of posterior, postero-lateral or lateral cord compression.

A wide posterior approach, giving better access than a laminectomy can be used for "all-round" decompression. (Posterior approaches are also referred to in Sect. 8.6.2.4.5 and 8.6.2.4.6).

8.6.2.3.2
STABILIZATION

For biomechanical reasons, the part of the spinal column which has failed should be restored (WHITE
and PANJABI 1990, p. 540). In particular, vertebral
body collapse should be treated by anterior reconstruction. [In this section *anterior* includes the *anterior* and the *middle* columns of DENIS (1983).]
Anterior Stabilization: Any form of spinal stabilization must take account of forces and possible movements in all six degrees of freedom. The most important are *flexion* and *compression* because the body's
centre of gravity lies anterior to the spine in the upright position. Compressive loads are transmitted
primarily by the vertebral body; both the cortical
shell and the end plates with the underlying cancellous core are important (WHITE and PANJABI 1990,
pp. 31–43).

Figure 8.19 illustrates how the anterior edge is
particularly important. Following destruction or removal of the vertebral body, the spine collapses into
kyphosis, pivoting about the still intact posterior elements. The kyphosis can be corrected by an upwards force F, which is most advantageously applied
at the anterior edge of the vertebral body. Fortunately, this anterior cortex is also the strongest part
of the cortical shell (MA et al. 1987).

Following insertion of a vertebral body prosthesis, the spine now tends to flex over a fulcrum (Fig.
8.19) created by the anterior edge of the prosthesis.
Any counterbalancing moment will be F' x B. To
achieve the maximum mechanical advantage, the
distance B must be as long as possible. Routine supplementary posterior instrumentation embodies
this principle but either necessitates an additional
posterior operation as described by HARMS (1992)
or an extensive posterior approach through which
the diseased vertebral body is also removed and replaced (STEFFEE et al. 1986; MAGERL and COSCIA
1988).

Similar calculations or mechanical investigations
and recommendations can be made for movements
in other directions. For example, following corporec-
tomy, rotation is also effectively resisted by the combination of an interbody spacer with an anterior
paravertebral rod and bone cement (FIDLER 1986b)
or, better still, the incorporation of a Kaneda device
(GURR et al. 1988). In the author's experience, except
at L4 and L5 (see Sect. 8.6.2.4.3), a supplementary
anterior paravertebral device has usually provided
sufficient mechanical fixation in the thoracic and
lumbar spine though, very occasionally, supplemen-

tary posterior instrumentation is necessary (see below). In certain circumstances (see Sect. 8.6.2.3.3),
posterior fusion is added for long-term security.

Vertebral body "prostheses" have been constructed
from metal, ceramic, high-density polyethylene and
hydroxyapatite (POLSTER and BRINCKMANN 1977;
FIDLER 1986a; MA et al. 1987; ONO et al. 1988; MOORE
and UTTLEY 1989; KANEDA 1991; HARMS 1992; MATSUI
et al. 1994; HOSONO et al. 1995).

Posterior Stabilization: Posterior stabilization alone
in the presence of anterior spinal destruction is an
unsound concept for resisting flexion/compression
forces (CUNNINGHAM et al. 1993). Long lever arms
and high moments will inevitably lead to failure of a
pedicle screw/plate implant when used in a "one
above to one below" configuration, though the risk
can be reduced by instrumenting multiple levels to
spread the loads. Laminar wiring or claw techniques
require fixation of two healthy vertebrae above and
below the diseased segment. Posterior stabilization
by means of pedicle screw/plate combinations
(GURR et al. 1988) or posterior rectangles/laminar
wires (FIDLER 1986c) is particularly effective in con-
trolling rotation, as well as, in varying degrees,
movements in the other directions. Despite the
biomechanical disadvantages with regard to flexion/
compression, there are circumstances where posterior stabilization alone is indicated and these will be
described in the following sections.

Posterior instrumentation to supplement anterior
stabilization is excellent biomechanically as described above. It is indicated if there is any doubt
about the efficacy of the anterior stabilization, particularly in large patients following resection of
three or more vertebrae or in the presence of osteo-

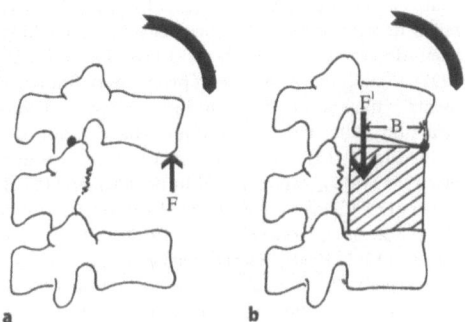

Fig. 8.19. The situation following (a) destruction and/or resection of a vertebral body and (b) the insertion of a vertebral body
prosthesis (see Sect. 8.6.2.3.2)

porosis. It is used routinely during reconstruction at L5 and frequently at L4 as described below (Sect. 8.6.2.4.3).

8.6.2.3.3
SUPPLEMENTARY POSTERIOR SPINAL FUSION

Rigid, stable fixation is essential for immediate relief of pain and early mobilization. However, as patients survive longer with better methods of treating their underlying tumours, so must the durability of spinal stabilization techniques improve. Where the prognosis is more than 1–2 years, posterior or postero-lateral spinal fusion is added for long-term security in the following situations:

1. Cervical spine and T1, or below T9, following replacement of two or more vertebral bodies
2. T2–T9, where the ribs add some measure of stability, following replacement of three or more vertebral bodies.

The availability of tumour-free autograft is assessed from the bone scan. If no such graft is available, homograft or irradiated autograft may be used, though with less certainty of success. Bone grafts are usually added after chemotherapy or radiotherapy, otherwise these treatments should be postponed for about 6 weeks. This is in keeping with the recent experimental work of EMERY et al. (1994) on the effect of irradiation on bone grafts.

8.6.2.4
Surgical Techniques for Metastases at Various Spinal Levels

The following techniques are those currently used by the author and have been developed during the course of 154 operations for spinal metastases. Detailed descriptions of the surgical techniques have been described previously (FIDLER 1985, 1986a, 1991), though there have been progressive improvements with regard to the techniques of spinal reconstruction. Alternative techniques have been described by: SALZER et al. (1973), VLAHOVITCH and FUENTÉS (1975), POLSTER and BRINCKMANN (1977), PRIVAT (1980), ROY-CAMILLE et al. (1981), CLARK et al. (1984), SUNDARESAN et al. (1985), SIEGAL and SIEGAL (1985, 1990), HARRINGTON (1986), ONIMUS et al. (1986) , STEFFEE et al. (1986) MA et al. (1987), KOSTUIK et al. (1988), MAGERL and COSCIA (1988), ONO et al. (1988), TURNER et al. (1988), MANABE et al. (1989), MOORE and UTTLEY (1989), CYBULSKI (1989), GALASKO (1991), KANEDA (1991), LAPRESLE

et al. (1991), HARMS (1992), HERTLEIN et al. (1992), COOPER et al. (1993), MATSUI et al. (1994), MALCOLM et al. (1994), MCAFEE et al. (1995), OLERUD and JÓNSSON (1996). Thoracoscopic techniques are now being developed (REGAN et al. 1995).

8.6.2.4.1
CERVICAL SPINE

The cervical spine may be approached anteriorly or posteriorly at any level for appropriate neural *decompression*. The direction will influence the choice of stabilization procedure, except where the transoral approach (FANG and ONG 1962; CROCKARD and RANSFORD 1991) is used for anterior cord decompression; the danger of infection makes this approach unsuitable for insertion of a permanent implant.

Stabilization: Although, as previously described, anterior reconstruction is biomechanically the most effective method for counteracting the important flexion and compression forces, in the cervical spine this is not always desirable or necessary. The flexion/compression forces are less than in the thoracic or, particularly, the lumbar spine, and control of rotation and translation is particularly important.

For *lesions involving the atlas or axis*, the occiput must be included and a special plate has been developed (Fig. 8.20). This is fixed to the thick part of the occiput with four screws and to the cervical spine with double laminar wires. Low-viscosity bone cement impregnated with gentamycin is added as a grout on both sides, or on one side if bone graft is to be added on the other. (The cement when used as a grout between bone and metal, is subjected to compression.)

For lesions at C3 and below, anterior reconstruction is the technique of choice after one or two vertebral bodies have been resected (Fig. 8.21). Posterior stabilization with a rectangle, laminar wires and cement, as a grout, is preferred when three or more vertebrae are involved as this probably provides better torsional stability, though at the expense of sacrificing an extra two motion segments (Fig. 8.22).

8.6.2.4.2
CERVICO-THORACIC JUNCTION

If anterior resection down to and including the body of T2 is required, the approach described by BIRCH et al. (1990) provides a good and safe exposure.

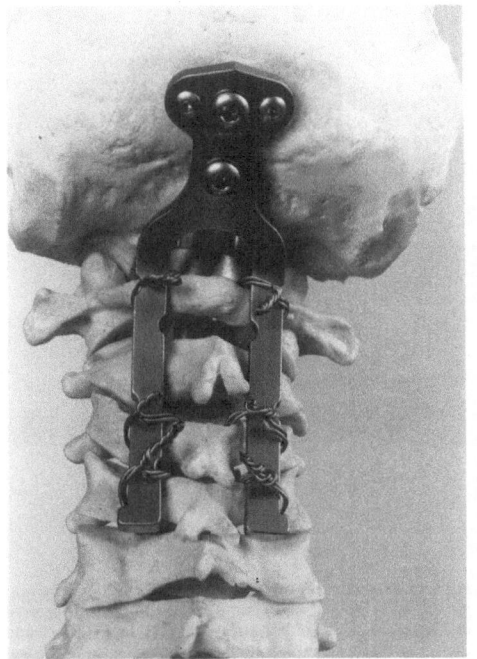

Fig. 8.20. The plate for occipito-cervical stabilization

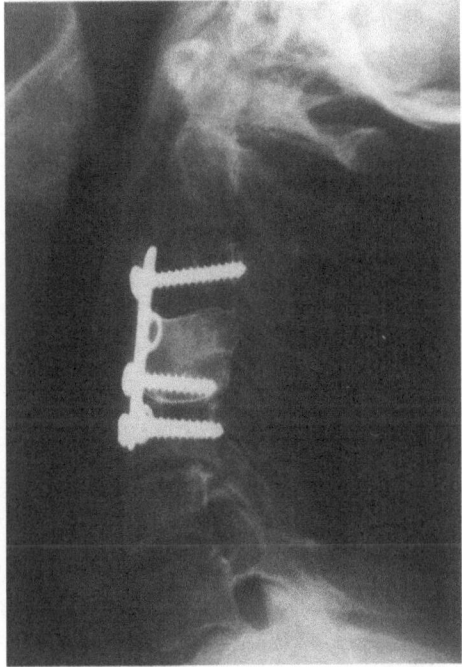

Fig. 8.21. Anterior reconstruction following resection of the severely involved vertebral body of C4

Other useful approaches have been described by AN et al. (1994) and DARLING et al. (1995). Anterior stabilization at this level is vulnerable as it bridges the well-supported thoracic spine and the highly mobile cervical spine. If there is any doubt about the quality of anterior reconstruction, posterior instrumentation (as in Fig. 8.22) or fusion should be added.

8.6.2.4.3
THORACIC AND LUMBAR SPINE

The spine may be approached from either side depending on the side of maximum cord compression, vertebral body destruction or the presence of important medullary feeder arteries. In general the left side is preferable so that the segmental arteries which supply the diseased vertebral bodies can be easily identified and ligated as they arise from the aorta. However, above T9, if the paravertebral device would press against the aorta, a right-side approach is chosen. The blood supply to the spinal cord (DOMMISSE 1980) must be safeguarded as well as possible.

Decompression: The diseased vertebral bodies and the neighbouring discs are removed except for a thin osteo-periosteal shell anteriorly and on the contralateral side. The posterior longitudinal ligament is removed partially or completely to ensure that no epidural tumour remains to cause compression.

Stabilization: Since the model first described (FIDLER 1986a), the interbody tumour jack has been gradually improved to facilitate its insertion. The present adjustable titanium tumour jack, in conjunction with cement and an adjustable paravertebral device, is used to replace one to four vertebral bodies. The construction resists movement in all six degrees of freedom and is particularly effective against the important flexion/compression forces (Figs. 8.23, 8.24). The anterior lips of the tumour jack's support plates ensure support of the important anterior edges of the vertebral bodies above and below. The addition of bone cement reinforces the telescopic connector, prevents the pegs from backing out and supports those parts of the vertebral end plates not directly supported by the tumour jack support

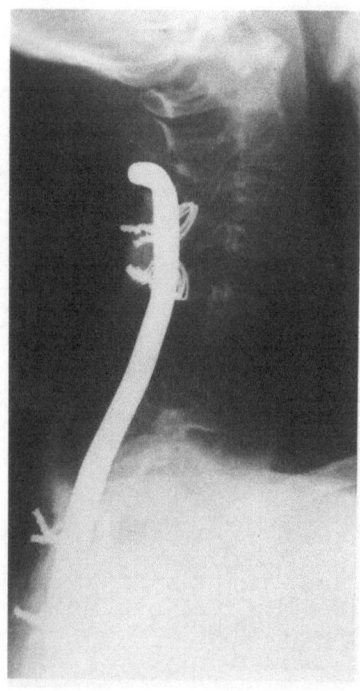

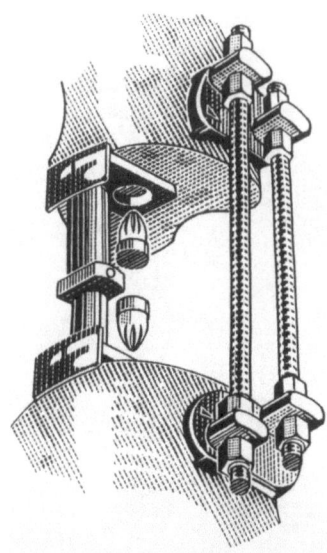

Fig. 8.23. Following resection of one or more vertebral bodies, the tumour jack is inserted and distracted. The studs prevent displacement. Addition of a paravertebral Kaneda device and then bone cement completes the reconstruction. Cross-bridges between the Kaneda rods are not necessary as the bone cement provides an effective substitute. (Reproduced from the *Tumour Jack Technique Manual* by kind permission of Acromed)

Fig. 8.22. Posterior stabilization of three severely involved vertebrae (C6, C7, T1)

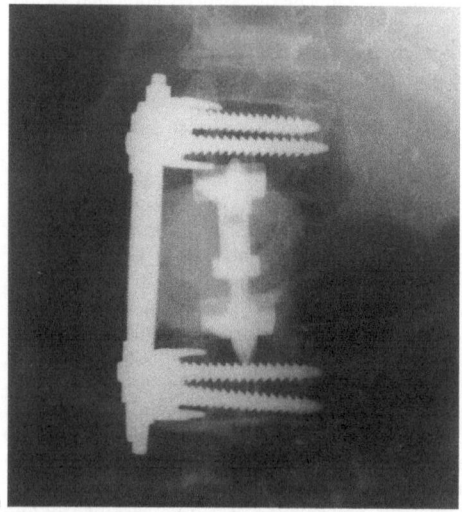

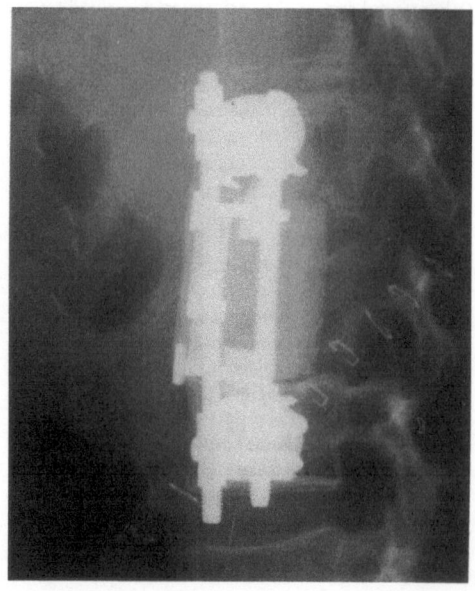

Fig. 8.24. A–P (a) and lateral (b) radiographs: stabilization following resection of the vertebral body of L2

plates. It also unites the tumour jack and paravertebral device. The central pegs, in combination with the paravertebral device, resist translation and rotation.

Any spinal malalignment can be corrected by adjusting the jack/paravertebral device combination prior to the addition of bone cement.

In the upper thoracic spine, where the forces are less and the vertebral bodies smaller, a single paravertebral rod is sufficient. Also, if the tumour jack is too large, it is omitted though the central studs are used to anchor the cement, which must reach the anterior edges of the vertebral bodies. An interbody Moss cage (HARMS 1992) is a possible alternative.

At L4, and especially at L5 where a supplementary paravertebral device might damage the iliac vessels, posterior pedicle screw/plate instrumentation is added instead (Fig. 8.25).

8.6.2.4.4
SACRUM

Destruction of the upper part of the sacrum is difficult to stablize. One can improvise using sacral bars, iliac wing screws, pedicle screws and contoured Isola rods. Secondary bone grafting is indicated if the tumour can be controlled in a patient with a reasonable life expectancy.

8.6.2.4.5
POSTERIOR AND POSTERO-LATERAL DECOMPRESSION/STABILIZATION OF THE THORACIC AND LUMBAR SPINE

When the MRI shows that cord or cauda equina compression is purely posterior or lateral, with involvement of the laminae, then decompression by laminectomy-facetectomy-(pedicle-ectomy) is indicated. If necessary, one or more thoracic nerve roots (except T1) may be ligatured or clipped and divided to aid gentle mobilization of the dura during removal of lateral epidural tumour.

The spine is stabilized with a pedicle screw/claw hook/laminar wire/plate/rod construction depending on the level: pedicle screws below the mid-thoracic level and hooks/wires above.

Occasionally, when the laminae are uninvolved and epidural tumour is causing compression, the laminae can be removed intact using a saw and an osteotome and, after removal of the epidural tumour, replaced (FIDLER and BONGARTZ 1988).

8.6.4.2.6
POSTERIOR APPROACH FOR (ANTERIOR) DECOMPRESSION AND POSTERIOR STABILIZATION OF THE THORACIC AND LUMBAR SPINE

A wide posterior approach for decompression, including anterior decompression, and posterior instrumentation is favoured by ROY-CAMILLE et al. (1981), STEFFEE et al. (1986), MAGERL and COSCIA (1988), PERRIN and McBROOM (1990), GALASKO (1991) and JÓNSSON et al. (1996) though STEFFEE et al. and MAGERL and COSCIA add interbody stabilization to the posterior instrumentation. Unless pre-operative embolization has been effective, there is always a danger of uncontrollable bleeding when performing anterior tumour resection from a posterior approach.

Although anterior decompression for anterior compression is more logical and anterior stabilization is mechanically superior, the posterior approach has a special appeal in the treatment of patients whose poor general condition or prognosis

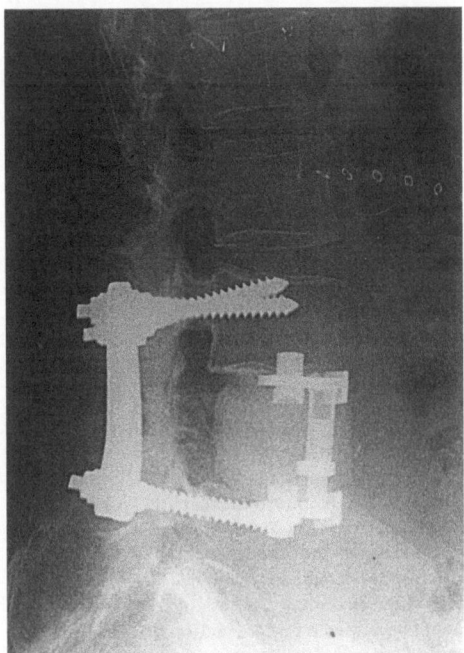

Fig. 8.25. A lateral radiograph: anterior stabilization and supplementary posterior stabilization following resection of the body of L4

weighs against the usual advantages of an anterior procedure. This is particularly true when treating metastases in the upper thoracic spine where the anterior approach is more difficult and time consuming. A large anterior, irresectable tumour mass strengthens the indication for this posterior approach.

Posterior stabilization alone is used to treat ill patients whose major problem is a painful metastasis/fracture rather than cord compression and, especially, if there are multiple non-contiguous lesions. The scoring system of Tokuhashi et al. (1990) can be helpful in assessing the prognosis.

8.6.2.5
Complications

The complications following "radical" resection of vertebral body tumours are described elsewhere (Fidler 1994). One patient who had an intralesional resection of a recurrent aggressive aneurysmal bone cyst of L4 and L5, developed a compartment syndrome of the leg, a delayed pressure sore (3 months), a deep infection and an iliac artery aneurysm. Emergency treatment of the aneurysm led to permanent dysfunction of the pelvic autonomic nerves. In this case it had been anticipated that the operation might cause autonomic dysfunction and the young man was referred to the sperm bank prior to the initial operation.

Regarding metastases, the following complications have occurred during 38 cervical and 111 thoracic and lumbar spine palliative operations carried out by the author.

8.6.2.5.1
Cervical Spine.

Pain due to degenerative changes subjacent to an occipito-cervical posterior plate/fusion was treated by anterior fusion (one patient). Loosening of the midline screws of an original occipito-cervical plate (Fidler 1985): re-fixation was successful. The plate was thereafter modified to take two additional postero-lateral angled screws (Fig. 8.20). One case of loose anterior cement: successful re-operation. One patient sustained a minor traction lesion of C8. Two cases of wound dehiscence following radiotherapy and during steroid treatment: one resutured, one treated conservatively.

Local tumour progression/recurrence occurred in eight patients: progressive destruction of neighbouring vertebrae following posterior stabilization and leading to mechanical failure in three cases. In one of these cases the construction was extended. Local tumour progression caused paraparesis in one patient due to circumferential cord compression. Re-operation was followed by progressive quadriparesis. In four patients further treatment was not indicated.

8.6.2.5.2
Thoracic and Lumbar Spine.

In case of anterior surgery there were two deaths, one due to ARDS and one due to a late post-operative haemorrhage. In two patients, 13 years ago, there was partial displacement of an L_4 prosthesis; additional posterior instrumentation is now routine at L_4 and L_5. In one elderly man, 12 years ago, there was indentation of an osteoporotic vertebral body for which supplementary posterior stabilization was effective. The tumour jack support plates were thereafter enlarged. There was one case of late infection in a patient who died of the systemic effects of the malignant disease. One patient had a chylothorax and the tip of the chest drain was infected. Treatment by ligation of the thoracic duct, nettoyage and long-term antibiotics was successful. In one patient who survived longer than expected progressive kyphosis was noted on routine radiographic follow-up at 2 years. Posterior instrumentation and fusion were effective. In one patient a left-sided Kaneda screw head impinged against the aorta at T7. The screw was replaced. Kaneda devices above T9 are now generally inserted from the right side of the spine. Haematothorax in one patient was evacuated.

Neurological complications: one patient with a circumferential lesion became paraplegic post-operatively; two patients did not improve following operation. Following posterior surgery, one posterior wound infection was treated by débridement and long-term antibiotics. Persistent cerebrospinal fluid fistula in one patient was related to the use of laminar wires following radiotherapy. There was one minor persistent sinus following a wound dehiscence.

Local tumour progression/recurrence occurred following 16 operations (11/84 anterior and 5/27 posterior operations). Re-decompression was possible in one patient and resection of the failed construction and re-reconstruction were carried out in two patients. Local tumour progression/recurrence

following anterior surgery is surprisingly uncommon considering the intralesional nature of the operation. The following factors may play a role:
- Virtually all macroscopic tumour is removed.
- The thermal effect of the cement.
- The possible effect of pre-operative embolization.
- Those patients with long post-operative survival are those with slow-growing tumours or whose tumours are responsive to conservative treatment.
- Those patients with short post-operative survival do not have the time available for a significant local recurrence to grow.

8.6.2.6
Expectations of Spinal Decompression and Reconstruction for Metastases

As to be expected from the stabilization of a (pathological) fracture, pain was diminished: almost completely in approximately 85% of cases and moderately in the remainder, except for one patient whose pain did not improve and one in whom pain relief was poor.

Neurological improvement occurred in 87% of patients; 85% of the patients became ambulant (FIDLER 1993). [These results are in keeping with other published data (COOPER et al. 1993; RACHBAUER et al. 1993; MORLEY et al. 1992; ONIMUS et al. 1996)]. The post-operative survival has so far ranged from 2 weeks to 9 years, with an average of more than 15 months. With improved general treatment, this survival time can be expected to improve, making these palliative spinal operations even more worthwhile. The best results are obtained when there is only one metastasis which is causing unbearable pain or when cord compression is caused by a bony fracture fragment which cannot itself be treated conservatively but where the general disease process is still amenable to conservative treatment.

Patients with breast and prostate metastases tend to fare best, followed by kidney and then lung metastases; stomach and melanoma metastases have a dismal prognosis.

8.6.2.7
Multi-disciplinary Approach

For these difficult problems a multi-disciplinary approach with close cooperation between radiologist, radiotherapist, neurologist, oncologist and spinal surgeon is essential.

8.6.2.8
Anterior Versus Posterior/Postero-lateral Surgery

There is still considerable controversy about which is the better approach to thoracic and lumbar spine metastases: the anterior or the posterior, including the postero-lateral. CYBULSKI (1989), in his review, found the overall success rates similar but pointed out that, for the individual case, such factors as tumour location, possible spinal instability, surgical skill and the patient's general health all need to be considered before deciding on the approach. It is clear that both approaches should be available. Some guidelines are possible:

Decompression: tumours lying purely posterior, postero-lateral and lateral to the dura can comfortably be removed *without cord retraction* via a posterior or postero-lateral approach. The more the tumour lies anterior to the dura, the more anterior must be the approach to ensure cord safety, so that finally the anterior (in fact antero-lateral) approach becomes logical. Of course there are exceptions, such as the anterior epidural tumour with minor destruction of the posterior part of the vertebral body, which is probably best approached from the postero-lateral direction with the aid of curved instruments to get around the dura. The safety margin is slightly greater at the level of the cauda equina as this is less vulnerable to pressure than the cord.

Stabilization: As a result of improved cancer therapy, patients are surviving longer and more durable reconstructions are necessary. As previously mentioned, posterior stabilization alone for anterior (and middle column) instability is unsound and in time will lead to stress fractures and breakage of posterior metal, possibly with serious consequences; the anterior (and middle) columns must be restored. For posterior and middle column collapse, at least one of these must be restored.

Armed with these biomechanical and anatomical facts, allied to the patient's general condition and life expectancy, one should be able to make the right choice, assuming of course that the surgeon is an all-round spinal surgeon, equally at home with the various approaches.

Acknowledgement: I wish to thank B. Walman and H. Maeijer for the photography.

References

Algra PR (1992) Magnetic resonance imaging and computed tomography of vertebral metastases. Thesis, Vrije Universiteit, Amsterdam, pp 107, 121

An HS, Vaccaro A, Cotler JM, Lin S (1994) Spinal disorders at the cervicothoracic junction. Spine 19:2557–2564

An HS, Andreshak TG, Nguyen C, Williams A, Daniels D (1995) Can we distinguish between benign versus malignant compression factures of the spine by magnetic resonance imaging? Spine 20:1776–1782

Arasil E, Erdem A, Yüceer N (1996) Osteochondroma of the upper cervical spine. Spine 21:516–518

Asumu TO, Williamson B, Hughes DG (1996) Symptomatic spinal hemangiomas in association with cutaneous hemangiomas. Spine (1996) 21:1082–1084

Babu NV, Titus VTK, Chittaranjan S, Abraham G, Prem H, Korula RJ (1994) Computed tomographically guided biopsy of the spine. Spine 19:2436–2442

Been HD, Fidler MW, Bras J (1994) Cellular hemangioma and angioblastoma of the spine, originally classified as hemangioendothelioma. A confusing diagnosis. Spine 19:990–995

Bennett CJ, Marcus RB, Million RR, Enneking WR (1993) Radiation therapy for giant cell tumor of bone. Int J Radiat Oncol Biol Phys 26:299–304

Bertoni F, Present D, Sudanese A, Baldini N, Bacchini P, Campanacci M (1988) Giant-cell tumor of bone with pulmonary metastases. Clin Orthop 237:275–285

Biagini R, De Cristofaro R, Ruggieri P, Boriani S (1990) Giant-cell tumor of the spine. J Bone Joint Surg Am 72:1102–1107

Birch R, Bonney G, Marshall RW (1990) A surgical approach to the cervicothoracic spine. J Bone Joint Surg Br 72:904–907

Black P (1997) Spinal metastases: current status and recommended guidelines for management. Neurosurgery 5:726–746

Bongioanni F, Assadurian E, Polivka M, George B (1996) Aneurysmal bone cyst of the atlas: operative removal through an anterolateral approach. J Bone Joint Surg Am 78:1574–1577

Boogerd W, van der Sande JJ (1993) Diagnosis and treatment of spinal cord compression in malignant disease. Cancer Treat Rev 19:129–150

Boriani S, Chevalley F, Weinstein JN, Biagini R, Campanacci L, De Iure F, Piccill P (1996a) Chordoma of the spine above the sacrum. Spine 21:1569–1577

Boriani S, Biagini R, De Iure F, Bertoni F, Malaguti MC, Di Fiore M, Zanoni A (1996b) En bloc resections of bone tumors of the thoracolumbar spine. Spine 21:1927–1931

Campanacci M (1990) Bone and soft tissue tumors. Springer, Berlin Heidelberg New York

Campanacci M, Boriani S, Giunti A (1990) Giant cell tumors of the spine. In: Sundaresan N, Schmidek HH, Schiller AL, Rosenthal DI (eds) Tumors of the spine, diagnosis and clinical management. Saunders, Philadelphia, pp 163–172

Clark CR, Keggi KJ, Panjabi MM (1984) Methylmethacrylate stabilisation of the cervical spine. J Bone Joint Surg Am 66:40–46

Cooper PR, Errico TJ, Martin R, Crawford B, DiBartolo T (1993) A systematic approach to spinal reconstruction after anterior decompression for neoplastic disease of the thoracic and lumbar spine. Neurosurgery 32:1-8

Crockard HA, Ransford AO (1991) Transoral approach to the cervical spine. In: Bentley G, Greer RB (eds) Operative surgery. Butterworth-Heinemann, London, pp 453–462

Cunningham BW, Sefter JC, Shono Y, McAfee PC (1993) Static and cyclical biomechanical analysis of pedicle screw spinal constructs. Spine 18:1677–1688

Cybulski GR (1989) Methods of surgical stabilization for metastatic disease of the spine. Neurosurgery 25:240–252

Dahlin DC (1977) Giant-cell tumor of vertebrae above the sacrum. Cancer 39:1350–1356

Darling GE, McBroom R, Perrin R (1995) Modified anterior approach to the cervicothoracic junction. Spine 20:1519–1521

Denis F (1983) The three column spine and its significance in the classification of acute thoracolumbar spinal injuries. Spine 8:817–831

Dickinson LD, Farhat SM (1991) Eosinophilic granuloma of the cervical spine. Surg Neurol 35:57–63

Dommisse GF (1980) The arteries, arterioles and capillaries of the spinal cord: surgical guidelines in the prevention of postoperative paraplegia. Ann R Coll Surg Engl 62:369–376

Edelstyn GA, Gillespie PJ, Grebbell FS (1967) The radiological demonstration of osseous metastases. Experimental observations. Clin Radiol 18:158–162

Emery SE, Brazinski MS, Koka A, Bensusan JS, Stevenson S (1994) The biological and biomechanical effects of irradiation on anterior spinal bone grafts in a canine model. J Bone Joint Surg Am 76:540–548

Enneking WF (1986) A system of staging musculoskeletal neoplasms. Clin Orthop 204:9–24

Fang HSY, Ong GB (1962) Direct anterior approach to the upper cervical spine. J Bone Joint Surg Am 44:1588–1604

Fidler MW (1985) Pathological fractures of the cervical spine: palliative surgical treatment. J Bone Joint Surg Br 67:352–357

Fidler MW (1986a) Anterior decompression and stabilisation of metastatic spinal fractures. J Bone Joint Surg Br 68:83–90

Fidler MW (1986b) Anterior and posterior stabilization of the spine following vertebral body resection. A postmortem investigation. Spine 11:362–366

Fidler MW (1986c) Posterior instrumentation of the spine. An experimental comparison of various possible techniques. Spine 11:367–372

Fidler MW (1991) Metastatic bone disease of the spine. In: Bentley G, Greer RB (eds) Operative surgery. Butterworth-Heinemann, London, pp 571–596

Fidler MW (1993) Thoracic and lumbar spine metastases: anterior surgery for pathological fracture, anterior spinal cord or cauda equina compression. Prospective study. Presented at the inaugural meeting of EFORT, Paris, April 1993. J Bone Joint Surg Br 75 [Suppl II]: 177

Fidler MW (1994) Radical resection of vertebral body tumours: A surgical technique used in ten cases. J Bone Joint Surg Br 76:765–772

Fidler MW (1996) Giant cell tumors of the spine: complete curative resection. International symposium: Bone tumors of the spine. Bologna, Italy

Fidler MW, Bongartz EB (1988) Laminar removal and replacement: a technique for the removal of epidural tumor. Spine 13:218–220

Fidler MW, Hoefnagel CA (1984) Lateral and computerized transverse ^{99m}Tc-Mdp bone scintigrams to supplement the anteroposterior bone scintigram for spinal hot spot localization. Spine 9:655–657

Fidler MW, Niers BBAM (1990) Open transpedicular biopsy of the vertebral body. J Bone Joint Surg Br 72:884–885

Findlay GFG (1987) The role of vertebral body collapse in the management of spinal cord compression. J Neurol Neurosurgery Psychiatry 50:151–154

Fox MW, Onofrio BM (1993) The natural history and management of symptomatic and asymptomatic vertebral hemangiomas. J Neurosurg 78:36–45

Galasko CSB (1986) Skeletal metastases. Butterworth, London

Galasko CSB (1991) Spinal instability secondary to metastatic cancer. J Bone Joint Surg Br 73:104–108

George B (1995) Management of the vertebral artery in excision of extradural tumors of the cervical spine. Neurosurgery 37:844–845

Goldenberg RR, Campbell CJ, Bonfiglio M (1970) Giant-cell tumor of bone. J Bone Joint Surg Am 52:619–664

Green NE, Robertson WW, Kilroy AW (1980) Eosinophilic granuloma of the spine with associated neural deficit. Report of three cases. J Bone Joint Surg Am 62:1198–1202

Grubb MR, Currier BL, Pritchard DJ, Ebersold MJ (1994) Primary Ewing's sarcoma of the spine. Spine 19:309–313

Gurr KR, McAfee PC, Shih CM (1988) Biomechanical analysis of anterior and posterior instrumentation systems after corpectomy. J Bone Joint Surg Am 70:1182–1191

Harms J (1992) Screw-threaded rod system in spinal fusion surgery. Spine State Art Rev 6:541–575

Harrington KD (1986) Metastatic disease of the spine. J Bone Joint Surg Am 68:1110–1115

Hay MC, Paterson D, Taylor TKF (1978) Aneurysmal bone cysts of the spine. J Bone Joint Surg Br 60:406–411

Hertlein H, Mittlmeier T, Piltz S, Schürmann M, Kauschke T, Lob G (1992) Spinal stabilization for patients with metastatic lesions of the spine using a titanium spacer. Eur Spine J 1:131–136

Hosono N, Yonenobu K, Fuji T, Ebara S, Yamashita K, Ono K (1995) Vertebral body replacement with a ceramic prosthesis for metastatic spinal tumors. Spine 20:2454–2462

Hug EB, Fitzek MM, Liebsch NJ, Munzenrider JE (1995) Locally challenging osteo- and chondrogenic tumors of the axial skeleton: results of combined proton and photon radiation therapy using three-dimensional treatment planning. Int J Radiat Oncol Biol Phys 31:467–476

Jackson RP, Reckling FW, Mantz FA (1977) Osteoid osteoma and osteoblastoma. Similar histologic lesions with different natural histories. Clin Orthop 128:303–313

Jaffe HL (1953) Giant-cell tumour (osteoclastoma) of bone: its pathologic delimitation and the inherent clinical implications. Ann R Coll Surg Engl 13:343–355

Jaffee HJ (1958) Tumors and tumorous conditions of the bones and joints. Lea and Febiger, Philadelphia, pp 30–32

Jaffe HJ, Lichtenstein L, Portis RB (1940) Giant cell tumor of bone. Arch Pathol 30:993–1031

Jelinek JS, Kransdorf MJ, Gray R, Aboulafia AJ, Malawer MM (1996) Percutaneous transpedicular biopsy of vertebral body lesions. Spine 21: 2035–2040

Jónsson B, Sjöström L, Olerud C, Andréasson I, Bring J, Rauschning W (1996) Outcome after limited posterior surgery for thoracic and lumbar spine metastases. Eur Spine J 5:36–44

Kaneda K (1991) Anterior approach and Kaneda instrumentation for lesions of the thoracic and lumbar spine. In: Bridwell KH, Dewald RL (eds) The textbook of spinal surgery. Lippincott, Philadelphia, pp 959–990

Kawahara N, Tomita K, Baba H, Toribatake Y, Fujita T, Mizuno K, Tanaka S (1996) Cadaveric vascular anatomy for total en bloc spondylectomy in malignant vertebral tumors. Spine 21:1401–1407

Kneisl JS, Simon MA (1992) Medical management compared with operative treatment for osteoid-osteoma. J Bone Joint Surg Am 74:179–185

Kos CB, Taconis WK, Fidler MW, ten Velden JJAM (1997) Multi-focal giant cell tumours in the spine. Spine 22:821–822

Kostuik JP, Errico TJ, Gleason TF, Errico CC (1988) Spinal stabilization of vertebral column tumors. Spine 13:250–256

Krajbich JI, Eldridge J (1991) Segmental spinal resection in patients with osteosarcoma. In: Brown KLB (ed) Complications of limb saving: prevention, management and outcome. ISOLS, Montreal, pp 391–394

Kreicbergs A, Bauer HCF, Brosjö O, Lindholm J, Skoog L, Söderlund V (1996) Cytological diagnosis of bone tumours. J Bone Joint Surg Br 78:258–263

Lapresle P, Roy-Camille R, Lazennec JY, Mariambourg G (1991) Traitement chirurgical des métastases vertébrales. Chirurgie 117:49–58

Ma, Y, Tang H, Chai B, Yeh Y, Jiang L, Zhou S, Chen W (1987) The treatment of primary vertebral tumors by radical resection and prosthetic vertebral replacement. Clin Orthop 215:78–90

Magerl F, Coscia MF (1988) Total posterior vertebrectomy of the thoracic or lumbar spine. Clin Orthop 232:62–69

Malcolm GP, Ransford AO, Crockard HA (1994) Treatment of non-rheumatoid occipitocervical instability. Internal fixation with the Hartshill-Ransford loop. J Bone Joint Surg Br 76:357–366

Manabe S, Tateishi A, Abe M, Ohno T (1989) Surgical treatment of metastatic tumours of the spine. Spine 14:41–47

Matsui H, Tatezaki S, Tsuji H (1994) Ceramic vertebral body replacement for metastatic spine tumors. J Spinal Disord 7:248–254

McAfee PC, Bohlman HH, Ducker TB, Zeidman SM, Goldstein JA (1995) One-stage anterior cervical decompression and posterior stabilization. J Bone Joint Surg Am 77:1791–1800

Meijer E (1977) Compression of the spinal cord due to vertebral metastases. Is a decompressive laminectomy worthwhile? (in Dutch) Thesis, Catholic University of Nijmegen, The Netherlands. Thieme, Nijmegen

Misaisi N, Cigala F, Iaccarino V, Cozzolino F, Sadile F, Marasco E (1982) Selective arterial embolisation in aneurysmal bone cysts. Int Orthop 6:123–128

Moore AJ, Uttley D (1989) Anterior decompression and stabilization of the spine in malignant disease. Neurosurgery 24:713–717

Morley TR, Thomas M, Smibert JG (1992) The management of spinal metastasis causing cord compression. Presented at the Annual Meeting of the European Spine Society, Rome, October 1991. J Bone Surg Br 74 [Suppl I]: 72

Murphy WA, Strecker WB, Schoenecker PL (1982) Transcatheter embolisation therapy of an ischial aneurysmal bone cyst. J Bone Joint Surg Br 64:166–168

Olerud C, Jónsson B (1996) Surgical palliation of symptomatic spinal metastases. Acta Orthop Scand 67:513–522

Onimus M, Schraub S, Bertin D, Bosset JF, Guidet M (1986) Surgical treatment of vertebral metastasis. Spine 11:883–891

Onimus M, Papin P, Gangloff S (1996) Results of surgical treatment of spinal thoracic and lumbar metastases. Eur Spine J 5:407–411

Ono K, Yonenobu K, Ebara S, Fujiwara K, Yamashita K, Fuji T, Dunn EJ (1988) Prosthetic replacement surgery for cervical spine metastasis. Spine 13:817–822

Osebold WR, Lester EL, Hurley JH, Vincent RL (1993) Intraoperative use of the mobile gamma camera in localizing and excising osteoid osteomas of the spine. Spine 18:1816–1828

Peimer CA, Schiller AL, Mankin HJ, Smith RJ (1980) Multi-centric giant-cell tumor of bone. J Bone Joint Surg Am 62:652–656

Perrin RG, McBroom RJ (1990) Surgical treatment for spinal metastases: the posterolateral approach. In: Sundaresan N, Schmidek HH, Schiller AL, Rosenthal DI (eds) Tumors of the spine, diagnosis and clinical management. Saunders, Philadelphia, pp 305–315

Pettine KA, Klassen RA (1986) Osteoid-osteoma and osteoblastoma of the spine. J Bone Joint Surg Am 68:354–361

Peyser AB, Makley JT, Callewart CC, Brackett B, Carter JR, Abdul-Karim FW (1996) Osteoma of the long bones and the spine. J Bone Joint Surg Am 78:1172–1180

Picard L, Bracard S, Roland J, Moreno A, Per A (1989) Embolisation des hémangiomes vertébraux. Technique-indications-résultats. Neurochirurgie 35:289–293

Polster J, Brinckmann P (1977) Ein Wirbelkörperimplantat zur Verwendung bei Palliativoperationen an der Wirbel-säule. Z Orthop Ihre Grenzgeb 115:118–122

Privat JM, Frerebeau P, Benezech J, Gros C (1980) Plaque occipito-rachidienne vissée. Indications et résultats. Neurochirurgie 26:391–399

Rachbauer F, Bauer R, Achammer T, Krismer M (1993) Surgi-cal treatment of tumors of the spine: principles and re-sults. Presented at the inaugural meeting of EFORT, Paris, April 1993. J Bone Joint Surg Br 75 [Suppl] II:177–178

Ransford AO, Pozo JL, Hutton PAN, Kirwan EOG. The behav-iour pattern of the scoliosis associated with osteoid os-teoma or osteoblastoma of the spine. J Bone Joint Surg Br 66:16–20

Regan JJ, Mack MJ, Picetti GD (1995) A technical report on video-assisted thoracoscopy in thoracic spinal surgery. Spine 20:831–837

Rock MG, Pritchard DJ, Unni KK (1984) Metastases from histologically benign giant-cell tumor of bone. J Bone Joint Surg Am 66:269–274

Rosenberg AE, Schiller AL (1990) Tumorous lesions of the spine: an overview. In: Sundaresan N, Schmidek HH, Schiller AL, Rosenthal DI (eds) Tumors of the spine, diag-nosis and clinical management. Saunders, Philadelphia, pp 82–85

Roy-Camille R, Saillant G, Bisserié M, Judet T, Hautefort E, Mamoudy P (1981) Résection vertébrale totale dans la chirurgie tumorale au niveau du rachis dorsal par voie postérieure pure. Technique – indications. Rev Chir Orthop Reparatrice Appar Mot 67:421–430

Roy-Camille R, Mazel C, Saillant G, Lapresle P (1990) Treat-ment of malignant tumors of the spine with posterior in-strumentation. In: Sundaresan N, Schmidek HH, Schiller AL, Rosenthal DI (eds) Tumors of the spine, diagnosis and clinical management. Saunders, Philadelphia, pp 473–487

Rupp RE, Ebraheim NA, Coombs RJ (1995) Magnetic reso-nance imaging differentiation of compression spine frac-tures or vertebral lesions caused by osteoporosis or tumor. Spine 20:2499–2504

Salzer M, Salzer G, Denck H, Brenner H, et al (1973) Operative Behandlung "solitärer" Metastasen der Brust- und Len-denwirbelkörper. Arch Orthop Unfallchir 15:249–254

Sanguinetti C, Specchia N, Gigante A, de Palma L, Greco F (1993) Clinical and pathological aspects of solitary spinal neurofibroma. J Bone Joint Surg Br 75:141–147

Sanjay BKS, Sim FH, Unni KK, McLeod RA, Klassen RA (1993) Giant-cell tumours of the spine. J Bone Joint Surg Br 75:148–154

Savini R, Gherlinzoni F, Morandi M, Neff JR, Picci P (1983) Surgical treatment of giant-cell tumor of the spine. J Bone Joint Surg Am 65:1283–1289

Schajowicz F (1994) Tumors and tumorlike lesions of bone. Pathology, radiology, and treatment, 2nd edn. Springer, Berlin Heidelberg New York

Schrijver JRN (1982) Giant cell-tumors of bone: classifica-tion, treatment, reconstruction. (in Dutch) Thesis, Univer-sity of Leiden, The Netherlands

Scully SP, Mott MP, Temple HT, O'Keefe RJ, O'Donnell RJ, Mankin HJ (1994) Late recurrence of giant-cell tumor of bone. J Bone Joint Surg Am 76:1231–1233

Sen C, Eisenberg M, Casden AM, Sundaresan N, Catalano PJ (1995) Management of the vertebral artery in excision of extradural tumors of the cervical spine. Neurosurgery 36:106–116

Siegal T, Siegal T (1985) Vertebral body resection for epidural compression by malignant tumors; results of forty-seven consecutive operative procedures. J Bone Joint Surg Am 67:375–382

Siegal T, Siegal T (1990) Surgical intervention for neoplastic involvement of the lumbar spine. In: Sundaresan N, Schmidek HH, Schiller AL, Rosenthal DI (eds) Tumors of the spine, diagnosis and clinical management. Saunders, Philadelphia, pp 380–390

Shikata J, Yamamuro T, Kotoura Y, Mikawa Y, Iida H, Maetani S (1988) Total sacrectomy and reconstruction for primary tumours. J Bone Joint Surg Am 70:122–125

Shives TC, Dahlin DC, Sim FH, Pritchard DJ, Earle JD (1986) Osteosarcoma of the spine. J Bone Joint Surg Am 68:660–668

Shives TC, McLeod RA, Unni KK, Schray MF (1989) Chondro-sarcoma of the spine. J Bone Joint Surg Am 71:1158–1165

Sim FH, McDonald DJ, McLeod RA, Unni KK (1990) Giant cell tumors of the spine and sacrum: Mayo Clinic experience. In: Sundaresan N, Schmidek HH, Schiller AL, Rosenthal DI (eds) Tumors of the spine, diagnosis and clinical manage-ment. Saunders, Philadelphia, pp 173–180

Smith D, Schmidek HH (1990) Tumors of the nerve sheath in-volving the spine. In: Sundaresan N, Schmidek HH, Schiller AL, Rosenthal DI (eds) Tumors of the spine, diag-nosis and clinical management. Saunders, Philadelphia, pp 226–234

Steffee AD, Sitkowsky DJ, Topham LS (1986) Total vertebral body and pedicle arthroplasty. Clin Orthop 203:203–208

Stener B (1971) Total spondylectomy in chondrosarcoma arising from the seventh thoracic vertebra. J Bone Joint Surg Br 53:288–295

Stener B (1989) Complete removal of vertebrae for extirpa-tion of tumors. Twenty year experience. Clin Orthop 245:72–82

Stener B, Gunterberg B (1978) High amputation of the sacrum for extirpation of tumors. Principles and tech-nique. Spine 3:351–366

Stener B, Johnsen OE (1971) Complete removal of three verte-brae for giant-cell tumour. J Bone Joint Surg Br 53:278–287

Sundaresan N (1986) Chordomas. Clin Orthop 204:135–142

Sundaresan N, Galicich JH, Lane JM, Bains MS, McCormack P (1985) Treatment of neoplastic epidural cord compression by vertebral body resection and stabilization. J Neurosurg 63:676–684

Sundaresan N, Rosen G, Huvos AG, Krol G (1988) Combined treatment of osteosarcoma of the spine. Neurosurgery 23:714–719

Sundaresan N, Digiacinto GV, Hughes JEO, Cafferty M, Vallejo A (1991) Treatment of neoplastic spinal cord compression: results of a prospective study. Neurosurgery 29:645–650

Sung HW, Shu WP, Wang HM, Yuai SY, Tsai YB (1987) Surgical treatment of primary tumors of the sacrum. Clin Orthop 215:91–98

Tatsui H, Onomura T, Morishita S, Oketa M, Inoue T (1996) Survival rates of patients with metastatic spinal cancer after scintigraphic detection of abnormal radioactive accumulation. Spine 21:2143–2148

Tokuhashi Y, Matsuzaki H, Toriyama S, Kawano H, Ohsaka S (1990) Scoring system for the preoperative evaluation of metastatic spine tumor prognosis. Spine 15:1110–1113

Tomita K, Tsuchiya H (1990) Total sacrectomy and reconstruction for huge sacral tumors. Spine 15:1223–1227

Tomita K, Kawahara N, Baba H, Tsuchiya H, Nagata S, Toribatake Y (1994) Total en bloc spondylectomy for solitary spinal metastases. Int Orthop 18:291–298

Turner PL, Prince HG, Webb JK, Sokal MPJW (1988) Surgery for malignant extradural tumours of the spine. J Bone Joint Surg Br 70:451–456

Vandertop WP, Pruijs JEH, Snoeck IN, van den Hout JHW (1994) Aneurysmal bone cyst of the thoracic spine: radical excision with use of the cavitron. J Bone Joint Surg Am 76:608–611

Vanel D, Contesso G, Rebibo G, Zafrani B, Masselot J (1983) Benign giant-cell tumours of bone with pulmonary metastases and favourable prognosis. Skeletal Radiol 10:221–226

Vlahovitch B, Fuentés JM (1975) Traitement chirurgical des métastases du rachis cervical. Nouv Presse Med 4:2493–2497

Ward JC, Jeanneret JB, Oehlschlegel C, Magerl F (1996) The value of percutaneous transpedicular vertebral bone biopsies for histological examination. Spine 21:2484–2490

Weinstein JN, McLain RF (1987) Primary tumors of the spine. Spine 12:843–851

White AA, Panjabi MM (1990) Clinical biomechanics of the spine. 2nd edn. Lippincott, Philadelphia

Wray CC, Macdonald AW, Richardson RA (1990) Benign giant cell tumour with metastases to bone and lung. J Bone Joint Surg Br 72:486–489

Wuisman P, Härle A, Matthiass HH, Roessner A, Erlemann R, Reiser M (1989) Two-stage therapy in the treatment of sacral tumors. Arch Orthop Trauma Surg 108:255–260

9 Current Concepts of Surgical Therapy of Intradural and Intramedullary Tumours

W.P. VANDERTOP, L.M.P. RAMOS, and C.A.F. TULLEKEN

CONTENTS

9.1
Introduction

Neoplasms of the spinal canal may be classified on the basis of their location into epidural, intradural-extramedullary and intramedullary tumours (Table 9.1). Whereas the majority of epidural neoplasms are metastatic in nature, the intradural tumours are often primary tumours. In neurosurgical practice, intraspinal neoplasms account for approximately 15% of all primary tumours of the central nervous system and its sheath elements (RUSSELL and RUBINSTEIN 1989). The relative frequency of epidural, intradural-extramedullary and intramedullary tumours is not

W.P. VANDERTOP, MD, PhD, Department of Neurosurgery, University Hospital Utrecht, P.O.Box 85500, 3508 GA Utrecht, The Netherlands
L.M.P. RAMOS, MD, Department of Neuroradiology, Department of Neurosurgery, University Hospital Utrecht, P.O.Box 85500, 3508 GA Utrecht, The Netherlands
C.A.F. TULLEKEN, MD, PhD, Department of Neurosurgery, University Hospital Utrecht, P.O. Box 85500, 3508 GA Utrecht, The Netherlands

exactly known. Based on available epidemiological data, metastatic spinal tumours are three to four times more common than primary spinal tumours (BYRNE and WAXMAN 1990). The average annual incidence of primary intraspinal neoplasms is reported to be 1.3 per 100,000 population, although figures ranging from 0.8 to 2.5 are quoted (FOGELHOLM et al. 1984). Metastatic disease to the spine is discussed in detail elsewhere in this book. This chapter will focus on the surgical treatment of intradural neoplasms.

Table 9.1. Classification of spinal neoplasms according to location

Epidural tumours
    Metastasis
    Multiple myeloma
    Osteogenic sarcoma
    Chordoma
    Chondrosarcoma
    Lipoma; teratoma
Intradural-extramedullary tumours
    Meningioma
    Nerve sheath tumour
    Vascular malformation and tumour
    Epidermoid and dermoid tumour
    Lipoma, teratoma
    Metastasis
Intramedullary tumours
    Ependymoma
    Astrocytoma
    Ganglioglioma
    Vascular malformation and tumour
    Metastasis

9.2
Intradural-Extramedullary Tumours

The first successful surgical removal of an intraspinal neoplasm was that of an intradural-extramedullary tumour by Sir Victor Horsley in 1888. Large series have been reported since by ELSBERG (1925), LIST (1941), SLOOFF et al. (1964), GIUFFRÉ (1966) and LEVY et al. (1982). Intradural-extramedullary tumours are usually the histologically benign meningiomas and nerve sheath tumours, although (epi)dermoid cysts, teratomas, lipomas and metastatic neoplasms to the leptomeninges also occur.

9.2.1
Meningiomas

Meningiomas constitute one of the most common forms of spinal tumour. The literature remains divided as to whether meningiomas or nerve sheath tumours head the list. The large series of 1322 primary intraspinal tumours described by SLOOFF et al. (1964) recorded an incidence of 29% of schwannomas, 25.5% of meningiomas, 22% of gliomas and almost 12% of sarcomas. In other series, meningiomas made up 33–47% of primary spinal tumours (BYRNE and WAXMAN 1990).

Meningiomas may arise from any of the cell elements that form the meninges but the majority stem from arachnoid cells. The tumour is usually firmly fixed to the lateral dura at the level of the dentate ligament and may extend anteriorly or posteriorly. In the cervical region an anterior location seems to be predominant. Meningiomas may occur at any level along the spinal axis, but it is generally accepted that the thoracic region is involved far more often than other levels. Occassionally the cervical segments are affected, whilst lumbar examples are rare. Spinal meningiomas are much more frequently encountered in women than in men. The most (approximately 80%) meningiomas in women occur in the thoracic region, whereas in men a nearly equal frequency of cervical (41%) and thoracic (47%) lesions has been reported (LEVY et al. 1982). The reason for this predilection for the thoracic spine in women is unknown. Multiple spinal meningiomas may occur in von Recklinghausen's disease.

The duration of symptoms arising from spinal meningiomas may be quite variable. Occasionally patients have an abrupt onset of symptoms, often precipitated by trauma. Usually, symptoms begin insidiously and progress over many months. As in most other spinal tumours, back pain is the most common presenting symptom and is usually progressive. Radicular pain is often a prominent complaint and may be present for months or years prior to diagnosis. In meningiomas the pain may be bilateral, contrary to neurofibromas where it is usually unilateral (BYRNE and WAXMAN 1990). Subjective complaints of radicular paraesthesia appear to be common in cases of meningioma, with frequencies of 23–37% reported (GUIDETTI and FORTUNA 1975). Sphincter disturbances are unusual early manifestations in intradural-extramedullary tumours unless the conus or cauda equina is involved. A meningioma en plaque, in which the tumour forms a diffuse collar-like mass around the cord, is rare. Occa-

sionally, the spinal meningiomas are separate from the dura and deeply embedded in the cord.

Epidural meningiomas have been known to occur in up to 10% of cases (BYRNE and WAXMAN 1990). It is noteworthy that epidural spinal meningiomas demonstrate a relatively high incidence in childhood and show a predominance in males (KEPES 1982). Epidural meningiomas are considered biologically more aggressive.

Abnormalities on plain spine radiographs occur in only 10% of patients with spinal meningiomas. The choice of further radiographic procedures may include myelography, CT scanning following intravenous contrast administration, CT myelography and MRI. The MRI scan is of course the most attractive because it is noninvasive, shows the entire spinal canal and surrounding structures in great detail, and can differentiate intramedullary neoplasms from syringomyelia, as well as demonstrate the relationship between the spinal cord and extramedullary lesions (Fig. 9.1). The characteristic radiographic features of meningiomas are discussed in detail elsewhere (Chap. 1).

9.2.2
Nerve Sheath Tumours

RUSSELL and RUBINSTEIN (1989) classified nerve sheath tumours into two main categories, which are usually readily distinguishable on both histological and electron microscopic grounds: the first, typified by a solitary encapsulated tumour of the nerve roots and peripheral nerves, is the *schwannoma*; the second is the *neurofibroma*, in which connective tissue fibres are a conspicuous element and nerve fibres within the substance of the tumour are often both more numerous and microscopically more obvious than in the schwannomas. This is not to say that neurofibromas are "unencapsulated" lesions, as previously thought. This characterisation was based upon histological discovery of nerve fibre elements within the tumour and not upon gross appearance or resectability. Most neurofibromas do have a capsule, and nerve fascicles are often peripherally enclosed in its layers (DONNER et al. 1994).

Alternative designations for schwannoma still used today include "neurinoma" and "neurilemoma" (often spelt "neurilemmoma"). The name schwannoma is preferable as it explicitly identifies the cell type involved (RUSSELL and RUBINSTEIN 1989). While these peripheral nerve sheath tumours are two distinct entities, their clinical appearance and

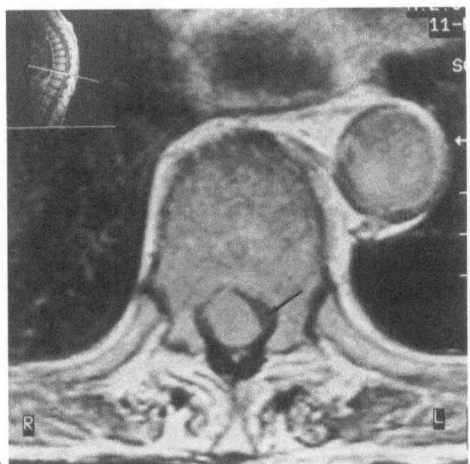 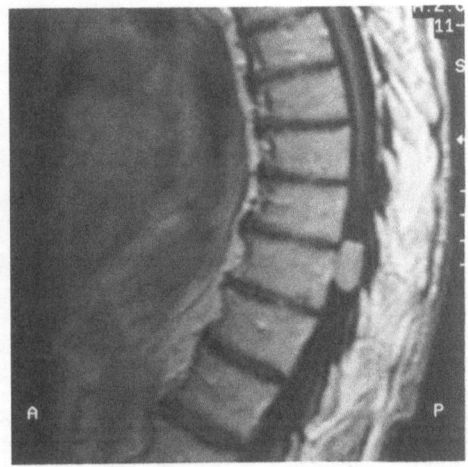

a   b

Fig.9.1a,b. Intradural-extramedullary thoracic meningioma. **a** An axial T1-weighted image without and **b** a sagittal T1-weighted image with gadolinium diethylene-triamine-pentaacetic acid (Gd-DTPA) show on the right an intradural hyperintense tumour with homogeneous enhancement which displaces and compresses the spinal cord to the left (*arrow*)

their treatment are similar and are therefore considered here under the title of (solitary) nerve sheath tumour.

The solitary intraspinal nerve sheath tumour is a common intrathecal neoplasm, competing with meningioma as the most common primary intraspinal tumour. There is a predominant tendency for nerve sheath tumours to involve the sensory roots, although occasional examples on motor nerve roots have been recorded (RUSSELL and RUBINSTEIN 1989). According to SLOOFF et al. (1964), the lumbar segments are the most frequently involved, but the thoracic and cervical regions do not lag far behind. Nerve sheath tumours are more evenly distributed along the spinal axis than meningiomas. Most nerve sheath tumours are completely intradural, but some are completely extradural. Occasionally an intrathecal tumour extends through the intervertebral foramen to expand into a further and even greater mass on the peripheral segment of the nerve: an "hourglass-" or "dumb-bell"-shaped nerve sheath tumour. These mostly arise in the cervical and thoracic region, and the extravertebral tumour is often the significant clinical feature (RUSSELL and RUBINSTEIN 1989). Rarely, nerve sheath tumours may be intramedullary (VAN DUIJNEN 1971).

Nerve sheath tumours affect both sexes equally. Like their intracranial counterparts, they are generally encountered in adults, but are occasionally seen in children. Unless associated with neurofibroma-

tosis, solitary neurofibromas are not considered familial.

When small, benign nerve sheath tumours are generally asymptomatic. The duration of symptoms prior to diagnosis averages 1–4 years. The shortest average course of symptoms is seen in cervical lesions and the longest among lumbar tumours. As they usually arise in the posterior spinal nerve roots, they first present with unilateral radicular pain. Pain is the initial symptom in a large majority of cases. Motor symptoms will develop if the cord or ventral roots become compressed. Motor and sensory symptoms and signs are occasionally presenting symptoms, but are frequently found at the time of diagnosis (BYRNE and WAXMAN 1990). Sphincter disturbance and sexual dysfunction is present in half of the cases.

Abnormalities on plain radiographs occur in 43–52% of patients with spinal nerve sheath tumours, contrary to the experience with spinal meningiomas where they occur in only 10% (BYRNE and WAXMAN 1990). Prior to the advent of CT and MRI, myelography was essential for the diagnosis. Nowadays, CT scanning following intravenous contrast medium administration, CT myelography and MRI are the modalities of choice to confirm the diagnosis and to accurately define the location, extent and relationships of the tumour with its surrounding structures (Fig. 9.2).

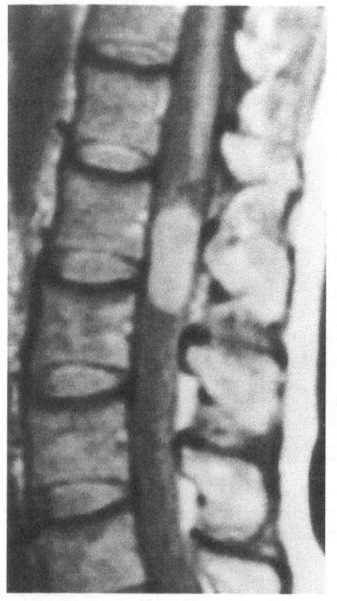 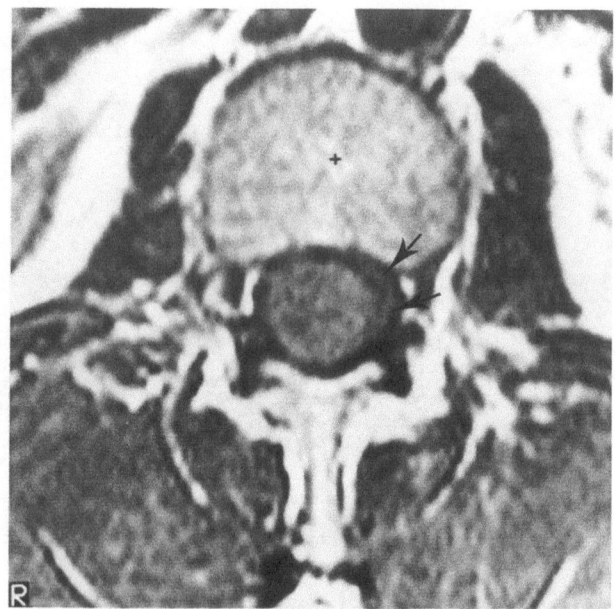

Fig.9.2a,b. Intradural-extramedullary low thoracic neurofibroma in a 53-year-old man with a history of back pain and pain in the right leg. a A sagittal T1-weighted image with Gd-DTPA and b an axial T1-weighted image without contrast show a well-defined, right-sided, brightly enhancing tumour with displacement of the nerve roots (*arrows*) at the level T12-L1

9.2.3
Epidermoid and dermoid cysts

Collectively, these tumours comprise approximately 1-2% of primary spinal tumours. It is generally agreed that both types of cyst arise from the inclusion of ectodermal elements at the time of closure of the neural groove, resulting in heterotopia of such elements (RUSSELL and RUBINSTEIN 1989). As a consequence, both show a tendency to be associated with congenital bony defects in the vertebral column. Non-congenital variants of epidermoid cysts have been reported to develop years following a lumbar puncture, whereas dermoids have been reported at the site of previous surgical repair of a myelomeningocele (SCOTT et al. 1986).

The majority of these lesions are intramedullary, but they may be located in the intradural-extramedullary space. While intracranially located dermoids are rarer than epidermoids, within the spinal canal dermoids are found to be more common than epidermoids. In the spinal canal most dermoids occur in the lumbosacral region, whereas epidermoids are more evenly distributed. This predominant distribution of intraspinal dermoid cysts in the caudal region is explained by certain distinctive features of development in the lower thoracic and lumbosacral segments.

Both dermoid and epidermoid cysts are slightly more common in males than in females. The average age at which symptoms appear from spinal dermoid cysts is within the first two decades of life. Spinal epidermoid cysts are slower to develop than dermoid cysts and may evoke symptoms at any time between the ages of 20 and 50 (LIST 1941). As most of these cysts occur in the lower part of the spinal canal, symptoms and signs referable to the cauda equina and conus medullaris usually develop. In cases associated with developmental anomalies, cutaneous stigmata may be present. Rarely, the lesions rupture, leading to an aseptic meningitis. More frequently, repeated bouts of septic meningitis lead to the discovery of a dimple with a sinus tract. Myelography and CT myelography may demonstrate dermoids and epidermoids, but again MRI will be the investigation of choice nowadays.

9.2.4
Teratomas

RUSSELL and RUBINSTEIN (1989) have separated the teratomas into mature teratomas, which are constituted by fully differentiated ectodermal, mesodermal and endodermal elements, and immature teratomas, which include more primitive elements derived from all or any of the three germinal layers. In the spinal canal, excluding the relatively common sacrococcygeal form, teratomas are very rare. A dorsal or dorsolateral location in the spine is usual, and the growth may be extra- or intradural, or intramedullary. Various levels are affected. Symptoms and signs are comparable to those seen in the dermoid and epidermoid cysts.

9.2.5
Lipomas

In the spinal canal, lipomas account for approximately 1% of all tumours and are distributed equally between the sexes. Lipomas are evidently of maldevelopmental origin, implicating both the leptomeninges and subjacent neural tissues. Most intraspinal lipomas are subpial, in the thoracic region, and never completely enclosed by neural tissue. Associated congenital abnormalities such as spina bifida or other forms of dysraphism are found in about a third of cases (RUSSELL and RUBINSTEIN 1989). Spinal lipomas tend to become intra- as well as extramedullary, provoking symptoms as a result (PIERRE-KAHN et al. 1986).

Two thirds of patients report symptoms before the age of 30 years (GIUFFRÈ 1966). Symptoms often are present for long periods of time prior to diagnosis. Although back pain has been reported as being the first symptom in the majority of cases, radicular pain seems to be less frequent: numbness and ataxia were the most common presenting complaints (GIUFFRÈ 1966). As spinal cord or cauda equina compression progress, symptoms and signs are those of other space-occupying lesions of the spine.

Abnormalities on plain radiographs are seen in approximately half of patients with an intradural lipoma. Again MRI will play the dominant role in diagnostic imaging in the future.

9.2.6
Surgical Intervention in Extramedullary Tumours

Laminectomy is the most flexible approach to intraspinal tumours. It can easily be extended in craniocaudal direction in order to totally encompass the tumour or, if necessary, to adjust if the initial localisation is not perfect. The latter can be largely avoided by preoperative or intraoperative radiographic localisation. A laminectomy can easily be extended to a transpedicular approach if the tumour is more laterally positioned than initially thought, or if a more lateral approach is necessary to avoid undue manipulation of the spinal cord in tumours situated entirely anteriorly or anterolaterally. Compared to the transthoracic approach, a posterolateral approach has fewer potential complications and eliminates the necessity of vertebrectomy when resecting ventrally located intradural thoracic tumours (STECK et al. 1994).

A disadvantage of laminectomy is the potential for spinal destabilisation, particularly in children. One must minimise the disturbance of the facet structure to avoid late kyphosis and still provide adequate access for complete tumour removal. A unilateral facetectomy in asymmetrically located tumours does not necessarily compromise vertebral column stability, whilst it does provide excellent access, even in anteriorly located tumours. Some authors have advocated the routine use of multiple level osteoplastic laminotomy (RAIMONDI et al. 1976; YASUOKA et al. 1982), but there is no definite proof that this policy prevents the occurrence of spinal instability or deformity.

Although some surgeons still prefer to have the patient in the sitting position for the access to cervical and upper thoracic area, the position typically used for the posterior or posterolateral approach to the spinal canal is prone. The risk of air embolism is thus avoided.

Anterior approaches can be useful for extradural, anteriorly located tumours, especially in the cervical region, and are obligatory for the complete removal of vertebral body tumours. Additional stabilisation procedures, however, are then mandatory. Access to the spinal canal is relatively simple from T4 to L2. The T2-4 area presents a major technical challenge. Multidisciplinary teams comprising neurosurgeons, thoracic, orthopaedic and general surgeons may be necessary. The obvious advantage of the anterior approach for tumours lying ventral to the spinal cord is the ability to excise them without manipulation of the spinal cord.The disadvantage is the relatively limited exposure, difficult haemostasis and the problem of dural closure in the case of intradurally located tumours. Control of bleeding through this limited exposure can be very challenging and necessitates the use of the operating microscope. Transthoracic approaches require postoperative chest tubes, which can promote cerebrospinal fluid (CSF) fistula. It is very important to attempt good dural closure and institute spinal drainage to avoid a CSF pleural fistula.

Following dural exposure at the appropriate level(s) we routinely perform an ultrasound examination in order to delineate exactly the level of the intradural lesion and its relation to the spinal cord. This allows us to remove additional bone from a lamina higher or lower before the dura is opened. We recommend using the microscope to open the dura, as this ensures careful and safe exposure of the intradural contents. In addition, dural traction sutures can be easily placed without any manipulation of the tumour or spinal cord. Unless the surgeon is sure that the tumour is completely located dorsal to the spinal cord, it is wise not to try to remove an intradural-extramedullary tumour "in one piece", for any excessive manipulation of the already compromised spinal cord can lead to additional neurological deficits. Piecemeal removal of an intradural tumour also allows for the spinal cord to re-expand in a far more gentle fashion than after "tumorectomy in toto".

After bipolar coagulation, the tumour capsule is opened and internal debulking is performed, with a variety of instruments available, i.e. a Cavitron ultrasonic surgical aspirator (CUSA), a laser or microsurgical instruments. During this phase it is crucial that the surgeon is constantly aware of the fact that every manipulation of or in the tumour indirectly results in manipulation of the spinal cord. This is particularly so when the tumour is so large that the spinal cord is not visible and only comes into view after a significant portion of the tumour has been removed. Frequent repeated coagulation of the capsule causes the residual tumour to shrink, thereby facilitating preparation of the plane of cleavage between tumour and spinal cord or between tumour and spinal nerve roots, and enables the surgeon to safely explore and interrupt any feeding arteries previously invisible. We have found that irrigation with isotonic mannitol during electrical coagulation, as advocated by SAKATANI et al. (1995), is far superior to irrigation with conventional physiological saline in reducing adherence of burned tissue and clots to the tips of bipolar diathermy forceps.

In case of a meningioma, one should not start with trying to find the place of dural attachment, which is usually quite far anterior, at the level of the dentate ligament. Although this does provide the possibility of interrupting important feeding arteries to the tumour, manipulation of the tumour can result in excessive indirect compression of the spinal cord. Only after significant debulking of the tumour is it easy to identify the site of dural attachment, which can then be coagulated and cut, and the dentate ligament divided. This will enable the surgeon to reach an anterior extension of the tumour without undue manipulation of the spinal cord and with full vision of any vessels or nerve roots attached to the residual tumour.

In case of a schwannoma, more or less the same applies as for the meningiomas. After significant debulking, it is usually quite easy to separate the dorsal roots (with the tumour attached) from the anterior motor roots. In this fashion the motor roots can be spared and thus it is not necessary to completely "sacrifice" the entire spinal nerve root.

Epidermoid and dermoid cyst can appear as "easy-to-resect" tumours. Whereas it is often very easy to remove the soft contents of these lesions by suction alone, creating a massive amount of space for the severely compressed spinal cord, the capsule of these tumours is usually very adherent to the surface of the spinal cord, spinal nerve roots or cauda equina. This often precludes total excision for fear of damaging these vulnerable structures. The same counts for lipomas. One is wiser to leave some (epi)dermoid capsule or lipoma tissue behind than to cause additional deficit, as recurrent tumour may take a decade or longer to develop.

After complete tumour removal has been accomplished one can close the dura using either the microscope or loupe magnification. We have no preference for interrupted or running sutures, or for absorbable or non-absorbable suture material.

Postoperative haematoma formation with spinal cord compression is a serious complication, but fortunately infrequent. Meticulous attention to haemostasis is the first line of defence. Suturing muscles is not necessary and carries the risk of significant arterial bleeding, whereas careful fascial closure is an extremely important step in wound closure. Preferably we use soft silicone wound drains in the epidural space which are not guided through the original incision. We avoid the use of (low) vacuum drains epidurally for fear of increasing the risk of a CSF leak. A careful dural repair combined with a multi-level wound closure should avoid the complication of CSF fistula. Any sign of progressive myelopathy postoperatively demands either rapid re-exploration or at least immediate appropriate radiographic studies to rule out the presence of a haematoma.

Lumbar drainage of CSF postoperatively can usually divert it sufficiently to allow for dural healing when complete dural closure has proved impossible. Few problems with infection are to be expected if lumbar spinal drains are limited to 5 or 6 days. Additional drainage time can be gained if necessary by simple replacement at a different level or by tunnelling the catheter.

9.2.7
Outcome

If the condition is diagnosed and treated early in its course, neurological function will be preserved and the patient usually cured. Even in patients with severe neurological deficit, removal of a benign, extramedullary neoplasm can be highly rewarding as significant recovery of function is often seen. However, if not recognised and surgically resected, these benign neoplasms will generally cause progressive neurological deficit and ultimately permanent loss of spinal cord function.

A totally resected meningioma or schwannoma is usually cured with no further adjuvant therapy. Only if histopathological examination reveals malignant features is postoperative radiotherapy warranted. Meningioma en plaque can hardly ever be resected totally and will have to be operated on several times in the course of years. Depending on the age of the patient and the neurological deficit incurred over time, radiotherapy may be considered. In cases of subtotal resection long-term follow-up is necessary, with frequent radiographic control for recurrent tumour.

In case of an epidermoid or dermoid cyst it is easy to remove the (soft) contents, thereby allowing the spinal cord to re-expand, but it is often not possible to completely remove the tumour capsule. In this case one must count on recurrence of the tumour, even if this does take 15-20 years. Lipomas are also very adherent to the spinal cord or cauda equina and often not completely resectable. Long-term follow-up in these cases is mandatory.

9.3
Intramedullary Tumours

In 1907, von Eiselberg reported the first successful removal of an intramedullary tumour (neurofibrosarcoma). In 1911, Elsberg commented on the operability of intramedullary tumours and subsequently gained a personal experience of 275 cases (ELSBERG 1925). It was he who developed the concept of "the extrusion of intramedullary tumours" (see Sect. 9.3.5). In 1954, Greenwood published findings in a series of patients with intramedullary tumours in whom he had accomplished a total removal. A follow-up study years later showed that the patients who had undergone an incomplete resection had all tumour progression and had become wheelchair dependent, whereas the patients who had undergone a total resection had all fared well (GREENWOOD 1963). At the end of the 1960s, the operating microscope, and with it the application of microsurgical techniques in neurosurgery, was introduced by YASARGIL et al. (YASARGIL 1970; YASARGIL et al. 1976). Since then reports have frequently been published on successful radical resection of intramedullary tumours, with acceptable operative morbidity and almost zero operative mortality. Most authors nowadays emphasise the need for primary total resection (MALIS 1977; STEIN 1979, 1983; GUIDETTI et al. 1981; COOPER and EPSTEIN 1985; COOPER 1989; EPSTEIN et al. 1990, 1992, 1993; VANDERTOP et al. 1991).

9.3.1
Clinical Signs and Symptoms

Typical radicular pain, characterised as a unilateral, lancinating dermatomal pain, is common with extradural growths but rare in cases of intramedullary tumour (BILLER and BRAZIS 1990; BYRNE and WAXMAN 1990). Funicular (central) pain, on the other hand, is common with intramedullary tumours but very unusual with extradural lesions. Funicular pain is described as deep, ill-defined dysaesthesia, usually distant from the affected spinal cord level (and thus of poor localising value) and is often bilateral. It is probably related to dysfunction of the spinothalamic tract or posterior columns (BILLER and BRAZIS 1990).

Motor disorders are second only to pain as the most common presenting manifestation of spinal cord tumours. Motor dysfunction will occur when either the lower motor neuron, upper motor neuron, or both are compromised. Upper motor neuron signs tend to occur early with intramedullary tumours and late with extramedullary lesions (BILLER and BRAZIS 1990). Weakness due to intramedullary tumours may characteristically spread in the limbs from proximal to distal. Intramedullary lesions in the cervical spine may cause unilateral or bilateral arm weakness with sparing of muscle strength of the legs early in their course. In cases of cervical intra-dural-extramedullary tumours, lower extremity strength is usually impaired to a degree comparable with that of the arms.

Paraesthesias are unusual presenting symptoms in patients with spinal neoplasms. Isolated sensory loss (with sacral sparing) and preservation of posterior column function with loss of spinothalamic functions is considered characteristic of intramedullary lesions (BYRNE and WAXMAN 1990). With intramedullary tumours, vibratory sense is usually more impaired than position sense.

9.3.2
Astrocytomas

Gliomas arise from neuroglia and may be classified into astrocytomas, oligodendrogliomas, ependymomas and anaplastic forms (RUSSELL and RUBINSTEIN 1989). Astrocytomas and ependymomas are the two most common tumours found in the spinal cord. Although the intraspinal gliomas constitute a majority of the intramedullary tumours, they account for only a minority of all intraspinal growths. In the large series of SLOOFF et al. (1964) 22% of all intraspinal tumours consisted of intramedullary gliomas (see Section 9.2.1). Series restricted to children alone show a relatively higher proportion of gliomas than in adults because of the low incidence of meningiomas and schwannomas in early life (RUSSELL and RUBINSTEIN 1989). The relative frequency of the types of spinal intramedullary gliomas encountered in childhood varies from that in adults and indicates a prevalence of astrocytomas over ependymomas.

Spinal cord astrocytomas are more frequently seen in men than in women. These tumours may arise at any age, but the average patient is middle aged. The mean duration of symptoms prior to diagnosis varies greatly, ranging from 1 month to 12 years, although this depends to some degree on the grade of malignancy of the astrocytoma. The thoracic spine is the most frequent location in adults for spinal cord astrocytomas, whereas in children and

adolescents the cervical segments seem to be the most frequently involved.

As in the brain, spinal astrocytomas are often histologically classified from grade I to IV. The less malignant grades I and II are much more frequently encountered in the spinal cord than the higher grade III and IV lesions.

Plain films of the spine are not helpful in diagnosing spinal astrocytomas. CT scanning following the administration of intrathecal contrast medium is sensitive, but the MRI scan will demonstrate the location and extent of these tumours in great detail, including the presence of any associated cysts (Fig.9.3). Areas of contrast enhancement after intravenous administration of paramagnetic contrast medium may identify regions of active neoplastic tissue, making MRI the initial imaging procedure of choice for intramedullary neoplasms (SZE et al. 1988).

9.3.3
Ependymoma

Spinal ependymomas arise from either ependymal cells lining the central cavity or from islands of ependymal cells in the region of the filum terminale. Approximately 50% occur at the level of the cauda equina and the other 50% within the substance of the spinal cord. When the group of filum terminale and cauda equina ependymomas is excluded, the distribution of intramedullary ependymomas at the various levels of the spinal cord is approximately even, with perhaps a slight preponderance for the thoracic region. They often extend over multiple segments and may occasionally metastasize throughout the neuraxis.

Spinal ependymomas are more frequent in men than in women. Unlike the intracranial ependymomas, spinal ependymomas appear to be rare in infancy and early childhood. The average age of patients with a spinal ependymoma is approximately 40 years. The interval of time between the onset of symptoms and diagnosis varies from days to years, with a shorter time period for more malignant ependymomas. Trauma often appears to precipitate symptoms.

Plain radiographs of the spine have been reported to appear abnormal in patients with ependymoma, but the MRI scan is nowadays clearly the imaging modality of choice in the evaluation of any patient suspected of harbouring an intramedullary neoplasm (ST AMOUR et al. 1994; Fig.9.4). As ependymomas

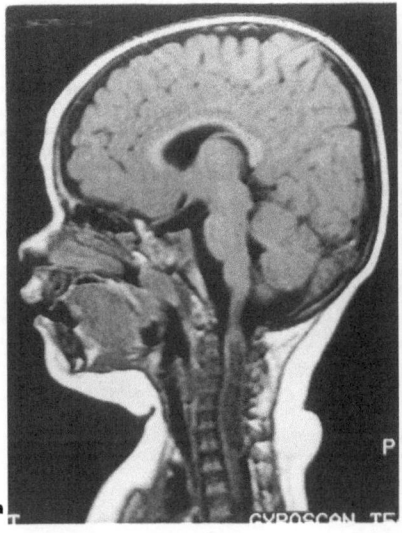 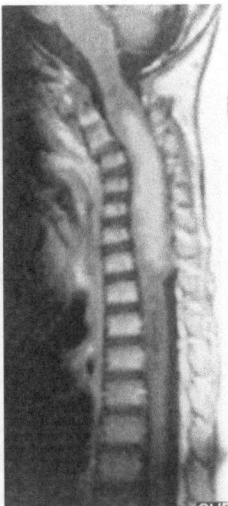

Fig. 9.3a.b. Intramedullary cervical astrocytoma in a 10-month-old-boy with nuchal pain and head tilt with torticollis. a A sagittal scout view shows abnormal enlargement of the cervical spinal cord with a low signal. b The T1-weighted image with Gd-DTPA shows an area of homogeneous enhancement surrounded by edema. Note the dislocation of C2 in relation to C3

have a tendency to seed through the CSF pathways, every patient with a spinal ependymoma should be evaluated for an intracranial ependymoma also.

9.3.4
Vascular Tumours

Vascular malformations and tumours have been estimated to account for approximately 5-10% of space-occupying lesions of the spine (BYRNE and WAXMAN 1990). The frequency of vascular malformations and tumours is not known, but vascular malformations are much more frequent than vascular tumours of the spine. A further discussion on vascular malformations is beyond the scope of this chapter. The neoplastic proliferations of the vasculature in the central and peripheral nervous system comprise the capillary *haemangioblastomas* and the *angiosarcomas*. The former constitute a well-documented entity in the spinal cord and are histologically benign; the latter are exceedingly rare (RUSSELL and RUBINSTEIN 1989).

Haemangioblastomas affect both sexes equally and are usually intramedullary. Extradural, intradural-extramedullary and intra-and extramedullary locations have been reported. The most common site seems to be the thoracic spine (almost 50%), followed by the cervical spine. In the spinal cord, the lesions are single in nearly 80% of cases (BYRNE

and WAXMAN 1990). Multiplicity of haemangioblastomas strongly suggests a genetic background of Lindau's syndrome.

Most haemangioblastomas are situated in the posterior part of the spinal cord and give rise to sensory loss and radicular pain at any early stage. With expansion of the tumour, motor symptoms and signs will develop. Spinal haemangioblastomas can remain silent throughout life and be found incidentally at autopsy.

Plain radiographs usually show no abnormalities. Myelography findings are reported to be abnormal in over 90% of cases. CT scanning may reveal a soft tissue mass with bright enhancement, and spinal angiography has been useful in the evaluation of these lesions, but MRI is the imaging modality of choice, showing clearly the nidus of the lesion and distinguishing it from the adjacent syrinx which is usually present (KAISER and RAMOS 1990) (Fig.9.5)

9.3.5
Surgical Intervention in Intramedullary Tumours

Elsberg, in 1911, developed the concept of "the extrusion of intramedullary tumours". During one of his operations he accidentally "nicked" the spinal cord when opening the dura and found that the tumour began to extrude. He closed the wound, re-operated 1 week later and achieved a gross total resection.

Nowadays, a vast array of technical equipment can assist in the safe removal of intramedullary neo-

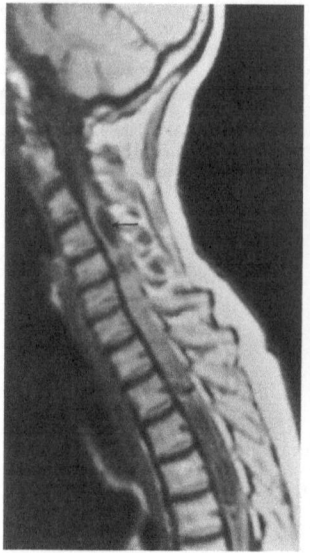
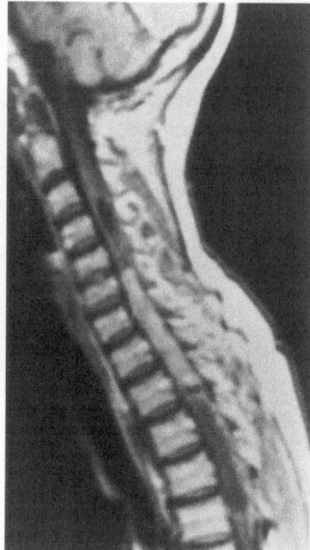

Fig. 9.4a,b. Intramedullary thoracic myxopapillary ependymoma in a 50-year-old woman with neck pain and pain in the right arm. Sagittal T1-weighted images without (a) and with (b) Gd-DTPA demonstrating enlargement of the cervical and upper thoracic spinal cord. Note the malignant intratumoral cyst (*arrow*)

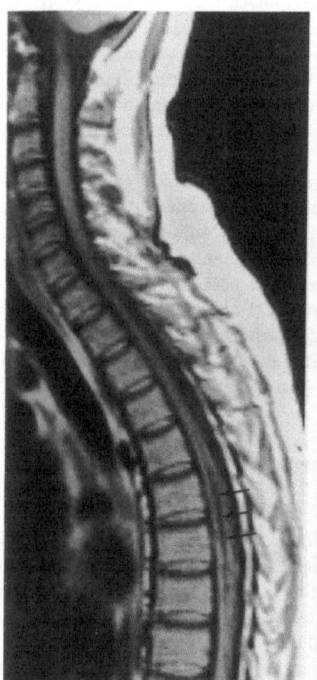
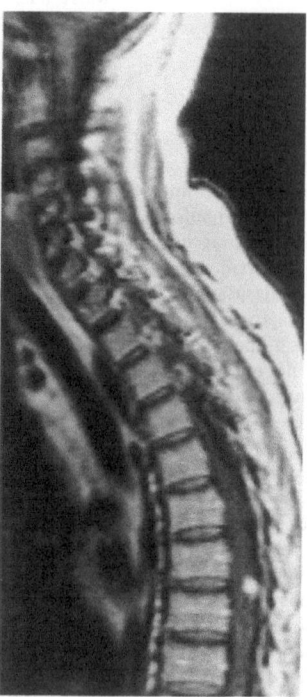

Fig. 9.5a,b. Intramedullary thoracic haemangioblastoma in a 52-year-old woman with von Hippel-Lindau disease. Sagittal T1-weighted images without (a) and with Gd-DTPA (b) demonstrating a small syrinx in the mid-thoracic spinal cord (*arrows*), with an enhancing nodule within the lower aspect of the syrinx

plasms: intraoperative neurophysiological monitoring, high-speed air drill, ultrasound scanning to help localise intramedullary tumours and establish their extent in order to avoid unnecessary bone removal or spinal cord dissection, bipolar cautery, laser and ultrasonic dissector and, last but not least, an operating microscope. Magnification and illumination provided by the operating microscope are essential for the safe removal of most intraspinal tumours: delineation of tumour from spinal cord tissue is greatly facilitated (ERICKSON 1988; EPSTEIN et al. 1990, 1993).

Following the induction of anaesthesia the patient is placed in the prone position. The posterior bony elements are removed at the appropriate level by either a laminectomy or an osteoplastic laminotomy. Intraoperative ultrasound prior to dural opening may ascertain that the rostral-caudal extent of the exposure is of sufficient length to expose the entire tumour and can delineate the site of maximum spinal cord swelling and the presence and extent of an intramedullary syrinx, when present. From now on the operating microscope is used. The dura is opened an stay sutures are placed. The spinal cord will appear swollen and pial vessels are tortuous or stretched (Fig. 9.6c).

Ependymomas characteristically form a cylindrical mass surrounded by normal spinal tissue so a clear interface can be found between the margins of the tumour and the surrounding spinal cord, often enabling the surgeon to perform a radical resection. Ependymomas are invariably adherent to the spinal cord in the region of the anterior median raphe where small branches of the anterior spinal artery enter the neoplasm (EPSTEIN et al. 1993). In cases of astrocytoma it may be far more difficult to define the tumour-spinal cord interface as astrocytomas tend to infiltrate the adjacent neural tissue. This is reflected in the far lower percentage of astrocytomas that can be radically resected (Fig. 9.7). In the presence of rostral or caudal cysts associated with an intramedullary neoplasm, the dissection in facilitated as the interface between tumour and normal spinal cord can be more easily identified. This is particularly the case in haemangioblastomas. After opening the cyst, one usually can see the protruding, cherry-red lesion attached to the wall of the cyst. Bipolar coagulation, facilitated by isotonic mannitol irrigation, will readily shrink the tumour, which is then easily completely removed (SAKATANI et al. 1995).

After resection, primary dural closure usually presents no problem as the intradural content is greatly reduced. Conventional closure of the wound in layers will lead to primary wound healing in virtually all patients.

9.3.6
The Utrecht Experience with Intramedullary Tumours

9.3.6.1
Patients and Methods

Forty-nine patients with an intramedullary tumour underwent surgery in the University Hospital and Wilhelmina Children's Hospital , Utrecht, The Netherlands, from 1981 to 1994. Of these, 45 patients (24 women and 21 men) had a primary intramedullary neoplasm. Age at diagnosis varied from 3 to 75 years (mean 45 years). The mean duration of symptoms at the time of surgery varied from 1 month to 12 years (mean 36 months).

Neurological function of upper and lower extremities was assessed both pre-and postoperatively, as well as 6 months postoperatively, according to the scale of COOPER and EPSTEIN (1985; Table 9.2).

Table 9.2. Grading according to COOPER and EPSTEIN (1985)

Arms
Grade 0: intact
Grade 1: sensory symptoms only
Grade 2: mild motor deficit with some functional impairment
Grade 3: major functional impairment in at least one arm but arms useful for simple tasks
Grade 4: no movement or flicker of movement in arms: no useful function

Legs
Grade 0: intact
Grade 1: walks independently but not normally
Grade 2: walks but needs cane or walker
Grade 3: stands but cannot walk
Garde 4: slight movement but cannot stand or walk
Grade 5: paralysis

9.3.6.2
Results

Histologically, the tumours were classified as follows: 17 ependymomas, 13 astrocytomas, 7 haemangioblastomas, 3 (epi)dermoid cysts and 1 ganglioglioma. In four patients a histopathological diagno-

W.P. Vandertop, L.M.P. Ramos, and C.A.F. Tulleken

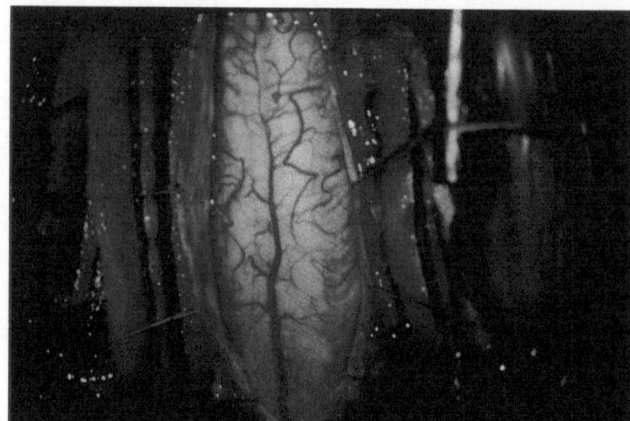

Fig. 9.6. a Operative view of the swollen cervical spinal cord in a 10-month-old boy (see also Fig.9.3). Note the tortuous and stretched pial vessels. b The same patient after midline myelotomy and pial traction sutures. c The same patient after gross total resection of the astrocytoma

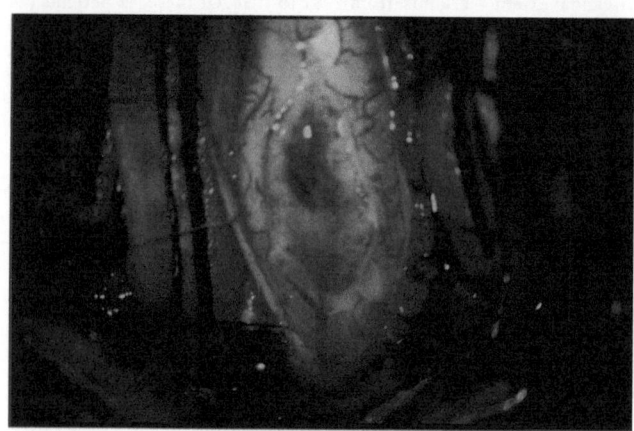

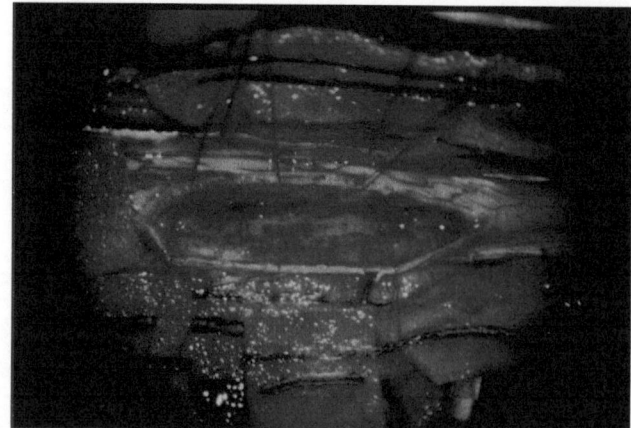

Fig. 9.7a,b. A 30-year-old woman with long-standing history of neck pain and slowly progressive sensibility loss and weakness of the right arm. **a** A preoperative sagittal T1-weighted image after Gd-DTPA administration demonstrates an enlarged spinal cord from C1 downwards, with extensive syrinx formation. Bright tumour enhancement is visible behind C2-4 and at the level of the foramen magnum. **b** A postoperative T1-weighted image after Gd-DTPA of the same patient after total resection of the tumour at the C2-4 level, but with residual tumour at C1 (*arrow*). The associated syrinx has completely collapsed

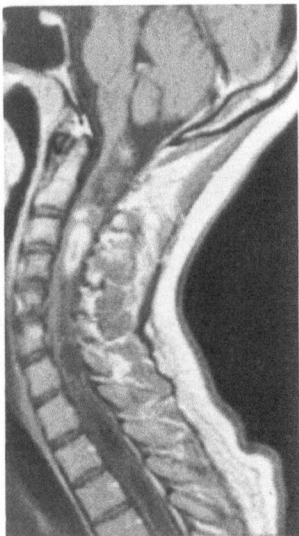

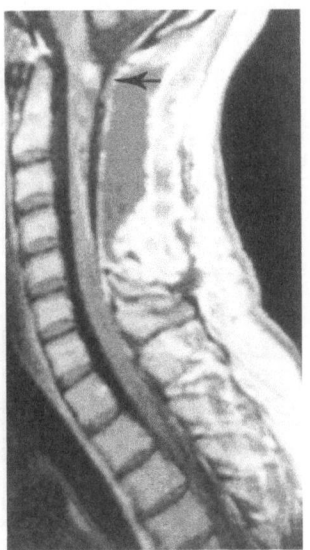

a

b

sis could not be made. The tumours were located in the cervical spine in 13 patients, cervicothoracic in 5 patients, thoracic in 15 patients and in the conus medullaris in 12 patients. In 20 of the 45 patients, cysts, extending cranially and/or caudally to the tumour, were found: in eight ependymomas, five astrocytomas, four haemangioblastomas and all three (epi)dermoids.

In 37 (82%) patients a total (23) or subtotal (14) resection could be performed. Total resection proved possible in 12/17 ependymomas (71%) in 3/13 astrocytomas (23%), in all seven haemangioblastomas and in 1 dermoid cyst. The surgical mortality was 0%. Three patients died within 6 month after the operation, and three patients were lost to long-term follow-up.

After the operation the neurological function of the *legs* in 32 patients had either improved (8) or remained unchanged (24; Fig 9.8). In 13 patients a deterioration had occurred, which proved temporary in 7 patients. After 6 months, neurological function could be assessed in 38 patients: in 32 this had either improved (12) or remained unchanged (20). In 6 patients the function of the legs had slightly deteriorated (Fig. 9.8a).

After the operation of a cervical or cervicothoracic tumour the neurological function of the *arms* in 15 of the 18 patients had either improved (12) or remained unchanged (3; Fig. 9.8b). In 3 patients a deterioration had occurred. After 6 months,

neurological function could be assessed in 16 patients: in 14 this had either improved (12) or remained unchanged (2). In 2 patients the function of the arms had slightly deteriorated compared to preoperatively (Fig. 9.8b).

Of the three patients who died within 6 months after the operation, one died as a result of an extensive obligodendroglioma with leptomeningeal seeding to cauda equina and brain stem. Another patient harboured a cervical astrocytoma leading to progressive ascending paralysis and respiratory insufficiency. The third patient died of internal causes unrelated to the spinal cord tumour.

In four patients a recurrent tumour developed, leading to progressive symptoms. The time between the first operation and the recurrence of tumour growth varied from 1 to 3 years. One patient with a subtotally resected ependymoma developed a recurrence after 3 years. The other three patients had an astrocytoma which recurred after 1, 2 and 3 years, respectively.

9.3.7
Outcome

The clinical picture after the operation is very much determined by the severity of the neurological deficit before the operation. If the neurological deficit before the operation is severe, a significant improve-

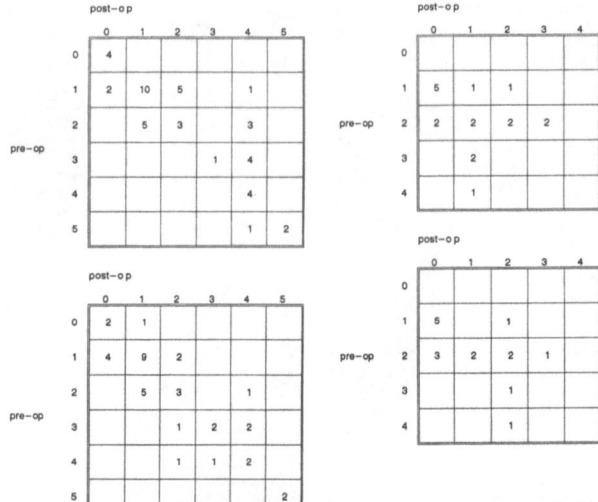

Fig. 9.8. a The relationship between preoperative and postoperative neurological function of the legs in 45 patients. The top diagram represents function directly postoperatively; the bottom diagram represents function 6 months after the operation. The numbers represent patients in each category. For functional grades see Table 9.2. **b** The relationship between preoperative and postoperative (6 months) neurological function of the arms in 38 patients. The top diagram represents the function directly postoperatively; the bottom diagram represents the function 6 months after the operation. The numbers represent patients in each category. For functional grades, see Table 9.2

ment is seldom achieved. Patients with only few neurological symptoms tolerate surgery well. Immediately after the operation a slight deterioration can be seen, especially of the function of the posterior columns, but this is often temporary.

The morbidity associated with the operation is strongly related to the segment of the spinal cord involved. Lesions in the conus medullaris usually lead to permanent loss of function. The relatively high content of grey matter in the conus probably accounts for its vulnerability to surgical manipulation. Operations on intramedullary tumours in the cervical spinal cord are better tolerated than previously thought and appear far less dangerous than resection in the lower thoracic segments. This is probably explained by the fact that the cervical cord contains a much higher percentage of white matter, which is much less vulnerable to surgical insults.

The clinical course after total resection is better than the natural course of a non-operated low-grade astrocytoma. It remains unclear whether the clinical course after total resection is also better than after subtotal resection. Controversy still exists over the question of whether radiotherapy is beneficial after subtotal resection (CONSTANTINI et al. 1994; MOTTOLESE et al. 1994; O'SULLIVAN et al. 1994). With or without radiotherapy, the natural course of low-grade astrocytomas remains very unpredictable (SANDLER et al. 1992). However, it must be clearly stated that there is no place for radiotherapy without

a histological diagnosis (BROTCHI et al. 1991). If the histological diagnosis is high-grade glioma, the prognosis in terms of morbidity and mortality is very poor, even in the short term, regardless of whether a total or subtotal resection has been performed, or whether radiotherapy is given (EPSTEIN et al. 1992).

Based on our own experience and the recent literature, it seems justified to be intent on performing a primary, radical microsurgical resection of intramedullary neoplasms in patients with *progressive* neurological symptoms and signs. If total, or subtotal, resection of a low-grade glioma has been achieved, postoperative radiotherapy seems to be warranted in only a few selected cases. If the tumour recurs, one may again try for a radical resection, this time often followed by radiotherapy. The key to success is to operate on patients before there is significant neurological deficit.

However, in patients with little or no progressive neurological deficit there is no absolute indication for operation. The decision to operate is based on the localisation and extent of the tumour, the age of the patient, the clinical symptoms and signs and the presumed diagnosis. Especially if one expects a haemangioblastoma or an (epi)dermoid cyst, operation will be strongly considered, as a radical resection will usually lead to complete cure. In the case of a suspected, or even histologically proven, low-grade glioma with little or no neurological deficit, the physician will have to decide for each individual patient between the feasibility and the desirability of a radical resection. An important factor in this is the personal experience of the surgeon.

References

Biller J, Brazis PW (1990) The localization of lesions affecting the spinal cord. In: Brazis PW, Masdeu JC, Biller J (eds) Localization in clinical neurology. Little, Brown, Boston, pp 69-92

Brotchi J, Dewitte O, Levivier M, Balériaux D, Vandesteene A, Raftopoulos C, Flament-Durand J, Noterman J (1991) A survey of 65 tumours within the spinal cord: surgical results and the importance of preoperative magnetic resonance imaging. Neurosurgery 29:651-657

Byrne TN, Waxman SG (1990) Spinal cord compression: diagnosis and principles of managment. Davis, Philadelphia

Constantini S, Ozek M, Nouten J, Freed D, Shiminski-Maher T, Miller D, Rorke L, Allen J, Epstein F (1994) Intramedullary spinal cord tumours in the first three years of life. Childs Nerv 10:482-483

Cooper PR (1989) Outcome after operative treatment of intramedullary spinal cord tumors in adults: intermediate and long-term results in 51 patients. Neurosurgery 25:855-859

Cooper PR, Epstein F (1985) Radical resection of intramedullary spinal cord tumors in adults. Neurosurg 63:492-499

Donner TR, Voorhies RM, Kline DG (1994) Neural sheath tumours of major nerves. Neurosurgery 81:362-373

van Duijnen MTA (1971) The intramedullary neurinoma. (in Dutch) Ned Tijdschr Geneesd 115:1070-1074

Elsberg CA (1925) Tumours of the spinal cord and the symptoms of irritation and compression of the spinal cord and the nerve roots: pathology, symptomatology, diagnosis and treatment. Hoeber, New York

Epstein FJ, Lassoff S, Wisoff JH, Allen JC, Freed D (1990) Primary intramedullary spinal cord tumour in children: the long-term follow-up. Neurosurg 72:358A

Epstein FJ, Farmer J-P, Freed D (1992) Adult intramedullary astrocytomas of the spinal cord. J Neurosurg 77:355-359

Epstein FJ, Farmer J-P, Freed D (1993) Adult intramedullary spinal cord ependymomas: the result of surgery in 38 patients. J Neurosurg 79:204-209

Erickson DL (1988) Recognition and surgical treatment of spinal cord tumours. In: Akbarnia BA (ed) Spine state of the art reviews: spinal tumours. Hanley and Belfus, Philadelphia, pp 313-324

Fogelholm R, Uutela T, Murros K (1984) Epidemiology of central nervous system neoplasms. A regional survey in central Finland. Acta Neurol Scand 69:129

Giuffrè R (1966) Intradural spinal lipomas: review of the literature (99 cases) and report of an additional case. Acta Neurochir (Wien) 14:69-95

Greenwood JJR (1963) Intramedullary tumours of the spinal cord. A follow-up study after total surgical removal. J Neurosurg 20:665-668

Guidetti B, Fortuna A (1975) Differential diagnosis of intramedullary and extramedullary tumours. In: Vinken PJ, Bruyn GW (eds) Handbook of clinical neurology, vol 19. North Holland, Amsterdam, pp 51-75

Guidetti B, Mercuri S, Vagnozzi R (1981) Long-term results of the surgical treatment of 129 intramedullary spinal gliomas. J Neurosurg 54:323-330

Kaiser MC, Ramos LMP (1990) MRI of the spine. Thieme, New York, pp 117-119

Kepes JJ (1982) Meningiomas. Biology, pathology and differential diagnosis. Masson, New York

Levy WJ, Bay J, Dohn D (1982) Spinal cord meningioma. J Neurosurg 57:804-812

List CF (1941) Intraspinal epidermoids, dermoids, and dermal sinuses. Surg Gynecol Obstet 73:525-538

Malis LI (1977) Intramedullary spinal cord tumours. Clin Neurosurg 25:512-539

Mottolese C, Pierre-Kahn A, Choux M, Roche JL, Marchal JC, Delhemmes P, Tremoulet M, Stilhart B, Chazal J, Caillaud P, Ravon R, Passagia JG, Bouffet E (1994) Spinal cord astrocytomas: a retrospective multicenter study of 60 cases. Childs Nerv Syst 10:483

O'Sullivan C, Jenkin RD, Doherty MA, Hoffman HJ, Greenberg ML (1994) Spinal cord tumours in children: long-term results of combined surgical and radiation treatment. J Neurosurg 81:507-512

Pierre-Kahn A, Lacombe J, Pichon J, Giudicelli Y, Renier D, Sainte-Rose C, Perrigot M, Hirsch J-F (1986) Intraspinal lipomas with spina bifida. Prognosis and treatment in 73 cases. J Neurosurg 65:756

Raimondi AJ, Guterriez FA, DiRocco C (1976) Laminotomy and total reconstruction of the posterior spinal arch for spinal canal surgery in childhood. J Neurosurg 45:555

Russell DS, Rubinstein LJ (1989) Pathology of tumours of the nervous system. Williams and Wilkins, Baltimore

Sakatani K, Ohtaki M, Morimoto S, Hashi K (1995) Isotonic mannitol and the prevention of local heat generation and tissue adherence to bipolar diathermy forceps during electrical coagulation. Neurosurg 82:669-671

Sandler HM, Papadopoulos SM, Thornton AF, Ross DA (1992) Spinal cord astrocytomas: results of therapy. Neurosurgery 30:490-493

Scott RM, Wolpert SM, Barthoshesky LE, Zimbler S, Klaubert GT (1986) Dermoid tumours occuring at the site of previous myelomeningocele repair. J Neurosurg 65:779

Slooff JL, Kernohan JW, MacCarty CS (1964) Primary intramedullary tumours of the spinal cord and filum terminale. Saunders, Philadelphia

St Amour TE, Hodges SC, Laakman RW (1994) MRI of the spine. Raven, New York, pp 305-315

Steck JC, Dietze DD, Fessler RG (1994) Posterolateral approach to intradural extramedullary thoracic tumours. J Neurosurg 81:202-205

Stein BM (1979) Surgery of intramedullary spinal cord tumours. Clin Neurosurg 26:529-542

Stein BM (1983) Intramedullary spinal cord tumours. Clin Neurosurg 30:717-741

Sze G, Krol G, Zimmerman RD, Deck MDF (1988) Intramedullary disease of the spne: diagnosis using gadolinium-DTPA-enhanced MR imaging. Am Neuroradiol 9:847-858

Vandertop WP, Wanroij van JL, Rosenberg WWJ, Tulleken CAF (1991) Resection as treatment for spinal intramedullary tumours. (in Dutch) Ned Tijdschr Geneesd 135:664-668

Yasargil MG (1970) Surgery of vascular lesions of the spinal cord with the microsurgical technique. Clin Neurosurg 17:257-265

Yasargil MG, Antic J, Laciga R, Preux de J, Fideler RW, Boone SC (1976) The microsurgical removal of intramedullary spinal hemangioblastomas: report of twelve cases and review of the literature. Surg Neurol 6:141-148

Yasuoka S, Peterson HA, MacCarty CS (1982) Incidence of spinal column deformity after multilevel laminectomy in children and adults. J Neurosurg 57:441

10 Current Concepts in Radiation Therapy of Spinal Tumours

J.W.H. LEER

CONTENTS

10.1
Introduction

Basically, there are two types of spinal cord malignancy for which radiotherapy is indicated: secondary deposits, which are the more frequent, and primary spinal cord tumours, which are very rare.

The incidence of primary spinal cord tumours ranges from 0,8 to 2.5 per 100.000 population (FOGELHOLM et al. 1984).

With respect to radiation oncology the spinal cord gliomas are the most important, accounting for about 20-25% of the primary spinal cord tumours (WHITAKER et al. 1991; BRADA and THOMAS 1995).

The most important spinal cord gliomas are ependymomas and astrocytomas. In most recent publications it is quoted that 50-60 % of the intramedullary spinal cord gliomas are ependymomas, the rest being astrocytomas. A special type of ependymoma, the myxopapillary ependymoma, is an extramedullary but still intradural lesion which originates from the cauda equina (WEN et al. 1991).

Most metastatic tumours are extradural. In this chapter we will, firstly, discuss the role of radiotherapy in the treatment of primary spinal cord tumours and, secondly , its importance in metastatic disease.

J.W.H. LEER, MD, Department of Clinical Oncology, University Hospital Leiden, P.O. Box 9600, Rijnsburgweg 10, 2300 Leiden, The Netherlands

10.2
Primary Spinal Cord Tumours

10.2.1
Ependymomas

Ependymomas are the most frequent pimary spinal cord tumours. The cellular-type ependymoma is an intramedullary tumour. The myxopapillary type is a low-grade tumour typical of the cauda equina, arising from the conus medullaris or filum terminale.

The primary treatment of these tumours is surgery. It is generally accepted that an attempt to do a complete en bloc resection is justified, but not at the expense of severe neurological deficit.

About half of the intramedullary ependymomas can be completely removed using modern microsurgical techniques (CHUN et al. 1990; BRADA and THOMAS 1995). In other, usually small, selected series the complete resection rate is lower (WEN et al. 1991), especially when these cellular ependymomas involve several segments of the cord. Most low-grade myxopapillary ependymomas can also be completely resected; however, growth around the nerve roots can prohibit a radical resection in this type of tumour, too.

With improving imaging and microsurgical techniques, the number of patients in whom a complete resection can be obtained will increase, and the role of postoperative radiotherapy in these patients must be questioned (McCORMICK et al. 1990; EPSTEIN et al. 1993). However, whenever a resection is incomplete or performed in a piecemeal fashion, postoperative radiotherapy is indicated.

It is generally accepted that, with postoperative irradiation, reasonably good survival and local control rates can be obtained. However, it is difficult to obtain a firm figure with respect to local control using postoperative irradiation because the published series are small, the tumours differ in histology, grade and size and also the surgical procedures are different. Nevertheless, the general picture is that a relapse-free or progression-free survival of about 70-80% at 5 years is to be expected (SHAW et al. 1986; LINDSTADT et al. 1989; WALDRON et al. 1993).

It is important to note that in almost all reports 10-year relapse-free survival rates are lower than the 5-year surviaval rates and even after 10 years incidental recurrences can still be observed. But most recurrences are seen within 3 years of initial treatment (WALDRON et al. 1993) and most curves tend to plateau, which indicates that radiotherapy can potentially control residual tumour.

The effectiveness of radiotherapy in this tumour type can also be concluded from reports of irradiation given following a diagnostic biopsy only, after which no relapses were seen (SHAW et al. 1986; WEN et al. 1991).

Several factors have been suggested to be of prognostic value for the local control rate, of which the most important seem to be extent of surgery, histological subtype and grade.

Of all these factors WEN et al. (1991) found that piecemeal removal of the tumour had the worst prognosis. Six out of 14 patients who underwent this treatment had a relapse. The authors especially observed a higher reccurence rate after this procedure in the thecal sac owing to drop metastases. Patients with myxopapillary subtype in general do better than those with the cellular type, but this probably also reflects the fact that the myxopapillary type is low grade and en bloc resection is more likely to be possible. However, not all reports show favourable outcome of myxopapillary ependymoma. In a small series described by CLOVER et al. (1993) half of the patients had a recurrence. A similar observation was made by SHAW et al. (1986).

The recurrence rate of intermediate or poorly differentiated ependymomas seems to be higher than that of the well-differentiated low grade tumours, for which reason WALDRON et al. (1993) advocate postoperative irradiation even after a so-called en bloc complete resection.

The target volume for radiotherapy is a subject for some debate but it is now generally accepted that it can be limited to the area of the tumour bed with a margin. Some authors advocate a margin of 1-2 cm, others of two vertebral bodies. This need for larger margins is based on the growth pattern (more diffuse) of the tumour and the precision with which the tumour (bed) can be identified by surgery, myelography or MRI. Following piecemeal resection, drop metastases to the thecal sac can be expected, and thecal sac irradiation is recommended by WEN

et al. (1991) where this procedure has been used. The main reason for not advocating larger target volumes or even total craniospinal irradiation is the observation that almost all recurrences are seen within the treatment field, which means that improving local control should be the most important objective and not the elective treatment of the whole craniospinal axis. There might be one exception to this rule, namely the rare anaplastic subtype ependymoma which might have a higher tendency for intracranial spread. WALDRON et al. (1993) had four such cases in a large series from the Princess Margaret Hospital in Toronto, Canada, and two of these four patients had cranial relapses, for which reason these authors advocate total craniospinal irradiation for this subtype.

The radiation dose advised by most authors is about 45-50 Gy, a dose which has an acceptable low risk of radiation myelitis.

A clear dose-response relationship could not be found by most authors because of the small numbers of patients in their series. However, there is a suggestion that lower doses are less effective and higher doses could still further reduce the local recurrence rate. SHAW et al. (1986) therefore recommend a slightly higher dose of 55 Gy. They suggest 50 Gy be applied to a large field and a boost of 5 Gy to the lesion only. The generally recommended fraction size is 1.5-1.8 Gy to be given five times a week. The fraction size should not exceed 2 Gy.

10.2.2
Astrocytomas

About 40-50% of the spinal gliomas are astrocytomas. They grow, in contrast to the ependymomas, more diffusely and are therefore less likely to be resected completely, although some authors claim complete resection in these cases also. There also is a great tendency in these tumours to grow at more than one site or more diffusely along the cord. As in brain, astrocytomas of the spinal cord can be graded and, although most are low grade, the highly anaplastic multiform glioblastoma can also be found in the spinal cord (LINDSTADT et al. 1989).

When complete resection of these tumours is impossible without hampering neurological function of the patient, the treatment of choice consists mostly of a biopsy or limited resection followed by postoperative irradiation. Because of the rarity of the tumour and consequently the few and small series found in the literature, the results of this treatment approach and the role of radiotherapy are even less well established than in the case of ependymomas.

LINDSTADT et al. (1989) describe a series of 15 astrocytomas. The relapse-free survival of the 12 patients with low-grade tumours was 66% at 5 years and 53% at 10 and 15 years. All failures (33%) were seen in the initially irradiated volume. The three patients with the highly anaplastic type tumour died within 1 year after diagnosis, all with a local recurrence and 2 with diffuse craniospinal axis metastases. CHUN et al. (1990) report 16 astrocytomas. The relapse-free survival at 5 years was 40% and at 10 years 25%. This is substantially worse than 80% relapse-free survival at 5 years of their patients with ependymomas. Nine of the 16 patients suffered a relapse, all inside the irradiated area, and there was no evidence of intracranial spread. Finally, HUDDART et al. (1993) describe a rather large series of 27 patients with spinal cord astrocytomas treated in the Royal Marsden Hospital in Sutton, UK. Eleven patients had histological eight grade I, grade II and six grade III or IV. Two had an unknown grading.

The progression-free survival at 5 years was 38% and at 10 years, 26%. The survival with low-grade tumours was better but there was no difference in progression-free survival, suggesting, according to the authors, a better salvage probability for the low grades. Therapy in 5 out of 16 patients with recurrent disease outside the initial treatment field failed; 3 of these patients had high-grade tumours.

Thus, it seems in general that the prognosis of spinal cord astrocytomas is worse than that of ependymomas. High-grade tumours especially have a bad outlook, mostly with a survival of less than 1 year. High-grade tumours also have a higher tendency to give rise to intracranial metastases. The contribution of radiotherapy to the treatment is difficult to prove. That radiotherapy at least gives a temporary disease control is, however, suggested by the reported local control rates and, especially, by the neurological improvement of patients after irradiation (HUDDART et al. 1993).

However, one can question the role of radiotherapy in the treatment of these tumours; as in brain gliomas the effect of radiotherapy for the low grades has not yet been conclusively proved, while the aggressive nature, in spite of radiotherapy, of the high-grade tumours could also be an argument against their treatment.

Nevertheless, most institutes nowadays still tend to irradiate the spinal cord astrocytomas.

As in ependymomas the target volume comprises the primary lesion with a margin of 2-4 cm.

Although these tumours, especially the high grades, have a high risk of dissemination, craniospinal radiotherapy is usually not recommended because its value is not proven and most if not all reccurences are found in the initally treated volume. The recommended dose is mostly 50 Gy using the same fraction size of 1.5-1.8 Gy in spinal cord ependymomas.

10.2.3
Other Primary Spinal Cord Tumours

There exists a variety of other primary spinal tumours, mostly extramedullary and extradural in which the role of radiotherapy is even less well established than in the case of ependymomas and astrocytomas. They include schwannomas, meningiomas and for example haemangioblastomas. These tumours are usually treated with surgical resection and not irradiated. As in the treatment of incompletely resected cranial meningiomas, postoperative irradiation can also be considered in the ones with a spinal localization, especially in case of a recurrence. The same is true for the other tumours. However, the dose to be given is high and close to spinal cord tolerance, and the possible advantages should be balanced against the risk of tumour induction and late radiation damage to the spinal cord. There are no studies available to indicate more precisely what the contribution of postoperative radiotherapy in these tumours could be.

10.3
Vertebral Metastases

A substantial percentage of cancer patients will develop bone metastases. Values ranging from 20-80% can be found in the literature depending on the selection of tumour types. Tumour types which most frequently spread to the bone are lung cancer, breast cancer and prostate cancer, bladder, cervix and colon cancer and malignant melanomas also can give rise to bone metastases.

Bone metastases are very frequently seen in the vertebrae. They can be lytic or blastic, e.g. in prostate cancer. Also, in the absence of severe destruction and collapse of the bone with nerve root compression, they can cause severe pain. In case of destruction and collapse, typical radiating pain will occur as a sign of nerve root compression and, eventually, destruction or growth of a soft tissue component of the metastases can lead to spinal cord compression.

There exists no doubt about the potential of radiotherapy in the palliative treatment of bone metastases and prevention of further destruction leading to cord compression.

Mostly, pain relief after irradiation is observed very quickly and can be partly or completely achieved in 60-80% of the patients, which is probably the result of an effect on the production of prostaglandins and bradykinins.

Recalcification of lytic lesions is observed after about 2 months and normalisation of the bone structure, of course in the absence of a collapse or fracture, takes about 6 months.

When no pain relief is achieved, one should consider a mechanical course due to instability of the spinal column or compression by bony fragments. Orthopaedic surgery, if possible, could be necessary in such cases in order to obtain an acceptable level of pain relief.

Although the average survival of patients with bone metastases is relatively short, with some tumour types, e.g. breast cancer and kidney cancer, many years of survival are not exceptional, because of effective systematic treatment or the natural course of the disease.

Partly for this reason, there is still debate in the literature about the optimal treatment schedule for radiotherapy for bone metastases.

The general rule in palliative treatment is that the best treatment is that which is short but effective for the expected life span of the patient and has the fewest side effects.

Several randomised studies have shown that short radiotherapy schedules, e.g. ten times 3 Gy, five times 4 Gy and five times 5 Gy are equally effective with respect to the incidence and duration of pain relief. A large study from the UK indicated that one fraction of 8 Gy was as effective as ten times 3 Gy. However, follow-up of the patients in these studies and their survival was limited. Thus, there is still doubt as to whether a single fraction or a low total dose will be effective enough for patients with a more favourable outlook.

The dilemma presented by these patients is obvious, either one applies a high dose close to spinal cord tolerance which might prevent the necessity of re-treating the same spot (which would be dangerous due to the limited repair capacity of the cord after these high doses) or one applies a low dose and accepts the possible necessity of re-treatment, which would be less dangerous because the repair chances of the cord would be more favourable.

Several large studies are presently underway to find an answer to these questions.

In our institution, we are inclined to treat patients with a favourable outlook with high doses in small fractions, e.g. 40-50 Gy with fractions of 2 Gy.

Because of the limited spinal cord tolerance, overlap of treated volumes for metastases at different levels of the spine should be avoided. Careful counting of vertebrae and documentation of areas already treated is therefore extremely important.

If one is applying treatment with one dorsal field, the dose should be specified at the depth of the spinal cord in order to prevent unwittingly exposing the cord to too high a dose with too high fractions. For the same reason, one should not use an opposed technique with specification of the dose in the middle of the body, giving only one portal a day.

10.3.1
Secondary Tumours Affecting the Spinal Cord

Tumours most frequently causing spinal cord compression are metastases of other primaries. Mostly these primaries are lung, prostate and breast cancer. In some series also lymphoproliferative tumours are found at a high frequency (LEVIOV et al. 1993). Other primaries can also cause spinal cord compression. Although bone metastases in the vertebral body are very frequent in metastatic disease, only about 5-15% of patients with systemic cancer will develop spinal cord compression. If untreated, almost all patients with spinal cord compression due to metastatic disease will become paraplegic and the treatment of this complication is considered to be one of the few emergencies in radiation oncology.

The thoracic spine is the most frequent site of compression, followed by lumbar and cervical compression. Cauda equina compression at the sacral level is very uncommon.

Patients are considered to have spinal cord compression if they have neurological symptoms. However, some authors advise further investigation with myelography, CT or MRI in patients with back pain and a positive bone scan or osteolytic lesions in the vertebral corpora but without neurological symptoms. This approach leads to an overestimation of the incidence of spinal cord compression. MARANZANO et al. (1992) found signs of spinal cord compression on myelography and

MRI in 38% of their patients with only pain and vertebral lysis. We are not in the habit of performing these diagnostic procedures in patients with only back pain and osteolytic metastases. Most of these patients, however, are irradiated according to conventional schedules and only seldom does their disease progress before the end of treatment to a clinical manifest cord compression.

Because some retrospective studies (GILBERT et al. 1978; GREENBERG and KIM 1988; SHAPIRO and POSNER 1983) and a prospective study (YOUNG et al. 1980) indicated that radiotherapy was as effective as laminectomy with or without postoperative radiotherapy, most centres nowadays use radiotherapy as the first treatment option in spinal cord compression. Surgery is only considered in case of a doubtful diagnosis, compression at a previously irradiated site, progression of neurological symptoms during irradiation and evidence of "bony impingement" of the spine (MARANZANO et al. 1991). Vertebral body collapse in itself is no reason for surgery. Finally, surgery can also be considered in relatively radioresistant tumours, e.g. melanoma, renal cell carcinoma and sarcoma (BRADA and THOMAS 1995). It is mostly recommended that the irradiation starts as soon as possible, in any case within 24h after the diagnosis has been established. When the clinical diagnosis is suspected, corticosteroids are administered, although there is no agreement about the dose. To obtain a rapid and sufficient cell kill in order to obtain a quick reduction of the compression, most radiotherapy schedules start with a few large fractions of 4 or 5 Gy. GREENBERG and KIM (1988) proposed a regimen starting with three times 5 Gy, to be continued after a 4-day rest with another five fractions of 3 Gy (total dose 30 Gy). We use three times 4 Gy, to be continued after 1 or 2 days with seven times 2.5 Gy (total dose 29.5 Gy).

Although not substantiated by the literature so far, it might well be that one fraction of 8 Gy as used in the treatment of bone metastases without spinal cord compression is as useful as three fractions of 5 Gy on 3 consecutive days, at least for pain relief (PODD et al. 1992). The use of large fractions, however, bears the disadvantage that re-treatment with radiotherapy at the same site becomes more difficult because repair of radiation damage to the cord is less likely and the biologically effective dose comes closer to the tolerance dose, above which spinal cord damage can be expected. For patients with a relatively fair outlook, therefore, one has to balance the advantage of a possibly quick reaction using a large fraction size against the disadvantage of exhausting the tolerance for radiation of the cord. Although the prognosis for most patients with spinal cord compression is bad, only 30% survive more than 1 year (MARANZANO et al. 1992) and the median survival in some series is even less than 3 months (PODD 1994), 29% of the patients with breast cancer in the series of Maranzano and co-workers had a survival probability of 3 years. So the fraction size has to take into account the need for speed, the prognosis of the patient and the expected sensitivity of the tumour. Large fraction sizes, therefore, are also considered unnecessary in (very) radiosensitive tumours, e.g. seminoma, lymphoproliferative tumours, Ewing's sarcoma and small lung cancers.

As in other bone metastases pain relief after irradiation is achieved in about 80% of the patients. Good or complete pain relief is observed in 60-70%. Apart from pain relief, however, functional improvement is the main aim of this treatment. About 50-70% of the patients with neurological motor deficits retain or regain the ability to walk with or without support. Most patients who are fully ambulatory at the time of diagnosis maintain ambulation. About 74% of the paraparetic patients in the series of MARANZANO et al. (1992) became ambulatory. In other series, however, only about 30% of non-ambulant paraparetic patients became ambulant (SÖRENSEN et al. 1990; LEVIOV et al. 1993). This difference is probably due to differences in patient selection and the definition of paraparesis. Patients with complete paraplegia seldom improve. Whatever the percentages of recovery are, it is clear from the literature that early treatment, before the patients become paraplegic, is mandatory because the degree of neurological impairment is the most important prognostic factor for the final outcome of the treatment. Also speed seems to be warranted because if the paralysis lasts for several hours the chances of recovery are poor.

However, if the compression of the cord is induced slowly, also a slow recovery from total paralysis can be expected, perhaps because the pathogenesis of a slowly progressive cord compression is different from a rapidly progressive compression (HELWEG-LARSEN et al. 1990). Also of interest is the effect of immediate radiotherapy on urinary dysfunction. About two thirds of the patients in the series of Maranzano no longer needed an indwelling catheter. This can be considered to be a very important palliative achievement because it facilitates the care of the patients and improves the quality of life even if the survival is short. The good palliative result of radiotherapy for cord compression is finally also illustrated by the fact that the relief of neurological symptoms mostly lasts until the time of death.

Special attention should be paid to spinal cord compression caused by ingrowth into the spinal canal of a paravertebral mass. This is mostly seen at the level of T1-6 by apical lung tumours and at the level of L1-5 by e.g. lymphomas and kidney tumours. It is found in approximately 10-15% of the patients with spinal cord compression (KIM et al. 1993). The outcome of these patients is usually less favourable than of patients without such a mass from lung cancer and an early recurrence of symptoms after treatment is often seen.

Because of the large tumour burden we, like others, tend to give these patients a higher dose (close to spinal cord tolerance), especially when they have a reasonably good general condition and no signs of distant metastases.

10.4
Radiotherapeutic Considerations

The spinal cord is considered to be a relatively sensitive structure for so-called late radiation damage and most radiation oncologists wish to avoid radiation myelitis at any price. The dose-response curve for spinal cord injury is steep, which means that a small increment in dose or fraction size leads to a substantial increase in the probability of spinal cord damage. Based on clinical and experimental data the tolerance dose of the spinal cord is mostly considered to be about 50 Gy using a conventional fractionation up to 2 Gy. At this level the incidence of myelopathy is probably less than 1% and the dose at which a 5% incidence of myelopathy can be expected is probably in the range between 55 and 60 Gy (BRADA and THOMAS 1995). However, most clinicans are very reluctant to surpass the clinically accepted threshold dose of 50 Gy.

How much can be gained by using even smaller fractions than 1.5 or 1.8 Gy is not yet clear. Some additional increase in tolerance can be expected owing to a larger cellular repair between the fractions, but the extent to which the total dose can be raised using this so-called hyperfractionation is not yet known. It might be worthwhile to test the tolerance of the spinal cord using smaller fraction sizes because, if the total dose could be raised, a better local control, especially of the primary spinal cord tumours, could be expected.

The spine is surrounded by other vulnerable structures, such as lung tissue at the thoracic part and by the kidneys and intestines at the lumbar level.

Before high-dose irradiation is given, the dose distribution in the surrounding tissues also should be carefully calculated. The treatment setup for primary spinal cord tumours is therefore especially critical. Opposed parallel anterior-posterior fields have the disadvantage of irradiating heart or stomach and small intestines above their tolerance level. Late cardiac toxicity and fatal ulcera could be the result. When oblique wedged fields are used the dose in the hilum or kidneys can become too high, using one dorsal field has the disadvantage of a dose inhomogeneity throughout the target volume and bears the risk of a high total dose given with too large fractions in the cord if the dose is specified at the wrong depth. Thus, careful computer planning, preferably using CT images, is mandatory when high total doses or a great number of large fractions have to be given.

Before any treatment starts a careful delineation of the target volume is obligatory. Modern imaging techniques can be very helpful; however, one should be sure that neurological symptoms, neuroanatomical information and abnormalities on the images are in agreement. Contrast medium-enhanced MRI has turned out to be a useful tool in planning the treatment of primary spinal cord tumours, CT scans also can be very helpful, especially in detecting bone destruction and paraspinal masses. However, CT is less useful in determining the length of a spinal cord compression. In these circumstances myelography is still advised.

The decision on whether and how to treat a spinal cord compression should be made by a team comprising at least a neurologist, a neurosurgeon, a neuroradiologist and a radiation oncologist.

References

Brada M, Thomas DGT (1995) Tumors of the brain and spinal cord in adults. In: Peckham M, Pinedo HM, Veronesi U (eda) Oxford textbook of oncology, vol 2. Oxford Medical, Oxford, pp 2063-2094

Chun HC, Schmidt-Ullrich RK, Wilfson A, Tercilla OF, Sagerman RH, Krug GA (1990) External beam radiotherapy for primary spinal cord tumors. J Neuroncology 9:211-217

Clover LL, Hazuka MB, Kinzie JJ (1993) Spinal cord ependymomas treated with surgery and radiation therapy. Am J Clin Oncol 16:350-353

Epstein FJ, Farmer JP, Freed D (1993) Adult inramedullary spinal cord ependymomas: the result of surgery in 38 Patients. J Neurosurg 79:204-209

Fogelholm R, Uutela T, Murros K (1984) Epidemiology of central nervous system neoplasms. A regional survey in Central Finland. Acta Neuro Scand 69:129-136

Gilbert PW, Kim JH, Posner JB (1978) Epidural spinal cord compression from metastatic tumor:diagnosis and treatment. Ann Neurol 3:40-51

Greenberg HS, Kim JH (1988) Epidural spinal cord compression from metastatic tumors. Results with a new treatment protocol. Ann Neurol 8:361-366

Helweg-Larsen S, Rasmusson B, Sörensen PS (1990) Recovery of gait after radiotherapy in paralytic patients with metastatic epidural spinal cord compression. Neurology 40: 1234-1236

Huddart R, Traish D, Ashley S, Moore A, Brada M (1993) Management of spinal astrocytoma with conservative surgery and radiotherapy. Br J Neurosurg 7:473-481

Kim RY, Smith JW, Spencer SA, Meredith RF, Salter MM (1993) Malignant epidural spinal cord compression associated with a paravertebral mass: its radiotherapeutic outcome on radiosensitivity. Int J Radiat Oncol Biol Phys 27:1079-1083

Leviov M, Dale J, Stein M, Ben-Shaker M. Ben-Arush M, Goldher D, Kuten A (1993) The management of metastatic spinal cord compression: a radiotherapeutic success ceiling. Int J Radiat Oncol Biol Phys 27:231-234

Lindstadt DE, Wara WM. Leibel SA, Gutin PH, Wilson CB, Sheline GE (1989) Postoperative radiotherapy of spinal cord tumors. Int J Radiat Oncol Biol Phys 16:1297-1403

Maranzano E, Latini P, Checcaglini F, Ricci S, Panizza BM, Aristei, C, Perrucci E, et al (1991) Radiation therapy in metastatic spinal cord compression. Cancer 67:1377-1417

Maranzano E, Latini P, Checcaglini F, Perrucci E, Aristei C, Panizza BM, Ricci S (1992) Radiation therapy of spinal cord compression caused by breast cancer:report of a prospective trial. Int J Radiat Oncol Biol Phys 24:301-306

McCormick PC, Torres R, Post KD, Stein BM (1990) Intramedullary ependymoma of the spinal cord. J Neurosurg 72: 523-532

Podd TJ (1994) Spinal cord compression:how best to treat. Radiother Oncol 32:128

Podd TJ, Carpenter DS, Banghon CA, Percival D, Dyson P (1992) Spinal cord compression:prognosis and implications for treatment fractination. Clin Oncol 4:341-344

Shapiro WR, Psoner JB (1983) Medical versus surgical treatment of metstatic spinal cord tumors. In: Thompson RA, Green JR (eds) Controversies in neurology. Raven, New York, pp 57-65

Shaw EG, Evans RG, Scheithauer BW, Ilstrup DM, Earle JD (1986) Radiotherapeutic management of adult intraspinal ependymomas. Int J Radiat Oncol Biol Phys 12:323-327

Sörensen PS, Borgeson SE, Rohde K, Rasmusson B, Bach F, Borde-Rasmussen T, Stjernholm P, et al (1990) Metastatic epidural spinal cord compression. Results of treatment and survival. Cancer 65:1502-1508

Waldron JN, Laperriere NJ, Jaakkimainen L, Simpson WJ, Payne d, Milosevic M, Wong CS (1993) Spinal cord ependymomas:a retrospective analysis of 59 cases. Int J Radiat Oncol Biol Phys 27:223-229

Wen BC, Hussey DH, Hitchon PW, Schelper RL, Vigliotti AP, Doornbos JT, Van Gilder JC (1991) The role of radiation therapy in the management of ependymomas of the spinal cord. Int J Radiat Oncol Biol Phys 20:781-786

Whitaker SJ, Bessell EM, Ashley SE, Bloom HJG, Bell BA, Brada M(1991) Postoperative radiotherapy in the management of the spinal cord ependymoma. J Neurosurg 53:741-748

11 Current Concepts of Systemic Therapy of Spinal Tumors

W. Boogerd

CONTENTS

11.1
Introduction

Tumors of the spinal column signify a serious risk of debilitating neurological complications, including paraplegia and loss of sphincter control through compression of the spinal roots and cord as the result of epidural extension from the neoplastic vertebral lesion or, more sporadically, due to bony impingement from a pathological vertebral fracture. By far the commonest type of neoplastic spinal cord compression is that caused by metastatic tumor. Vertebral metatstases are particularly common in breast cancer, lung cancer, and cancer of the prostate and occur in the majority of these patients with advanced disseminated disease (STOLL 1983). Metastases develop usually in multiple vertebral bodies, esepcially in breast and prostate cancer (STARK et al. 1982). Analogous to the occurence of bone metastases, epidural metastases may present at any stage of metastatic disease. Epidural spinal cord compression can also result from an extradural extension of a paravertebral tumor through the intervertebral foramina. This occurs in 10-15% of patients with epidural cord compression. Lymphoma accounts for about 75% of this kind of epidural invasion in adults, whereas in children neuroblastoma is the most common cause (CH'IEN et al. 1982).

Multiple epidural metastases are reported occasionally, but have been found to occur in 9-30% of patients with epidural tumor (BERNAT et al. 1983; RUFF and LANSKA 1989; VAN DER SANDE et al. 1990).

W. BOOGERD, MD, PhD, Department of Neurology, The Netherlands Cancer Institute/Antoni van Leeuwenhoekhuis, Plesmanlaan 121, 1066 CX Amsterdam, The Netherlands

A high proportion of these multiple epidural lesions appeared (still) asymptomatic. Presumably, (still) asymptomatic epidural tumor occurs more frequently than generally realized. In a study on asymptomatic patients with cancer, 17% of the patients with pathological bone scan, but unremarkable plain films, and 47% of those with vertebral metastases on plain films were reported to have epidural tumor on CT scan combined with myelography (O'ROURKE et al. 1986).

The functional outcome in a patient with epidural tumor and, as a consequence, the quality of the rest of that patients life is primarily related to the ambulatory status at the time treatment is started (STARK et al. 1982; GILBERT et al. 1978; BOOGERD et al. 1992). Although serious neurological deficit may develop suddenly, resulting in an already nonambulatory status at presentation, the clinical course, even after the first neurological symptoms, is often long enough to institute adequate treatment in time. Nearly all patients complain for weeks or months of local back pain at the site of the spinal tumor before the first signs of neurological involvement occur. Initial neurological symptoms usually are indicative of involvement of the spinal roots, followed by the first signs of myelopathy before paraparesis develops. The interval between the onset of radicular symptoms and those of myelopathy lasted less than 1 week in 21% of the patients, but more than 1 month in 55% (SHAW et al. 1980). The interval between the onset of signs of myelopathy and complete paraplegia may be less than 1 day, but on the average amounts to a few weeks (STARK et al. 1982). Nevertheless, in most studies the majority of the patients have developed paraparesis by the time the diagnosis is established (BOOGERD and VAN DER SANDE 1993).

11.2
Treatment

The aim of treatment of neoplastic epidural spinal cord compression is to maintain or restore neurological function and spinal stability, to relieve pain, and to achieve local tumor control. Neurological recovery after treatment of spinal cord compression depends on the rate of progression of spinal cord dysfunction (HELWEG-LARSEN et al. 1990; TARLOV and KLINER 1954). Rapid progression of cord compression is often observed in patients with lung cancer and renal cell cancer, whereas a more protracted course is seen in breast cancer and prostate cancer.

Standard treatment of epidural tumor consists of radiation therapy (RT) alone or in combination with surgical decompression. Corticosteroids are considered important for adjuvant therapy, particularly in the first days of treatment.

Surgical resection of the offending tumor mass will decompress the spinal cord immediately. RT alone may result in substantial tumor reduction in exquisitely radiosensitive tumors at best in a number of days. In combination with steroids, given for their antiedemic effect, it appears to be an adequate therapy to preserve an ambulatory status in the majoroty of the treated patients, even in those with less radiosensitive tumors. The reported incidence of local relapse after an initial response to RT is approximately 10% (BOOGERD et al. 1992; KAMINSKI et al. 1991; LOEFFLER et al. 1983). Notably, median survival in patients with treated epidural metastasis is about 6 months. However, probably most of the patients surviving 2 years or more will eventually suffer recurrent epidural tumor (J.J. VAN DER SANDE and W. BOOGERD, in preparation). Usually re-irradiation is contraindicated in these patients because of the risk of radiation-induced myelopathy.

Systemic therapy, including corticosteroids, is usually given as adjuvant therapy, but in metastatic epidural tumor it has occasionally also been given as an effective primary treatment alternative to surgery and RT.

11.2.1
Corticosteroids

Corticosteroids play an important role in the management of epidural cord compression for their antiedemic effect. Clinical studies demonstrated a significant reduction of neurological deficit and pain during and after treatment with dexamethasone, sometimes even starting within a few hours (GREENBERG et al. 1980; SÖRENSEN et al. 1994). Experimental studies showed that dexamethasone can reduce spinal cord edema and delay the onset of paraplegia (DELATTRE et al. 1989). These effects appeared to be dose dependent. Clinically, a high dose of 100 mg dexamethasone a day may be superior to a dose of 10 mg a day in relieving pain, but a significant difference in neurological outcome was not demonstrated (GREENBERG et al. 1980; VECHT et al. 1989).

Generally, dexamethasone is given as an initial bolus of 10 or 16 mg, followed by 4 mg orally four times a day during the first 3 to 7 days, and then tapered off over the following 2 weeks. An intravenous bolus of 100 mg followed by 24 mg four times a day for 3 days can be reserved for patients with serious and rapidly progressive cord dysfunction. The well-known side effcts of steroids frequently complicate the treatment of patients with epidural tumor (WEISSMAN 1988). However, the chance of major morbidity is relatively small when steroids can be stopped within a few weeks, even when a dose of 100 mg dexamenthasone is given during the first 3 days (GREENBERG et al . 1980; MARTENSON et al. 1985). On the other hand, clinicans should be aware of the significant risk of (fatal) intestinal perforation from the use of steroids, in combination with constipation and diminished pain sensation due to myelopathy and/or use of morphine.

Corticosteroids have specific antineoplastic activity in lymphoma. Regression of epidural lymphoma itself was observed within several days following treatment with corticosteroids alone (POSNER et al. 1977). To enhance the antitumor effect and to obtain tumor reduction as rapidly as possible, also in lymphoma corticosteroids are used adjuvantly to RT and/or systemic chemotherapy. Specific oncolytic efficacy of corticosteroids was also suggested after observation of neurological improvement following administration of steroids alone in patients with epidural metastasis from thymoma, seminoma and Ewing's sarcoma (POSNER et al. 1977). The duration of improvement in these patients lasted, however, only from 4 days to 6 weeks.

11.2.2
Hormonal Therapy

Nonsteroid hormonal therapy may be of value as additional treatment but it is regarded insufficient as primary treatment of metastatic epidural tumor because of uncertainty whether a significant antineoplastic effect can be achieved rapidly enough to prevent irreversible neurological deficits.

Breast cancer and prostate cancer are the hormone-responsive tumors that are frequently complicated by epidural metastatic disease. Epidural metastasis of these primaries is often characterized by a protracted course. Early recognition of epidural tumor may make hormonal therapy as single treatment possible in selected cases, as we observed in a patient with epidural metastasis from breast cancer (BOOGERD et al. 1989). But even paraparesis and a complete myelographic epidural block do not exclude a favorable outcome following hormonal therapy alone. In three patients with paraparesis and paraplegia, prostate cancer was diagnosed at presentation of the neurological deficit. Orchidectomy and treatment with diethylstilbestrol resulted in relief of pain within a few days and in neurological and radiological remission within a few weeks (EDELMAN 1949; SASAGAWA et al. 1991). Sustained neurological improvement was observed in a patient with prostate cancer following stilbestrol treatment for a clinical relapse of a previously irradiated metastasis (MARSHALL and LANGFITT 1977).

11.2.3
Chemotherapy

In general, systemic chemotherapy is considered inadequate as a single treatment of epidural metastatic spinal cord compression. Though usually more effective than hormonal therapy, it is assumed that it will take at least a few weeks to induce reduction of a chemosensitive epidural tumor. Although some exquisitely sensitive tumors, like lymphoma, may respond within days, it is generally recommended that chemotherapy be combined with RT or surgery in order to avoid any risk of irreversible neurological deficit.

In primary malignant spinal bone tumors surgical removal of the tumor mass with postoperative RT is the principal approach. Chemotherapy has been used accidently for recurrent lesions but was hardly ever beneficial. Neurological improvement was observed in a patient with a recurrent chordoma at the cervical spine following treatment with vincristine and high-dose methotrexate with leukovorin rescue (FULLER and BLOOM 1988). For patients with a mesenchymal less well-differentiated chondrosarcoma doxorubicin, but also a regimen including high-dose methtrexate as used for patients with osteosarcoma, may be of some benefit (HUVOS 1991). Repeated courses of intra-arterial doxorubicin through the intercostal artery, followed by a systemic chemotherapy regimen including vincristine, methotrexate, phenylalanine mustard and doxorubicin

resulted in a complete and sustained remission of an unresectable osteosarcoma proved by biopsy, originating in the body of a thoracic vertebra in a 15-year-old boy (OGIHARA et al. 1984).

Substantial responses of spinal epidural metastases to chemotherapy alone have been described occasionally, but series including more than a few patients are still not available. Chemotherapy as first-line treatment of epidural tumor was employed systematically in small series of patients with lymphoma, myeloma, germ cell tumors and neuroblastoma. Particularly in children with epidural cord compression from neuroblastoma or Hodgkin's lymphoma, chemotherapy appears to offer an alternative method of primary treatment avoiding long-term complications like progressive spinal deformities, instability and growth disturbances that develop in about half of the children following laminectomy or spinal RT (TRAGGIS et al. 1977; KING et al. 1975; ROBERTSON et al. 1989).

About half of the patients with neuroblastoma present with localized tumor and have a good prognosis. Approximately 10-15% of localized neuroblastomas infiltrate the epidural space via the intervertebral foramina (LEWIS et al. 1986; PLANTAZ et al. 1996). HAYES and colleagues treated a sequent series of nine children with epidural extension from neuroblastoma and a series of four children with epidural metastasis from Ewing's sarcoma with chemotherapy (HAYES et al. 1984). All patients showed neurological improvement after the first 8-day course of cyclophosphamide and doxorubicin. Steroids were not given in most of these patients. The patients with Ewing's sarcoma received local RT after induction of remission with chemotherapy.

SANDERSON et al. (1989) reported a similar beneficial effect in four consecutive patients with neuroblastoma: all patients showed a complete and permanent neurological recovery within 1-3 weeks after chemotherapy alone including vincristine, cisplatin, teniposide and cyclophosphamide. Thirty-two patients with intraspinal extension from nonmetastatic neuroblastoma received chemotherapy as first-line treatment. Complete regression of the intraspinal component was observed in 13 patients and partial regression of more than 50% in 5 patients. Only one patient developed neurological deterioration during chemotherapy including carboplatin, etoposide, cyclophosphamide, vincristine and doxorubicin (PLANTAZ et al. 1996). In a retrospective analysis of children with spinal epidural metastasis no difference was found in outcome between patients with neuroblastoma, Hodgkin's lymphoma, and germ cell tumors treated with chemotherapy alone or in combination with other treatment modalities (KLEIN et al. 1991). In children with sarcoma chemotherapy as a single treatment has not demonstrated a beneficial effect on spinal epidural metastasis. Successful preoperative chemotherapy was reported in a patient with osteosarcoma, one with Ewing's sarcoma, and one with rhabdomyosarcoma (SUNDARESAN et al. 1983).

In the case of adults, a few consecutive patients with epidural compression from germ cell tumor (COOPER et al. 1990) and a small sequent series of myeloma patients (SINOFF and BLUMSOHN 1989) were successfully treated with chemotherapy alone. In addition, efficacy of chemotherapy alone on epidural metastasis from some chemosensitive primary tumors was reported in a few case studies (Table 11.1). In our institute, we have treated several adults with epidural metastais from Hodgkin's disease or non-Hodgkin's lymphoma successfully with chemotherapy and dexamethasone.

It can be concluded that, in chemosensitive tumors, chemotherapy will usually work quickly enough to prevent permanent neurological deficit from epidural metastasis. Similarly, in experimental spinal cord compression from a chemosensitive tumor, chemotherapy appeared more effective than RT in relieving neurological symptoms (USHIO et al. 1977).

Also in less chemosensitive tumors, such as carcinomas, chemotherapy may be valuable as primary treatment of epidural metastasis. We used chemotherapy as single treatment in a number of patients with epidural metastases from breast carcinoma (BOOGERD et al. 1989, 1992). Usually it was given for recurrence after RT. As stated above, relapse of epidural tumor after RT is a well-known feature in breast cancer. Awareness of this phenomenon and, as a consequence, early recognition of recurrence often appears to render enough time for chemotherapy to prevent serious neurological deficit. But also a complete spinal block due to recurrent epidural metastasis from breast cancer was treated successfully with chemotherapy alone, consisting of cyclophosphamide, doxorubicin and flourouracil (Fig. 11.1). In addition, a diagnosis of epidural metastasis made when the patient is not in an emergency status allows suc-

Table 11.1. Successful treatment of spinal epidural metastasis with systemic therapy

Primary tumor	Systemic therapy	No. of patients	Duration of response[a]	Reference
Acute leukemia	Chemotherapy	1	8.5 Years	Pui et al. 1985
Hodgkin's lymphoma	Chemotherapy	1	13 Months	Marshall and Langfitt 1977
Non-Hodgkin's lymphoma	Corticosteroids	2	2-4 Months	Clarke and Saunders 1975
	Chemotherapy	11	8-24+ Months	Posner et al. 1977; Irvine and Robertson 1964; Oviatt et al. 1982; Wong et al. 1996
Myeloma	Chemotherapy	5	2+-12+ Months	Sinoff and Blumsohn 1989
Neuroblastoma	Chemotherapy	18	12+-28+ Months	Hayes et al. 1984; Sanderson et al. 1989; Klein et al. 1991; Raina et al. 1993
Paraganglioma	Chemotherapy	1		Mertens et al. 1993
Germ cell tumor	Chemotherapy	5	5+-24+ Months	Cooper et al. 1990; Gale et al. 1986; Itoyama et al. 1993
Seminoma	Corticosteroids	1	1 Month	Posner et al. 1977
Ewing's sarcoma	Corticosteroids	1	4+ Days	Posner et al. 1977
	Chemotherapy	4[b]		Hayes et al. 1984
Thymoma	Corticosteroids	1	6 Weeks	Posner et al. 1977
Leiomyoma	Hormone therapy	1	60+ Months	Hekster et al. 1994
Prostate cancer	Hormone therapy	5	2.5+-12+ Months	Edelman 1949; Sasagawa et al. 1991; Marshall and Langfitt 1977
Breast cancer	Chemotherapy	11	2-22 Months	Boogerd et al. 1989, 1992; Marshall and Langfitt 1977
	Hormone therapy	2	7-13 Months	Boogerd et al 1989,1992
Colorectal cancer	Chemotherapy	1	17+ Months	Present study (Sect.11.2.3)

[a] +Neurologically improved at last day of follow-up or until death
[b] Radiotherapy of the residual bone lesion after remission with chemotherapy

cessful treatment with systemic therapy of de novo epidural lesions. In nine patients with epidural metastasis from breast cancer treated with chemotherapy alone we noticed a response rate and duration that did differ significantly from the response following RT (BOOGERD et al. 1992).

Chemotherapy may occasionally be successful in epidural metastasis from tumors showing little chemosensitivity, as we observed in a patient with recurrent epidural metastasis from colorectal cancer. The patient was a 69-year-old woman who, 2 years after resection of the primary tumor (Dukes C2) developed bone metastasis in C7 and T1 with evident epidural extension. Neck pain and radiculopathy subsided gradually in 4 weeks following RT (20 Gy in five fractions). Five months later neck pain recurred, radiating into both arms. Neurological examination revealed paresis of the right hand, negative triceps jerk at the right side, sensory disturbances in T1 and pathological plantar reflexes. In addition, pathological lymph nodes were found in the supraclavicular region. A CT scan with contrast showed metastases in C7 and T1, with evident epidural extension. It was decided to treat the patient with weekly cycles of flourouracil and leukovorin. Dexamethasone treatment was started. During the first three weeks of this treatment neurological deficit still increased while the patient was bedridden because of severe pain when sitting and standing. From the 4th week paresis and pain gradually diminished. CT repeated after 2 months showed disappearance of the epidural tumor extension. From that time chemotherapy was given at 2-week intervals and eventually stopped after 10 months because of adverse effects. The patient remained neurologically well and stable. Repeat CT scan after 12 months showed recalcification and absence of epidural tumor. The patient died of rectal bleeding due to local tumor progression 17 months after the start of chemotherapy for epidural metastasis.

In conclusion, it has been demonstrated convincingly that chemotherapy can be applied successfully as principal treatment of epidural extension from chemosensitive tumors. It is recommended as primary and single treatment in young children with epidural spinal cord compression from neuroblastoma, lymphoma or germ cell tumors, thus avoiding serious late spinal deformation caused by surgery or RT. Surgery or RT might be reserved in the case of these primaries for patients with serious neurological deficit like paraplegia and for neurological deterioration during chemotherapy. In adults the choice between systemic therapy or local RT as principal therapy for epidural metastasis from chemosensitive

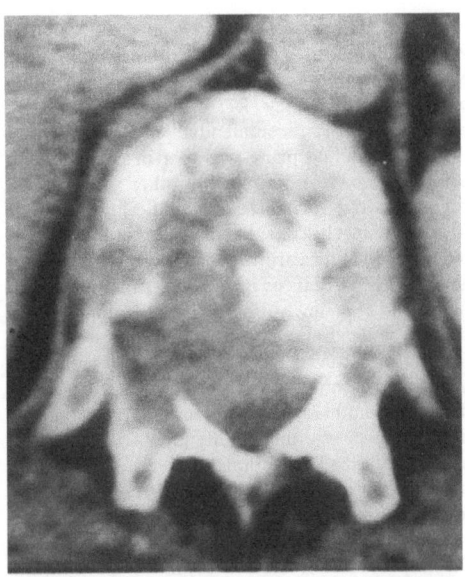

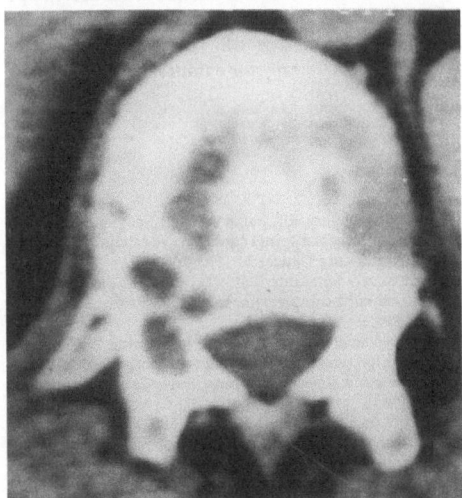

Fig.11.1. a A CT scan after intravenous contrast medium administration in a patient with breast cancer shows tumorous involvement of the body and pedicle of T12 with epidural extension. A previous myelogram had shown a complete block at this level. The patient was treated with chemotherapy consisting of cyclophosphamide, doxorubicin, and flourouracil. No dexamethasone was given. b Repeat Ct scan after intravenous contrast medium administration 4 months later showed disappearance of the epidural tumor. Eight cycles of chemotherapy were given over 6 months. The patient remained free of neurologic symptoms until her death 22 months after systemic therapy of the epidural tumor

tumors (lymphoma, myeloma, germ cell tumors) will depend on the status of the disease and on the extent of neurological deficit; in rapidly evolving paraplegia emergency RT in combination with corticosteroids is recommended. In breast cancer, the most common primary tumor in patients with epidural metastases, but also in other more or less chemosensitive primaries chemotherapy as single treatment must be considered in cases of local recurrence in which retreatment with RT or surgery is regarded as hazardous or impossible. In patients with minor and only slowly progressive neurological deficit or in asymptomatic epidural metastasis, systemic therapy might even be used as primary treatment instead of RT, thus reserving RT for deterioration during chemotherapy. The risk of recurrence of epidural metastasis, either locally after RT because of excessively small radiation ports or distantly because of outgrowth of asymptomatic non-irradiated lesions, might be reduced by using systemic therapy.

It may be expected that increased awareness of the importance of early recognition of epidural tumor and the increased incidence of recurrent epidural metastasis due to longer survival of patients with metastatic disease will result in an increased use of systemic therapy for epidural spinal tumor.

References

Bernat JL, Greenberg ER, Barte J (1983) Suspected epidural compression of the spinal cord and cauda equina by metastatic carcinoma. Cancer 51:1953-1957

Boogerd W, van der Sande JJ (1993) Diagnosis and treatment of spinal cord compression in malignant disease. Cancer Treat Rev 19:129-150

Boogerd W, van der Sande JJ, Kröger R, Bruning PF, Somers R (1989) Effective systemic therapy for spinal epidural metastases from breast carcinoma. Eur J Cancer Clin Oncol 25:149-153

Boogerd W, van der Sande JJ, Kröger R (1992) Early diagnosis and treatment of spinal epidural metastasis in breast cancer: a prospective study. J Neurol Neurosurg Psychiatry 55:1188-1193

Ch'ien LT, Kalwinsky DK, Peterson G, Pratt CB, Murphy SB, Hayes FA, Green AA, Hustu H (1982) Metastatic epidural tumors in children. Med Pediatr Oncol 10:455-462

Clarke PRR, Saunders M (1975) Steroid-induced remission in spinal canal reticulum cell sarcoma. J Neurosurg 42:346-348

Cooper K, Bajorin D, Shapiro W, Krol G, Sze G, Bosl GJ (1990) Decompression of epidural metastasis from germ cell tumors with chemotherapy. J Neurooncol 8:275-280

Delattre JY, Arbit E, Thaler HT, Rosenblum MK, Posner JB (1989) A dose-response study of dexamethasone in a model of spinal cord compression caused by epidural tumor. J Neurosurg 70:920-925

Edelman IS (1949) Paraplegia secondary to metastatic prostatic carcinoma treated with stilbestrol. Ann Intern Med 31:1098-1102

Fuller DB, Bloom JG (1988) Radiotherapy for chordoma. Int J Radiat Oncol Biol Phys 15:331-339

Gale GB, O'Connor DM, Chee JY (1986) Succesful chemotherapeutic decompression of epidural malignant germ cell tumor. Med Pediatr Oncol 14:97-99

Gilbert LW, Kim JH, Posner JB (1978) Epidural spinal cord compression from metastatic tumour:diagnosis and treatment. Ann Neurol 3:40-51

Greenberg HS, Kim JH, Posner JB (1980) Epidural spinal cord compression from metastatic tumour: results with a new treatment protocol. Ann Neurol 8:361-366

Hayes FA, Thompsom EI, Hvidzala E, O`Connor D, Green AA (1984) Chemotherapy as an alternative to laminectomy and radiation in the management of epidural tumor. J Pediatr 104:221-224

Hekster REM, Lambooy N, van Hall EV, Kazzaz BA, van Rijssel EJC (1994) Hormone-dependent spinal leiomyoma. Surg Neurol 41:330-333

Helweg-Larsen S, Rasmussen B, Sörensen PS (1990) Recovery of gait after radiotherapy in paralytic patients with metastatic epidural spinal cord compression. Neurology 40: 1234-1236

Huvos AG (1991) Bone tumors. Diagnosis, treatment, and prognosis. Saunders, Philadelphia, pp 343-394

Irvine RA, Robertson WB (1964) Spinal cord compression in the malignant lymphomas. Br Med J 1:1354-1356

Itoyama Y, Kochi M, Yamashiro S, Yoshizato K, Kuratsu J, Ushio Y (1993) Combination chemotherapy with cisplatin and etoposide for hematogenous spinal metastasis of intracranial germinoma. Neurol Med Chir (Tokyo) 33:28-31

Kaminski HJ, Diwan VG, Ruff RL (1991) Second occurrence of spinal epidural metastases. Neurology 41:744-746

King D, Goodman J, Hawk T, Boles T, Sayers M (1975) Dumbbell neuroblastomas in children. Arch Surg 10:888-892

Klein SL, Sanford RA, Muhlbauer MS (1991) Pediatric spinal epidural metastases. J Neurosurg 74:70-75

Lewis DW, Packer RJ, Raney B, Rak JW, Belasco J, Lange B (1986) Incidence, presentation and outcome of spinal cord disease in children with systemic cancer. Pediatrics 78: 438-443

Loeffler JS, Glicksman AS, Teft M, Gelch M (1983) Treatment of spinal cord compression: a retrospective analysis. Med Pediatr Oncol 11:347-351

Marshall LF, Langfitt TW (1977) Combined therapy for metastatic extradural tumor of the spine. Cancer 40:2067-2070

Martenson JA, Evans RG, Lie MR, Ilstrup DM, Dinapoli R, Ebersold MJ, Early JD (1985) Treatment outcome and complications in patients treated for malignant epidural spinal cord compression (SCC). J Neurooncol 3:77-84

Mertens WC, Grignon DJ, Romano W (1993) Malignant paraganglioma with skeletal metastases and spinal cord compression: response and palliation with chemotherapy. Clin Oncol 5:126-128

Ogihara Y, Sekigucki K, Tsuruta T (1984) Osteogenic sarcoma of the fourth thoracic vertebra. Cancer 53:2615-2618

O'Rourke T, George CB, Redmond J, Davidson H, Cornett P, Fill WL, Spring DB, Sobel D, Dabe IB, Karl RD, Cromwell LD (1986) Spinal computed tomography and computed tomographic metrizamide myelography in the early diagnosis of metastatic disease. J Clin Oncol 4:576-583

Oviatt DL, Kirshner HS, Stein RS (1982) Successful chemotherapeutic treatment of epidural compression in non-Hodgkin's lymphoma. Cancer 49:2446-2448

Plataz D, Rubie M, Michon J, Mechinaud F, Coze C, Chastagner P, Frappaz D, Gigond M, Passagia JG, Hartmann O (1996) The treatment of neuroblastoma with intraspinal extension with chemotherapy followed by surgical removal of residual disease. Cancer 78:311-319

Posner JB, Howieson J, Cvitkovic E (1977) 'Disappearing' spinal cord compression: oncolytic effect of glucocorticoids (and other chemotherapeutic agents) on epidural metastases. Ann Neurol 2:409-413

Pui C, Dahl GV, Hustu HA, Murphy SB (1985) Epidural cord compression as the initial finding in childhood acute leukemia and non-Hodgkin's lymphoma. J Pediatr 106:788-792

Raina V, Kamble R, Tanwar R, Singh SP, Sharma S (1993) Spinal ganglioneuroblastoma: complete response to chemotherapy alone. Postgrad Med J 69:746-748

Robertson W, Schnauferd B, Drummond D, Brockmeyer T, D'Angio G (1989) Prevention of kyphosis in the management of intrathoracic neuroblastoma with intraspinal protrusion. Med Pediatr Oncol 17:291

Ruff RL, Lanska DJ (1989) Epidural metastases in prospectively evaluated veterans with cancer and back pain. Cancer 63:2234-2241

Sanderson IR, Pritchard J, Marsh MT (1989) Chemotherapy as the initial treatment of spinal cord compression due to disseminated neuroblastoma. J Neurosurg 70:688-690

Sasagawa J, Guton H, Miyabayashi H, Yamaquchi O, Shiraiara Y (1991) Hormonal treatment of symptomatic spinal cord compression in advanced prostate cancer. Int Urol Nephrol 21:351-356

Shaw MDM, Rose JE, Paterson A (1980) Metastatic extradural malignancy of the spine. Acta Neurochir (Wien) 52:113-120

Sinoff CL, Blumsohn A (1989) Spinal cord compression in myelomatosis: response to chemotherapy alone. Eur J Cancer Clin Oncol 25:197-200

Sörensen PS, Helweg-Larsen S, Mouridsen H, Hansen HH (1994) Effect of high-dose dexamethasone in carcinomatous metastatic spinal cord compression treated with radiotherapy: a randomized trail. Eur J Cancer 30:22-27

Stark RJ, Henson RA, Evans JW (1982) Spinal metastases: a retrospective survey from a general hospital. Brain 105:189-213

Stoll BA (1983) Natural history, prognosis, and staging of bone metastases. In: Stoll BA, Parbhoo S (eds) Bone metastases: monitoring and treatment. Raven, New York, pp 1-4

Sundaresan N, Rosen G, Fortner JG, Lane JM, Hilaris BS (1983) Preoperative chemotherapy and surgical resection in the managment of posterior paraspinal tumors. Report of three cases. J Neurosurg 58:446-450

Tarlov IM, Kliner H (1954) Spinal cord compression studies. II Time limits for recovery after acute compression in dogs. Arch Neurol Psychiatry 71:271-290

Traggis D, Filler R, Druckman H, Jaffe N, Cassady JR (1977) Prognosis for children with neuroblastoma presenting with paralysis. J Pediatr Surg 12:419-425

Ushio Y, Posner R, Kim J, Shapiro WK, Posner JB (1977) Treatment of experimental spinal cord compression caused by extradural neoplasms. J Neurosurg 47:380-390

Van der Sande JJ, Kröger R, Boogerd W (1990) Multiple spinal epidural metastases: an unexpectedly frequent finding. J Neurol Neurosurg Psychiatry 53:1001-1003

Vecht CJ, Haaxma-Reiche H, van Putten WLJ, de Visser M, Vries EP, Twijnstra A (1989) Initial bolus of conventional versus high-dose dexamethasone in metastatic spinal cord compression. Neurology 39:1255-1257

Weissman DE (1988) Glucocorticoid treatment for brain metastases and epidural cord compression: a review. J Clin Oncol 6:543-551

Wong ET, Portlock CS, O'Vrien JP, DeAngelis LM (1996) Chemosensitive epidural spinal cord disease in non-Hodgkin's lymphoma. Neurology 46:1543-1547

Subject Index

List of Contributors

P.R. ALGRA, MD, PhD
Department of Radiology
Medical Center Alkmaar
P.O. Box 501
1800 AM Alkmaar
The Netherlands

J.L. BLOEM, MD
Department of Radiology
Leiden University Medical Center
Albinusdreef 2
2333 AA Leiden
The Netherlands

W. BOOGERD, MD, PhD
Department of Neurology
The Netherlands Cancer Institute
Antoni van Leeuwenhoekhuis
Plesmanlaan 121
1066 CX Amsterdam
The Netherlands

M.J. DONOVAN POST, MD
Department of Radiology
University of Miami School of
Medicine
P.O. Box 016960 (R-109)
Miami, FL 33101
USA

C.F. DOWD, MD
Neurovascular Medical Group
Department of Radiology
UCSF Medical Center
505 Parnasus Avenue
San Francisco, CA 94143-0628
USA

M.W. FIDLER, MS, FRCS
Orthopaedic Department
Onze Lieve Vrouwe Gasthuis
le Oosterparkstraat 179
1091 HA Amsterdam
The Netherlands

K.W. FRASER, MD
St. Francis Medical Center
Department of Radiology
530 NE Glen Oak Avenue
Peoria, IL 61637
USA

J.J. HEIMANS, MD, PhD
Department of Neurology
Free University Hospital
P.O. Box 7057
1007 MB Amsterdam
The Netherlands

J.W.H. LEER, MD
Department of Clinical Oncology
University Hospital Leiden
P.O. Box 9600
Rijnsburgweg 10
2300 RC Leiden
The Netherlands

P.M. PARZIEL, MD, PhD
Professor, Department of Radiology
Universitair Ziekenhuis Antwerpen
(University of Antwerp)
Wilrijkstraat 10
B-2520 Edegem
Belgium

L.M.P. RAMOS, MD
Department of Neuroradiology
University Hospital Utrecht
P.O. Box 85500
3508 GA Utrecht
The Netherlands

J. RATCLIFFE, MD, PhD
Department of Radiological Sciences
Royal Children´s Hospital Brisbane
Herston Q 4029
Brisbane
Australia

C.A.F. TULLEKEN, MD, PhD
Department of Neurosurgery
University Hospital Utrecht
P.O. Box 85500
3508 GA Utrecht
The Netherlands

J. VALK, MD, PhD
Department of Radiology
Free University Hospital
Academisch Ziekenhuis
P.O. Box 7057
1007 MB Amsterdam
The Netherlands

M.A. Van Buchem, MD
Department of Radiology
University Medical Center
Albinusdreef 2
2333 AA Leiden
The Netherlands

V.P.M. Van der Hulst, MD
Department of Radiology
Onze Lieve Vrouwe Gasthuis
1e Oosterparkstraat 179
1090 HM Amsterdam
The Netherlands

W.P. Vandertop, MD, PhD
Department of Neurosurgery
University Hospital Utrecht
P.O. Box 85500
3508 GA Utrecht
The Netherlands

J. Weerts, MD
Department of Radiology
Free University Hospital
Academisch Ziekenhuis
P.O. Box 7057
1007 MB Amsterdam
The Netherlands

J.T. Wilmink, MD, PhD
Department of Radiology
Academisch Ziekenhuis Maastricht
P. Debeyelaan 25
P.O. Box 5800
6202 AZ Maastricht
The Netherlands

MEDICAL RADIOLOGY
Diagnostic Imaging and Radiation Oncology

Titles in the series already published

DIAGNOSTIC IMAGING

Innovations in Diagnostic Imaging
Edited by J.H. Anderson

Radiology of the Upper Urinary Tract
Edited by E.K. Lang

The Thymus - Diagnostic Imaging, Functions, and Pathologic Anatomy
Edited by E. Walter, E. Willich, and W.R. Webb

Interventional Neuroradiology
Edited by A. Valavanis

Radiology of the Pancreas
Edited by A.L. Baert, co-edited by G. Delorme

Radiology of the Lower Urinary Tract
Edited by E.K. Lang

Magnetic Resonance Angiography
Edited by I.P. Arlart, G.M. Bongartz, and G. Marchal

Contrast-Enhanced MRI of the Breast
S. Heywang-Köbrunner and R. Beck

Spiral CT of the Chest
Edited by M. Rémy-Jardin and J. Rémy

Radiological Diagnosis of Breast Diseases
Edited by M. Friedrich and E.A. Sickles

Radiology of the Trauma
Edited by M. Heller and A. Fink

Biliary Tract Radiology
Edited by P. Rossi

Radiological Imaging of Sports Injuries
Edited by C. Masciocchi

Modern Imaging of the Alimentary Tube
Edited by A. R. Margulis

Diagnosis and Therapy of Spinal Tumors
Edited by P. R. Algra, J. Valk, and J. J. Heimans

Interventional Magnetic Resonance Imaging
Edited by J. F. Debatin and G. Adam

RADIATION ONCOLOGY

Lung Cancer
Edited by C.W. Scarantino

Innovations in Radiation Oncology
Edited by H.R. Withers and L.J. Peters

Radiation Therapy of Head and Neck Cancer
Edited by G.E. Laramore

Gastrointestinal Cancer – Radiation Therapy
Edited by R.R. Dobelbower, Jr.

Radiation Exposure and Occupational Risks
Edited by E. Scherer, C. Streffer, and K.-R. Trott

Radiation Therapy of Benign Diseases - A Clinical Guide
S.E. Order and S.S. Donaldson

MEDICAL RADIOLOGY
Diagnostic Imaging and Radiation Oncology

Titles in the series already published